IARC MONOGRAPHS
ON THE
EVALUATION OF THE CARCINOGENIC RISK
OF CHEMICALS TO MAN:

Some Fumigants, the Herbicides 2,4-D and 2,4,5-T,
Chlorinated Dibenzodioxins and
Miscellaneous Industrial Chemicals

Volume 15

This publication represents the views of an
IARC Working Group on the
Evaluation of the Carcinogenic Risk of Chemicals to Man
which met in Lyon,
8-15 February 1977

1977

IARC WORKING GROUP ON THE EVALUATION OF THE CARCINOGENIC RISK OF CHEMICALS TO MAN: SOME FUMIGANTS, THE HERBICIDES 2,4-D AND 2,4,5-T, CHLORINATED DIBENZODIOXINS AND MISCELLANEOUS INDUSTRIAL CHEMICALS

Lyon, 8-15 February 1977

Members[1]

Dr A. Abbondandolo, Laboratorio di Mutagenesi e Differenziamento - C.N.R., Via Cisanello 147/B, 56100 Pisa, Italy

Dr F. Berrino, Istituto Nazionale per lo Studio e la Cura dei Tumori, Servizio di Epidemiologia, Via Venezian 1, 20133 Milan, Italy

Professor E. Boyland, London School of Hygiene and Tropical Medicine, Keppel Street, London WC1E 7HT, UK (*Chairman*)

Dr I. Chernozemsky, Institute of Oncology, Medical Academy, Sofia 1156, Bulgaria

Dr L. Fishbein, Assistant to the Director for Environmental Surveillance, National Center for Toxicological Research, Jefferson, Arkansas 72079, USA

Dr R. Gingell, Assistant Professor, The Eppley Institute for Research in Cancer, University of Nebraska Medical Center, 42nd and Dewey Avenue, Omaha, Nebraska 68105, USA

Dr H.C. Grice, Director, Bureau of Chemical Safety, Health and Welfare Canada, Health Protection Branch, Tunney's Pasture, Ottawa, Ontario K1A 0L2, Canada

Dr J.E. Huff[2], Director, Biomedical Science Section, Information Center Complex, Information Division, Oak Ridge National Laboratory, PO Box X, Oak Ridge, Tennessee 37830, USA

Dr P.F. Infante, Industry-Wide Studies Branch, Division of Surveillance, Hazard Evaluation and Field Studies, National Institute for Occupational Safety and Health, Robert A. Taft Laboratories, 4676 Columbia Parkway, Cincinnati, Ohio 45226, USA

---

[1]Unable to attend: Dr B. Paccagnella, Università di Padova, 11° Istituto di Igiene, Policlinico Borgo Roma, 37100 Verona, Italy

[2]Present address: Unit of Chemical Carcinogenesis, International Agency for Research on Cancer, 150 Cours Albert Thomas, 69372 Lyon Cédex 2, France

Professor D. Neubert, Institut für Toxikologie und Embryonal-Pharmakologie der Freien Universität Berlin, Garystrasse 1-9, 1000 Berlin 33, FRG

Professor G. Prodi, Director, Istituto di Cancerologia, Università degli Studi di Bologna, Via S. Giacomo 14, 40138 Bologna, Italy

Dr G. Saint-Ruf, C.N.R.S., Centre Marcel Delépine, Service Saint-Ruf, Département de Chimie Organique-Biologique, 45045 Orléans Cedex, France

Professor C. Schlatter, Director, Institut für Toxikologie der Eidgenössischen Technischen Hochschule und der Universität Zürich, Schorenstrasse 16, CH-8603 Schwerzenbach bei Zürich, Switzerland

Dr V.F. Simmon, Manager, Microbial Genetics, Stanford Research Institute, Menlo Park, California 94025, USA

Dr B. Teichmann, Akademie der Wissenschaften der DDR, Zentralinstitut für Krebsforschung, Lindenberger Weg 80, 1115 Berlin-Buch, DDR

Dr V.S. Turusov, Cancer Research Center, USSR Academy of Medical Sciences, Karshirskoye Shosse 6, Moscow 115478, USSR (*Vice-Chairman*)

Professor V. Vojvodic, Bulevar Revolucije 257/III, 11000 Belgrade, Yugoslavia

Observers[1]

Dr O.H. Johnson, Senior Industrial Economist, Chemical-Environmental Program, Chemical Industries Center, Stanford Research Institute, Menlo Park, California 94025, USA (*Rapporteur sections 2.1 and 2.2*)

Mrs M.-T. van der Venne, Commission of the European Communities, Health and Safety Directorate, Bâtiment Jean Monnet, Avenue Alcide-de-Gasperi, Kirchberg/Luxembourg, Great Duchy of Luxembourg

Dr S. Villa-Trevino, Professor and Chairman, Centro de Investigacion y de Estudios Avanzados del Instituto Politecnico Nacional, Department of Cellular Biology, Apartado Postal 14-740, Mexico 14, D.F., Mexico

---

[1]Unable to attend: Dr L. Rinzema, Dow Chemical Europe S.A., 8810 Horgen, Switzerland; Dr E.E. Turtle, Pesticides Specialist, Plant Protection Service, Plant Production and Protection Division, Food and Agriculture Organization of the United Nations, Via delle Terme di Caracalla, 00100 Rome, Italy

Representative from the National Cancer Institute

Dr S. Siegel, Coordinator, Technical Information Activities, Room C-216, Landow Building, Bioassay and Carcinogenesis Program, Division of Cancer Cause and Prevention, National Cancer Institute, Bethesda, Maryland 20014, USA

Secretariat

    Dr C. Agthe, Chief, Food Additives Unit, WHO, Geneva

    Dr H. Bartsch, Unit of Chemical Carcinogenesis (*Rapporteur section 3.2*)

    Dr L. Griciute, Chief, Unit of Environmental Carcinogens

    Mrs D. Mietton, Unit of Chemical Carcinogenesis (*Library assistant*)

    Dr R. Montesano, Unit of Chemical Carcinogenesis (*Rapporteur section 3.1*)

    Mrs C. Partensky, Unit of Chemical Carcinogenesis (*Technical editor*)

    Mrs I. Peterschmitt, Unit of Chemical Carcinogenesis, WHO, Geneva (*Bibliographic researcher*)

    Dr V. Ponomarkov, Unit of Chemical Carcinogenesis

    Dr R. Saracci, Unit of Epidemiology and Biostatistics (*Rapporteur section 3.3*)

    Dr L. Tomatis, Chief, Unit of Chemical Carcinogenesis (*Head of the Programme and Secretary*)

    Dr M. Vandekar, Medical Officer/Toxicologist, Division of Vector Biology and Control, WHO, Geneva

    Mr E.A. Walker, Unit of Environmental Carcinogens (*Rapporteur sections 1 and 2.3*)

    Mrs E. Ward, Montignac, France (*Editor*)

    Mr J.D. Wilbourn, Unit of Chemical Carcinogenesis (*Co-secretary*)

Note to the reader

Every effort is made to present the monographs as accurately as possible without unduly delaying their publication. Nevertheless, mistakes have occurred and are still likely to occur. In the interest of all users of these monographs, readers are requested to communicate any errors observed to the Unit of Chemical Carcinogenesis of the International Agency for Research on Cancer, Lyon, France, in order that these can be included in corrigenda which will appear in subsequent volumes.

Since the monographs are not intended to be a review of the literature and contain only data considered relevant by the Working Group, it is not possible for the reader to determine whether a certain study was considered or not. However, research workers who are aware of important published data that may change the evaluation are requested to make them available to the above-mentioned address, in order that they can be considered for a possible re-evaluation by a future Working Group.

CONTENTS

BACKGROUND AND PURPOSE OF THE IARC PROGRAMME ON THE EVALUATION OF THE CARCINOGENIC RISK OF CHEMICALS TO MAN 11

SCOPE OF THE MONOGRAPHS 11

MECHANISM FOR PRODUCING THE MONOGRAPHS 12

GENERAL PRINCIPLES FOR THE EVALUATION 13

EXPLANATORY NOTES ON THE MONOGRAPHS 16

GENERAL REMARKS ON THE SUBSTANCES CONSIDERED 27

THE MONOGRAPHS

    1,2-Bis(chloromethoxy)ethane 31

    1,4-Bis(chloromethoxymethyl)benzene 37

    Chlorinated dibenzodioxins 41

    Copper 8-hydroxyquinoline 103

    2,4-D and esters 111

    1,2-Dibromo-3-chloropropane 139

    trans-1,4-Dichlorobutene 149

    Dihydroxybenzenes 155
        Catechol
        Resorcinol
        Hydroquinone

    Dimethoxane 177

    Eosin and eosin disodium salt 183

    Ethylene dibromide 195

    Hexamethylphosphoramide 211

    Isopropyl alcohol and isopropyl oils 223

    Methyl iodide 245

    para-Quinone 255

    Succinic anhydride 265

    2,4,5-T and esters 273

    1,2,3-Tris(chloromethoxy)propane 301

APPENDIX A 307

SUPPLEMENTARY CORRIGENDA TO VOLUMES 1-14 341

CUMULATIVE INDEX TO MONOGRAPHS 343

BACKGROUND AND PURPOSE OF THE IARC PROGRAMME ON THE EVALUATION OF THE CARCINOGENIC RISK OF CHEMICALS TO MAN

The International Agency for Research on Cancer (IARC) initiated in 1971 a programme to evaluate the carcinogenic risk of chemicals to man. This programme was supported by a Resolution of the Governing Council at its Ninth Session concerning the role of IARC in providing government authorities with expert, independent scientific opinion on environmental carcinogenesis.

In view of the importance of the project and in order to expedite production of monographs, the National Cancer Institute of the United States has provided IARC with additional funds for this purpose.

The objective of the programme is to elaborate and publish in the form of monographs critical reviews of carcinogenicity and related data in the light of the present state of knowledge, with the final aim of evaluating the data in terms of possible human risk, and at the same time to indicate where additional research efforts are needed.

SCOPE OF THE MONOGRAPHS

The monographs summarize the evidence for the carcinogenicity of individual chemicals and other relevant information on the basis of data compiled, reviewed and evaluated by a Working Group of experts. No recommendations are given concerning preventive measures or legislation, since these matters depend on risk-benefit evaluations, which seem best made by individual governments and/or international agencies such as WHO and ILO.

Since 1971, when the programme started, fourteen previous volumes have been published[1-14]. As new data on chemicals for which monographs have already been prepared and new principles for evaluation become available, re-evaluations will be made at future meetings, and revised monographs will be published as necessary.

The monographs are distributed to international and governmental agencies, are available to industries and scientists dealing with these chemicals and are offered to any interested reader through their world-wide distribution as WHO publications. They also form the basis of advice from IARC on carcinogenesis from these substances.

MECHANISM FOR PRODUCING THE MONOGRAPHS

As a first step, a list of chemicals for possible consideration by the Working Group is established. IARC then collects pertinent references regarding physico-chemical characteristics*, production and use*, occurrence and analysis* and biological data** on these compounds. The material on biological aspects is summarized by an expert consultant or an IARC staff member, who prepares the first draft, which in some cases is sent to another expert for comments. The drafts are circulated to all members of the Working Group about one month before the meeting. During the meeting, further additions to and deletions from the data are agreed upon, and a final version of comments and evaluation on each compound is adopted.

Priority for the preparation of monographs

Priority is given mainly to chemicals belonging to particular chemical groups and for which there is at least some suggestion of carcinogenicity from observations in animals and/or man and evidence of human exposure. However, *the inclusion of a particular compound in a volume does not necessarily mean that it is considered to be carcinogenic. Equally, the fact that a substance has not yet been considered does not imply that it is without carcinogenic hazard.*

Data on which the evaluation is based

With regard to the biological data, only published articles and papers already accepted for publication are reviewed. The monographs are not intended to be a full review of the literature, and they contain only data

---

*Data provided by Chemical Industries Center, Stanford Research Institute, Menlo Park, California, USA

**In the collection of original data reference was made to the series of publications 'Survey of Compounds which have been Tested for Carcinogenic Activity'[15-20]. Most of the information on mutagenicity was provided by the Environmental Mutagen Information Center, Oak Ridge, TN, USA.

considered relevant by the Working Group. Research workers who are aware of important data (published or accepted for publication) that may influence the evaluation are invited to make them available to the Unit of Chemical Carcinogenesis of the International Agency for Research on Cancer, Lyon, France.

The Working Group

The tasks of the Working Group are five-fold: (1) to ascertain that all data have been collected; (2) to select the data relevant for the evaluation; (3) to determine whether the data, as summarized, will enable the reader to follow the reasoning of the committee; (4) to judge the significance of results of experimental and epidemiological studies; and (5) to make an evaluation of carcinogenicity.

The members of the Working Group who participated in the consideration of particular substances are listed at the beginning of each publication. The members serve in their individual capacities as scientists and not as representatives of their governments or of any organization with which they are affiliated.

GENERAL PRINCIPLES FOR THE EVALUATION

The general principles for evaluation of carcinogenicity were elaborated by previous Working Groups and also applied to the substances covered in this volume.

Terminology

The term 'chemical carcinogenesis' in its widely accepted sense is used to indicate the induction or enhancement of neoplasia by chemicals. It is recognized that, in the strict etymological sense, this term means the induction of cancer; however, common usage has led to its employment to denote the induction of various types of neoplasms. The terms 'tumourigen', 'oncogen' and 'blastomogen' have all been used synonymously with 'carcinogen', although occasionally 'tumourigen' has been used specifically to denote the induction of benign tumours.

Response to carcinogens

In general, no distinction is made between the induction of tumours and the enhancement of tumour incidence, although it is noted that there may be fundamental differences in mechanisms that will eventually be elucidated. The response of experimental animals to a carcinogen may take several forms: a significant increase in the incidence of one or more of the same types of neoplasms as found in control animals; the occurrence of types of neoplasms not observed in control animals; and/or a decreased latent period for the production of neoplasms as compared with that in control animals.

Purity of the compounds tested

In any evaluation of biological data with respect to a possible carcinogenic risk, particular attention must be paid to the purity of the chemicals tested and to their stability under conditions of storage or administration. Information on purity and stability is given, when available, in the monographs.

Qualitative aspects

In many instances, both benign and malignant tumours are induced by chemical carcinogens. There are so far few recorded instances in which only benign tumours are induced by chemicals that have been studied extensively. Their occurrence in experimental systems has been taken to indicate the possibility of an increased risk of malignant tumours also.

In experimental carcinogenesis, the type of cancer seen may be the same as that recorded in human studies, e.g., bladder cancer in man, monkeys, dogs and hamsters after administration of 2-naphthylamine. In other instances, however, a chemical may induce other types of neoplasms at different sites in various species, e.g., benzidine induces hepatic carcinoma in rats but bladder carcinoma in man.

Quantitative aspects

Dose-response studies are important in the evaluation of human and animal carcinogenesis: the confidence with which a carcinogenic effect can be established is strengthened by the observation of an increasing incidence of neoplasms with increasing exposure. In addition, such studies form the only basis on which a minimal effective dose can be established, allowing some comparison with data for human exposure.

Comparison of compounds with regard to potency can only be made when the substances have been tested simultaneously.

Animal data in relation to the evaluation of risk to man

At the present time no attempt can be made to interpret the animal data directly in terms of human risk, since no objective criteria are available to do so. The critical assessments of the validity of the animal data given in these monographs are intended to assist national and/or international authorities in making decisions concerning preventive measures or legislation. In this connection, attention is drawn to WHO recommendations in relation to food additives[21], drugs[22] and occupational carcinogens[23].

Evidence of human carcinogenicity

Evaluation of the carcinogenic risk to man of suspected environmental agents rests on purely observational studies. Such studies must cover a sufficient variation in levels of human exposure to allow a meaningful relationship between cancer incidence and exposure to a given chemical to be established. Difficulties arise in isolating the effects of individual agents, however, since people are usually exposed to multiple carcinogens.

The initial suggestion of a relationship between an agent and disease often comes from case reports of patients with similar exposures. Variations and time trends in regional or national cancer incidences, or their correlation with regional or national 'exposure' levels, may also provide valuable insights. Such observations by themselves cannot, however, in most circumstances be regarded as conclusive evidence of carcinogenicity.

The most satisfactory epidemiological method is to compare the cancer risk (adjusted for age, sex and other confounding variables) among groups of cohorts, or among individuals exposed to various levels of the agent in question, and among control groups not so exposed. Ideally, this is accomplished directly, by following such groups forward in time (prospectively) to determine time relationships, dose-response relationships and other aspects of cancer induction. Large cohorts and long observation periods are required to provide sufficient cases for a statistically valid comparison.

An alternative to prospective investigation is to assemble cohorts from past records and to evaluate their subsequent morbidity or mortality by means of medical histories and death certificates. Such occupational carcinogens as nickel, 2-naphthylamine, asbestos and benzidine have been confirmed by this method. Another method is to compare the past exposures of a defined group of cancer cases with those of control samples from the hospital or general population. This does not provide an absolute measure of carcinogenic risk but can indicate the relative risks associated with different levels of exposure. Indirect means (e.g., interviews or tissue residues) of measuring exposures which may have commenced many years before can constitute a major source of error. Nevertheless, such 'case-control' studies can often isolate one factor from several suspected agents and can thus indicate which substance should be followed up by cohort studies.

EXPLANATORY NOTES ON THE MONOGRAPHS

In sections 1, 2 and 3 of each monograph, except for minor remarks, the data are recorded as given by the author, whereas the comments by the Working Group are given in section 4, headed 'Comments on Data Reported and Evaluation'.

Chemical and Physical Data (section 1)

The Chemical Abstracts Services Registry Number and the latest Chemical Abstracts Name are recorded in this section. Other synonyms and trade names are given, but this list is not intended to be comprehensive.

It should also be noted that some of the trade names are those of mixtures in which the compound being evaluated is only one of the active ingredients.

Chemical and physical properties include, in particular, data that might be relevant to carcinogenicity (for example, lipid solubility) and those that concern identification. All chemical data in this section refer to the pure substance, unless otherwise specified.

Production, Use, Occurrence and Analysis (section 2)

The purpose of this section is to indicate the extent of possible human exposure. With regard to data on production, use and occurrence, IARC has collaborated with the Stanford Research Institute, USA, with the support of the National Cancer Institute of the USA. Since cancer is a delayed toxic effect, past use and production data are also provided.

The United States, Europe and Japan are reasonably representative industrialized areas of the world, and if data on production or use are available from these countries they are reported. It should *not*, however, be inferred that these nations are the sole or even the major sources of any individual chemical.

Production data are obtained from both governmental and trade publications in the three geographic areas. In some cases, separate production data on chemicals manufactured in the US were not available, for proprietary reasons. However, the fact that a manufacturer acknowledges production of a chemical to the US International Trade Commission implies that annual production of that chemical is greater than 450 kg or that its annual sales exceed $1000. Information on use and occurrence is obtained by a review of published data, complemented by direct contact with manufacturers of the chemical in question; however, information on only some of the uses is available, and this section cannot be considered to be comprehensive. In an effort to provide estimates of production in some European countries, the Stanford Research Institute in Zurich sent general questionnaires to some of those European companies thought to produce the compounds being evaluated. Information from the replies to these questionnaires has been compiled by country and included in the individual monographs.

Statements concerning regulations in some countries are mentioned as examples only. They may not reflect the most recent situation, since such legislation is in a constant state of change; nor should it be taken to imply that other countries do not have similar regulations. In the case of drugs, mention of the therapeutic uses of such chemicals does not necessarily represent presently accepted therapeutic indications, nor does it imply judgement as to their clinical efficacy.

The purpose of the section on analysis is to give the reader a general indication, rather than a complete review, of methods cited in the literature. No attempt is made to evaluate the methods quoted.

Biological Data Relevant to the Evaluation of Carcinogenic Risk to Man (section 3)

The monographs are not intended to consider all reported studies. Some studies were purposely omitted (a) because they were inadequate, as judged from previously described criteria$^{24-27}$ (e.g., too short a duration, too few animals, poor survival or too small a dose); (b) because they only confirmed findings which have already been fully described; or (c) because they were judged irrelevant for the purpose of the evaluation. However, in certain cases, reference is made to studies which did not meet established criteria of adequacy, particularly when this information was considered a useful supplement to other reports or when it was the only data available. Their inclusion does not, however, imply acceptance of the adequacy of their experimental design.

In general, the data recorded in this section are summarized as given by the author; however, certain shortcomings of reporting or of experimental design that were commented upon by the Working Group are given in square brackets.

Carcinogenicity and related studies in animals: Mention is made of all routes of administration by which the compound has been adequately tested and of all species in which relevant tests have been carried out. In most cases, animal strains are given (general characteristics of mouse strains have been reviewed^{28}). Quantitative data are given to indicate the order of magnitude of the effective doses. In general, the doses are indicated as they appear in the original paper; sometimes conversions have been made for better comparison. When the carcinogenicity of known metabolites has been tested this also is reported.

Other relevant biological data: LD_{50} data are given when available, and other data on toxicity are included when considered relevant. The metabolic data included is restricted to studies showing the metabolic fate of the chemical in animals and man, and comparisons of animal and human data are made when possible. Other metabolic information (e.g., absorption, storage and excretion) is given when the Working Group considered that it would be useful for the reader to have a better understanding of the fate of the compound in the body.

Teratogenicity data from studies in experimental animals and in humans are included for some of the substances considered; however, they are not mean to represent a thorough review of the literature.

Mutagenicity data are also included; the reasons for including them and the principles adopted by the Working Group for their selection are outlined below.

Many, but not all, mutagens are carcinogens and *vice versa*; the exact level of correlation is still under investigation. Nevertheless, practical use may be made of the available mutagenicity test procedures that combine microbial, mammalian or other animal cell systems as genetic targets with an *in vitro* or *in vivo* metabolic activation system. The results of relatively rapid and inexpensive mutagenicity tests on non-human organisms may help to pre-screen chemicals and may also aid in the selection of the most relevant animal species in which to carry out long-term carcinogenicity tests on these chemicals.

The role of genetic alterations in chemical carcinogenesis is not yet fully understood, and therefore consideration must be given to a variety of changes. Although nuclear DNA has been defined as the main cellular target for the induction of genetic changes, other relevant targets have been recognized, e.g., mitochondrial DNA, enzymes involved in DNA synthesis, repair and recombination, and the spindle apparatus. Tests to detect the genetic activity of chemicals, including gene mutation, structural and numerical chromosomal changes and mitotic recombination, are available for non-human models; but not all such tests can be applied at present to human cells.

Ideally, an appropriate mutagenicity test system would include the full metabolic competency of the intact human. Since the development or application of such a system appears to be impossible, a battery of test systems is necessary in order to establish the mutagenic potential of chemicals. There are many genetic indicators and metabolic activation systems available for detecting mutagenic activity; they all, however, have individual advantages and limitations.

Since many chemicals require metabolism to an active form, test systems which do not take this into account may fail to reveal the full range of genetic damage. Furthermore, since some reactive metabolites with a limited lifespan may fail to reach or to react with the genetic indicator, either because they are further metabolized to inactive compounds or because they react with other cellular constituents, mutagenicity tests in intact animals may give false negative results.

It is difficult in the present state of knowledge to select specific mutagenicity tests as being the most appropriate for the pre-screening of substances for possible carcinogenic activity. However, greater reliance may be placed on data obtained from those test systems which (a) permit identification of the nature of induced genetic changes, and (b) demonstrate that the changes are transmitted to subsequent generations. Mutagenicity tests using organisms that are well-understood genetically, e.g., *Escherichia coli*, *Salmonella typhimurium*, *Saccharomyces cerevisiae* and *Drosophila melanogaster*, meet these requirements.

Although a correlation has often been observed between the ability of a chemical to cause chromosome breakage and its ability to induce gene mutation, data on chromosomal breakage alone do not provide adequate evidence for mutagenicity, and therefore less weight should be given to pre-screening that is based on the use of peripheral leucocyte cultures.

Because of the complexity of factors that can contribute to reproductive failure, as well as the insensitivity of the method, the dominant lethal test in the mammal does not provide reliable data on mutagenicity.

A large-scale systematic screening of compounds to assess a correlation between mutagenicity and carcinogenicity has so far been carried out only with the bacterial/mammalian liver microsome system. Notwithstanding the demonstration of the mutagenicity of many known carcinogens to *Salmonella typhimurium* in the presence of liver microsomal systems, the possibility of false-negative and false-positive results must not be overlooked. False negatives might arise as a consequence of mutagen specificity or from failure to achieve optimal conditions for activation *in vitro*. Alternative test systems must be used if there appear to be substantial reasons for suspecting that a chemical which is apparently non-mutagenic in a bacterial test system may nevertheless be potentially carcinogenic. Conversely, some chemicals found to be mutagenic in this test may not in fact have mutagenic activity in other systems.

For more detailed information, see references 29-36.

Observations in man: Case reports of cancer and epidemiological studies are summarized in this section.

Comments on Data Reported and Evaluation (section 4)

This section gives the critical view of the Working Group on the data reported.

Animal data: The animal species mentioned are those in which the carcinogenicity of the substances was clearly demonstrated. The route of administration used in experimental animals that is similar to the possible human exposure (ingestion, inhalation and skin exposure) is given particular mention. Tumour sites are also indicated.

Experiments involving a possible action of the vehicle or a physical effect of the agent, such as in studies by subcutaneous injection or bladder implantation, are included, however, the results of such tests require careful consideration, particularly if they are the only ones raising a suspicion of carcinogenicity. If the substance has produced tumours after prenatal exposure or in single-dose experiments, this also is indicated. This sub-section should be read in the light of comments made in the section, 'Animal Data in Relation to the Evaluation of Risk to Man' of this introduction.

Human data: In some cases, a brief statement is made on possible human exposure. The significance of epidemiological studies and case reports is discussed, and the data are interpreted in terms of possible human risk.

References

1. IARC (1972) *IARC Monographs on the Evaluation of Carcinogenic Risk of Chemicals to Man, 1*, Lyon

2. IARC (1973) *IARC Monographs on the Evaluation of Carcinogenic Risk of Chemicals to Man, 2, Some Inorganic and Organometallic Compounds*, Lyon

3. IARC (1973) *IARC Monographs on the Evaluation of Carcinogenic Risk of Chemicals to Man, 3, Certain Polycyclic Aromatic Hydrocarbons and Heterocyclic Compounds*, Lyon

4. IARC (1974) *IARC Monographs on the Evaluation of Carcinogenic Risk of Chemicals to Man, 4, Some Aromatic Amines, Hydrazine and Related Substances, N-Nitroso Compounds and Miscellaneous Alkylating Agents*, Lyon

5. IARC (1974) *IARC Monographs on the Evaluation of Carcinogenic Risk of Chemicals to Man, 5, Some Organochlorine Pesticides*, Lyon

6. IARC (1974) *IARC Monographs on the Evaluation of Carcinogenic Risk of Chemicals to Man, 6, Sex Hormones*, Lyon

7. IARC (1974) *IARC Monographs on the Evaluation of Carcinogenic Risk of Chemicals to Man, 7, Some Anti-thyroid and Related Substances, Nitrofurans and Industrial Chemicals*, Lyon

8. IARC (1975) *IARC Monographs on the Evaluation of Carcinogenic Risk of Chemicals to Man, 8, Some Aromatic Azo Compounds*, Lyon

9. IARC (1975) *IARC Monographs on the Evaluation of Carcinogenic Risk of Chemicals to Man, 9, Some Aziridines, N-, S- and O-Mustards and Selenium*, Lyon

10. IARC (1976) *IARC Monographs on the Evaluation of Carcinogenic Risk of Chemicals to Man, 10, Some Naturally Occurring Substances*, Lyon

11. IARC (1976) *IARC Monographs on the Evaluation of Carcinogenic Risk of Chemicals to Man, 11, Cadmium, Nickel, Some Epoxides, Miscellaneous Industrial Chemicals and General Considerations on Volatile Anaesthetics*, Lyon

12. IARC (1976) *IARC Monographs on the Evaluation of Carcinogenic Risk of Chemicals to Man, 12, Some Carbamates, Thiocarbamates and Carbazides*, Lyon

13. IARC (1977) *IARC Monographs on the Evaluation of Carcinogenic Risk of Chemicals to Man, 13, Some Miscellaneous Pharmaceutical Substances*, Lyon

14. IARC (1977) *IARC Monographs on the Evaluation of Carcinogenic Risk of Chemicals to Man, 14, Asbestos*, Lyon

15. Hartwell, J.L. (1951) *Survey of Compounds which have been Tested for Carcinogenic Activity*, Washington DC, US Government Printing Office (Public Health Service Publication No. 149)

16. Shubik, P. & Hartwell, J.L. (1957) *Survey of Compounds which have been Tested for Carcinogenic Activity*, Washington DC, US Government Printing Office (Public Health Service Publication No. 149: Supplement 1)

17. Shubik, P. & Hartwell, J.L. (1969) *Survey of Compounds which have been Tested for Carcinogenic Activity*, Washington DC, US Government Printing Office (Public Health Service Publication No. 149: Supplement 2)

18. Carcinogenesis Program National Cancer Institute (1971) *Survey of Compounds which have been Tested for Carcinogenic Activity*, Washington DC, US Government Printing Office (Public Health Service Publication No. 149: 1968-1969)

19. Carcinogenesis Program National Cancer Institute (1973) *Survey of Compounds which have been Tested for Carcinogenic Activity*, Washington DC, US Government Printing Office (Public Health Service Publication No. 149: 1961-1967)

20. Carcinogenesis Program National Cancer Institute (1974) *Survey of Compounds which have been Tested for Carcinogenic Activity*, Washington DC, US Government Printing Office (Public Health Service Publication No. 149: 1970-1971)

21. WHO (1961) Fifth Report of the Joint FAO/WHO Expert Committee on Food Additives. Evaluation of carcinogenic hazard of food additives. *Wld Hlth Org. techn. Rep. Ser., No. 220*, pp. 5, 18, 19

22. WHO (1969) Report of a WHO Scientific Group. Principles for the testing and evaluation of drugs for carcinogenicity. *Wld Hlth Org. techn. Rep. Ser., No. 426*, pp. 19, 21, 22

23. WHO (1964) Report of a WHO Expert Committee. Prevention of cancer. *Wld Hlth Org. techn. Rep. Ser., No. 276*, pp. 29, 30

24. WHO (1958) Second Report of the Joint FAO/WHO Expert Committee on Food Additives. Procedures for the testing of intentional food additives to establish their safety and use. *Wld Hlth Org. techn. Rep. Ser., No. 144*

25. WHO (1961) Fifth Report of the Joint FAO/WHO Expert Committee on Food Additives. Evaluation of carcinogenic hazard of food additives. *Wld Hlth Org. techn. Rep. Ser., No. 220*

26. WHO (1967) Scientific Group. Procedures for investigating intentional and unintentional food additives. <u>Wld Hlth Org. techn. Rep. Ser.</u>, No. 348

27. Berenblum, I., ed. (1969) Carcinogenicity testing. <u>UICC techn. Rep. Ser.</u>, <u>2</u>

28. Committee on Standardized Genetic Nomenclature for Mice (1972) Standardized nomenclature for inbred strains of mice. Fifth listing. <u>Cancer Res.</u>, <u>32</u>, 1609-1646

29. Bartsch, H. & Grover, P.L. (1976) <u>Chemical carcinogenesis and mutagenesis</u>. In: Symington, T. & Carter, R.L., eds, <u>Scientific Foundations of Oncology</u>, Vol. IX, <u>Chemical Carcinogenesis</u>, London, Heinemann Medical Books Ltd, pp. 334-342

30. Holländer, A., ed. (1971) <u>Chemical Mutagens: Principles and Methods for Their Detection</u>, Vols 1-3, New York, Plenum Press

31. Montesano, R. & Tomatis, L., eds (1974) <u>Chemical Carcinogenesis Essays</u>, Lyon (<u>IARC Scientific Publications No. 10</u>)

32. Ramel, C., ed. (1973) Evaluation of genetic risks of environmental chemicals: report of a symposium held at Skokloster, Sweden, 1972. <u>Ambio Special Report</u>, No. 3

33. Stoltz, D.R., Poirier, L.A., Irving, C.C., Stich, H.F., Weisburger, J.H. & Grice, H.C. (1974) Evaluation of short-term tests for carcinogenicity. <u>Toxicol. appl. Pharmacol.</u>, <u>29</u>, 157-180

34. WHO (1974) Report of WHO Scientific Group. Assessment of the carcinogenicity and mutagenicity of chemicals. <u>Wld Hlth Org. techn. Rep. Ser.</u>, No. 546

35. Montesano, R., Bartsch, H. & Tomatis, L., eds (1976) <u>Screening Tests in Chemical Carcinogenesis</u>, Lyon (<u>IARC Scientific Publications No. 12</u>)

36. Committee 17 (1975) Environmental mutagenic hazards. <u>Science</u>, <u>187</u>, 503-514

GENERAL REMARKS ON SUBSTANCES CONSIDERED

This volume includes monographs on a number of miscellaneous compounds not belonging to a particular chemical class. Some fumigants, certain industrial chemicals and chemical intermediates, the herbicides 2,4-D and 2,4,5-T and the chlorinated dibenzodioxins have been considered.

Of the compounds considered by the Working Group, seven do not appear in this volume. Monographs on four, dimethoate[1], fluorescein, fluorescein disodium[2] and trichlorphon, were postponed for consideration because the data available to the Working Group were judged insufficient to permit evaluations of their carcinogenicity. These compounds will be reconsidered when the results of current studies are published or when adequate data are made available. Two other compounds, polyvinyl pyrrolidone and polypropylene, will be reconsidered by a future Working Group and will be published in a subsequent volume that will include monographs on other, more closely related chemicals or classes of chemicals. Similarly, 5-nitroacenaphthene will be reconsidered with other aromatic amines by another Working Group in June 1977.

With regard to the herbicides 2,4-D and 2,4,5-T, the Working Group noted that confusion may possibly arise from the use of trade names for these substances, since both compounds may occur as active ingredients in a single formulation. For this reason, a representative list of trade names for 2,4-D and 2,4,5-T is given in Appendix A. The composition of such formulations may vary considerably in that a product may contain one or both of the parent compounds, its salts or its esters, together with other active compounds or inert ingredients.

---

[1] The Working Group was aware of carcinogenicity tests in progress in mice and rats involving oral administration of dimethoate (IARC, 1976a).

[2] The Working Group was aware of carcinogenicity tests in progress in newborn mice and rats involving subcutaneous injection of fluorescein disodium (IARC, 1976b).

Isopropyl oils and the chlorinated dibenzodioxins are not produced commercially but occur as contaminants of isopropyl alcohol and 2,4,5-T, respectively. Chlorodibenzo-*para*-dioxins may also occur in chlorophenols and products derived from them (see also monograph on chlorinated dibenzodioxins, p. 41).

Production of those compounds that are manufactured commercially varies considerably. Total annual production in three representative areas of the world, the US, Europe and Japan, estimated from the latest figures available, and the year of first commercial production are shown in Table 1. For many of these compounds total annual production was 5-10 million kg or more.

The Working Group noted that in the US pesticide regulations exist for some of the compounds considered. The 1972 Federal Environmental Pesticide Control Act gave the Environmental Protection Agency (EPA) authority over registration requirements for the use of new pesticides and provided for reconsideration of currently registered pesticide uses and a decision regarding their registration by a deadline date, now established at October 1977.

At present, a pesticide is registered for use only if labelling requirements are satisfied and only if its use according to directions causes no unreasonable risk to man or to the environment, taking into account economic, social and environmental costs and benefits of the use of the pesticide. To cope more adequately with the processes of registration and re-registration, the EPA implemented a 'rebuttable presumption' system. If the EPA determines that the use of a pesticide meets or exceeds any of several published risk criteria that are designed to identify unreasonable adverse effects in the environment, a notice of a 'rebuttable presumption against registration (RPAR)' is made. The prospective registrant has 45 days, extendable by 60 days for valid reasons, in which to challenge this notice, by submitting information that the evidence supporting the RPAR is not valid, that the risk is not real or that potential benefits exceed potential risks. If the notice is successfully rebutted, re-registration occurs without a hearing; if the new information is insufficient or if none is supplied, the EPA issues a notice of intent to deny or to cancel registration or to hold a hearing.

TABLE 1

Chemical	Year of first commercial production	Estimated annual production
1,2-Bis(chloromethoxy)-ethane	-	-
1,4-Bis(chloromethoxymethyl)benzene	-	-
Catechol	1920	>5 million kg
Copper 8-hydroxyquinoline	1949	>350,000 kg
2,4-D	1944	>30 million kg
1,2-Dibromo-3-chloropropane	1955	>3 million kg
trans-1,4-Dichlorobutene	1963	unknown but >450 kg[a]
Dimethoxane	1962	unknown but >450 kg[a]
Eosin and eosin disodium salt	1918	>9 million kg
Ethylene dibromide	1923	>150 million kg
Hexamethylphosphoramide	unknown	>150,000 kg
Hydroquinone	1918	>15 million kg
Isopropyl alcohol	1921	>1000 million kg
Methyl iodide	1943	>2 million kg
para-Quinone	1919	>3 million kg
Resorcinol	1918	>20 million kg
Succinic anhydride	1921	unknown but >450 kg[a]
2,4,5-T	1944	>10 million kg
1,2,3-Tris(chloromethoxy)-propane	-	-

[a] See preamble, p. 17.

References

IARC (1976a) *IARC Information Bulletin on the Survey of Chemicals Being Tested for Carcinogenicity*, No. 6, Lyon, p. 217

IARC (1976b) *IARC Information Bulletin on the Survey of Chemicals Being Tested for Carcinogenicity*, No. 6, Lyon, p. 93

THE MONOGRAPHS

1,2-BIS(CHLOROMETHOXY)ETHANE

1. Chemical and Physical Data

1.1 Synonyms and trade names

Chem. Abstr. Services Reg. No.: 13483-18-6

Chem. Abstr. Name: 1,2-Bis(chloromethoxy)ethane

Bis-1,2-(chloromethoxy)ethane; ethylene glycol bis(chloromethyl)ether

1.2 Chemical formula and molecular weight

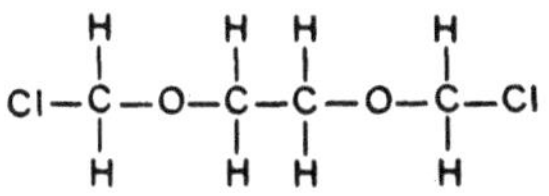

$$Cl-\underset{H}{\overset{H}{C}}-O-\underset{H}{\overset{H}{C}}-\underset{H}{\overset{H}{C}}-O-\underset{H}{\overset{H}{C}}-Cl$$

$C_4H_8Cl_2O_2$ Mol. wt: 159.0

1.3 Chemical and physical properties of the pure substance

(a) Description: Viscous liquid (Lichtenberger & Martin, 1947)

(b) Boiling-point: 99-100°C at 22 mm (Lichtenberger & Martin, 1945, 1947); 97-99°C at 13 mm (Walker, 1933)

(c) Density: d_{15}^{14} 1.2879 (Lichtenberger & Martin, 1945)

(d) Refractive index: n_D^{14} 1.4659; n_D^{15} 1.4657 (Lichtenberger & Martin, 1945, 1947)

(e) Spectroscopy data: Nuclear magnetic resonance spectra are given by Van Duuren et al. (1975).

(f) Solubility: Insoluble in water (Walker, 1933)

(g) Stability: Decomposes in moist air (Lichtenberger & Martin, 1947)

(h) Reactivity: Reacts as an alkylating agent with water and glutathione (Van Duuren et al., 1975)

1.4 Technical products and impurities

No data were available to the Working Group.

2. Production, Use, Occurrence and Analysis

For background information on this section, see preamble, p. 17.

2.1 Production and use

(a) Production

1,2-Bis(chloromethoxy)ethane was prepared in 1933 by the reaction of ethylene glycol, formaldehyde and hydrochloric acid (Walker, 1933).

(b) Use

Although 1,2-bis(chloromethoxy)ethane does not appear to have been used commercially, it has been investigated for potential commercial use on cellulosic textiles for imparting crease resistance (Anon., 1966; Kocher, 1959; Tesoro, 1963), improving wet strength (Kocher, 1958a) and facilitating dyeing (Kocher, 1958b); as a stabilizer for vulcanized rubbers (Pokonova & Mamedova, 1968); as a curing agent for epoxy resins (Anon., 1971); in the preparation of light-sensitive polymers for lithographic plates (Borden *et al.*, 1970); and in the synthesis of ion-exchange resins.

2.2 Occurrence

1,2-Bis(chloromethoxy)ethane is not known to occur in nature.

2.3 Analysis

No data were available to the Working Group.

3. Biological Data Relevant to the Evaluation of Carcinogenic Risk to Man

3.1 Carcinogenicity and related studies in animals

(a) Skin application

Mouse: Fifty 6-8-week old female ICR/Ha Swiss mice were administered 1 mg 1,2-bis(chloromethoxy)ethane in 0.1 ml cyclohexane on the dorsal skin thrice weekly for up to 502 days, at which time more than half the animals were still alive. Four mice developed skin papillomas, the first of which appeared after 320 days, and 4 animals had local squamous-cell carcinomas ($P<0.05$). In 50 control mice treated with cyclohexane only, the median survival time was greater than 504 days; no tumours occurred at the site of administration (Van Duuren *et al.*, 1975).

(b) Subcutaneous and/or intramuscular administration

Mouse: Fifty 6-8-week old female ICR/Ha Swiss mice were given weekly s.c. injections of 0.3 mg 1,2-bis(chloromethoxy)ethane in 0.05 ml tricaprylin. The test lasted 569 days, and the median survival time of treated mice was 362 days. Nine mice had local sarcomas ($P<0.01$). In 50 control animals treated with tricaprylin alone, the median survival time was 436 days; no local malignant tumours occurred (Van Duuren *et al.*, 1975).

(c) Intraperitoneal administration

Mouse: Thirty 6-8-week old female ICR/Ha Swiss mice were given weekly i.p. injections of 0.3 mg 1,2-bis(chloromethoxy)ethane in 0.05 ml tricaprylin. The test lasted 546 days, and the median survival time of treated mice was 481 days. Two mice developed undifferentiated malignant tumours at the injection site, and 2 had local sarcomas ($P<0.05$). In 30 controls treated with tricaprylin alone, the median survival time was 513 days; no local malignant tumours occurred (Van Duuren *et al.*, 1975).

3.2 Other relevant biological data

No data were available to the Working Group.

3.3 Case reports and epidemiological studies

No data were available to the Working Group.

4. Comments on Data Reported and Evaluation[1]

4.1 Animal data

1,2-Bis(chloromethoxy)ethane is carcinogenic in mice, the only species tested, following its application to the skin or its subcutaneous or intraperitoneal administration; it produced malignant tumours at the sites of administration.

4.2 Human data

No case reports or epidemiological studies were available to the Working Group.

---

[1]See also the section, 'Animal Data in Relation to the Evaluation of Risk to Man' in the introduction to this volume, p. 15.

5. References

Anon. (1966) Crease-resistant cellulosic textiles. <u>French Patent</u> 1,434,107, 8 April, to Traitements Chimiques des Textiles

Anon. (1971) Catalytic polymerization and/or hardening of epoxy resins. <u>Netherlander Application</u> 70 05,967, 26 October, to Nederlandse Organisatie voor Toegepast-Natuurwetenschappelijk Onderzoek ten behoeve van Nijverheid, Handel en Verkeer

Borden, D.G., Williams, J.L.R. & Laakso, T.M. (1970) Light-sensitive polymers. <u>Def. Publ.</u>, <u>US Patent</u> 872,003, 10 March

Kocher, F. (1958a) Treatment of cellulosic textiles. <u>French Addition</u> 68,167, 9 April, to Etablissements Schaeffer & Cie

Kocher, F. (1958b) Improving the dyeability of cellulosic textiles. <u>French Addition</u> 68,993, 26 August, to Etablissements Schaeffer & Cie

Kocher, F. (1959) Imparting permanent wrinkle resistance to cellulosic textiles by chemical treatment. <u>French Patent</u> 1,171,153, 22 January, to Traitements Chimiques des Textiles

Lichtenberger, J. & Martin, L. (1945) Chlorométhylation des diols. <u>Bull. Soc. chim. Fr.</u>, <u>12</u>, 114-115

Lichtenberger, J. & Martin, L. (1947) Etude sur les éthers chlorométhyliques des polyols. <u>Bull. Soc. chim. Fr.</u>, <u>14</u>, 468-476

Pokonova, Y.V. & Mamedova, M.M. (1968) Stabilization of rubbers. <u>USSR Patent</u> 231,790, 28 November, to Azerbaidzhan Institute of Petroleum and Chemistry

Tesoro, G.C. (1963) Treating cellulosic material with polyquaternary ammonium derivatives of bis halomethyl ethers. <u>US Patent</u> 3,115,383, 24 December, to J.P. Stevens & Co., Inc.

Van Duuren, B.L., Goldschmidt, B.M. & Seidman, I. (1975) Carcinogenic activity of di- and trifunctional α-chloro ethers and of 1,4-dichlorobutene-2 in ICR/HA Swiss mice. <u>Cancer Res.</u>, <u>35</u>, 2553-2557

Walker, F. (1933) Methylene ether esters. <u>Plastic Products</u>, <u>9</u>, 187-188

1,4-BIS(CHLOROMETHOXYMETHYL)BENZENE

1. Chemical and Physical Data

1.1 Synonyms and trade names

Chem. Abstr. Services Reg. No.: 56894-91-8

Chem. Abstr. Name: 1,4-Bis(chloromethoxymethyl)benzene

Bis-1,4-(chloromethoxy)-*para*-xylene; 1,4-bis(chloromethoxy)-*para*-xylene

1.2 Chemical formula and molecular weight

$$ClCH_2-O-CH_2-\langle C_6H_4 \rangle-CH_2-O-CH_2Cl$$

$C_{10}H_{12}Cl_2O_2$ Mol. wt: 235.1

1.3 Chemical and physical properties of the pure substance

(a) *Spectroscopy data*: Nuclear magnetic resonance spectra are given by Van Duuren *et al.* (1975).

(b) *Reactivity*: Reacts as an alkylating agent with water and glutathione (Van Duuren *et al.*, 1975)

1.4 Technical products and impurities

No data were available to the Working Group.

2. Production, Use, Occurrence and Analysis

For background information on this section, see preamble, p. 17.

2.1 Production and use

1,4-Bis(chloromethoxymethyl)benzene has been investigated in the US for use in the preparation of ion-exchange resins.

2.2 Occurrence

1,4-Bis(chloromethoxymethyl)benzene is not known to occur in nature.

2.3 Analysis

No data were available to the Working Group.

3. Biological Data Relevant to the Evaluation of Carcinogenic Risk to Man

3.1 Carcinogenicity and related studies in animals

(a) Skin application

Mouse: Fifty 6-8-week old female ICR/Ha Swiss mice were administered 0.3 mg 1,4-bis(chloromethoxymethyl)benzene in 0.1 ml cyclohexane on the dorsal skin thrice weekly for up to 502 days. The median survival time of treated animals was 484 days. Seven mice developed skin papillomas, the first of which was observed after 328 days; one mouse had an 'undifferentiated malignant tumour in the treatment area', and 7 animals had local squamous-cell carcinomas ($P<0.01$). In 50 control mice treated with cyclohexane alone, the median survival time was greater than 504 days; no tumours occurred at the site of administration (Van Duuren et al., 1975).

(b) Subcutaneous and/or intramuscular administration

Mouse: Fifty 6-8-week old female ICR/Ha Swiss mice were given weekly s.c. injections of 0.3 mg 1,4-bis(chloromethoxymethyl)benzene in 0.05 ml tricaprylin. The test lasted 569 days, and the median survival time of treated mice was 401 days. One mouse had a squamous-cell carcinoma at the injection site, and 11 animals developed local sarcomas ($P<0.01$). In 50 control animals treated with tricaprylin alone, the median survival time was 436 days; no local malignant tumours occurred (Van Duuren et al., 1975).

3.2 Other relevant biological data

No data were available to the Working Group.

3.3 Case reports and epidemiological studies

No data were available to the Working Group.

4. Comments on Data Reported and Evaluation[1]

4.1 Animal data

1,4-Bis(chloromethoxymethyl)benzene is carcinogenic in mice, the only species tested, following its application to the skin or its subcutaneous administration; it produced malignant tumours at the sites of application.

4.2 Human data

No case reports or epidemiological studies were available to the Working Group.

---

[1] See also the section, 'Animal Data in Relation to the Evaluation of Risk to Man' in the introduction to this volume, p. 15.

5. References

Van Duuren, B.L., Goldschmidt, B.M. & Seidman, I. (1975) Carcinogenic activity of di- and trifunctional α-chloro ethers and of 1,4-dichlorobutene-2 in ICR/HA Swiss mice. Cancer Res., 35, 2553-2557

CHLORINATED DIBENZODIOXINS

1. Chemical and Physical Data

1.1 Synonyms and trade names

Dibenzo-*para*-dioxin

Chem. Abstr. Services Reg. No.: 262-12-4

Chem. Abstr. Name: Dibenzo[*b,e*](1,4)dioxin

Dibenzodioxin; dibenzo(1,4)dioxin; dibenzo-*para*-dioxin; diphenylene dioxide; oxanthrene; phenodioxin

1-Chlorodibenzo-*para*-dioxin

Chem. Abstr. Services Reg. No.: 39227-53-7

Chem. Abstr. Name: 1-Chlorodibenzo[*b,e*](1,4)dioxin

1-Chlorodibenzodioxin

2-Chlorodibenzo-*para*-dioxin

Chem. Abstr. Services Reg. No.: 39227-54-8

Chem. Abstr. Name: 2-Chlorodibenzo[*b,e*](1,4)dioxin

2-Chlorodibenzodioxin

1,3-Dichlorodibenzo-*para*-dioxin

Chem. Abstr. Services Reg. No.: 50585-39-2

Chem. Abstr. Name: 1,3-Dichlorodibenzo[*b,e*](1,4)dioxin

1,3-Dichlorodibenzodioxin

1,6-Dichlorodibenzo-*para*-dioxin

Chem. Abstr. Services Reg. No.: 38178-38-0

Chem. Abstr. Name: 1,6-Dichlorodibenzo[*b,e*](1,4)dioxin

1,6-Dichlorodibenzodioxin

2,3-Dichlorodibenzo-*para*-dioxin

Chem. Abstr. Services Reg. No.: 29446-15-9

Chem. Abstr. Name: 2,3-Dichlorodibenzo[*b,e*](1,4)dioxin

2,3-Dichlorodibenzodioxin

2,7-Dichlorodibenzo-*para*-dioxin

Chem. Abstr. Services Reg. No.: 33857-26-0

Chem. Abstr. Name: 2,7-Dichlorodibenzo[*b,e*](1,4)dioxin

2,7-Dichlorodibenzodioxin; DCDD

2,8-Dichlorodibenzo-*para*-dioxin

Chem. Abstr. Services Reg. No.: 38964-22-6

Chem. Abstr. Name: 2,8-Dichlorodibenzo[*b,e*](1,4)dioxin

2,8-Dichlorodibenzodioxin

1,2,4-Trichlorodibenzo-*para*-dioxin

Chem. Abstr. Services Reg. No.: 39227-58-2

Chem. Abstr. Name: 1,2,4-Trichlorodibenzo[*b,e*](1,4)dioxin

1,2,4-Trichlorodibenzodioxin

2,3,7-Trichlorodibenzo-*para*-dioxin

Chem. Abstr. Services Reg. No.: 33857-28-2

Chem. Abstr. Name: 2,3,7-Trichlorodibenzo[*b,e*](1,4)dioxin

2,3,7-Trichlorodibenzodioxin

1,2,3,4-Tetrachlorodibenzo-*para*-dioxin

Chem. Abstr. Services Reg. No.: 30746-58-8

Chem. Abstr. Name: 1,2,3,4-Tetrachlorodibenzo[*b,e*](1,4)dioxin

1,2,3,4-Tetrachlorodibenzodioxin

1,2,3,8-Tetrachlorodibenzo-*para*-dioxin

Chem. Abstr. Services Reg. No.: 53555-02-5

Chem. Abstr. Name: 1,2,3,8-Tetrachlorodibenzo[b,e](1,4)dioxin

1,2,3,8-Tetrachlorodibenzodioxin

1,3,6,8-Tetrachlorodibenzo-*para*-dioxin

Chem. Abstr. Services Reg. No.: 33423-92-6

Chem. Abstr. Name: 1,3,6,8-Tetrachlorodibenzo[b,e](1,4)dioxin

1,3,6,8-Tetrachlorodibenzodioxin

1,3,7,8-Tetrachlorodibenzo-*para*-dioxin

Chem. Abstr. Services Reg. No.: 50585-46-1

Chem. Abstr. Name: 1,3,7,8-Tetrachlorodibenzo[b,e](1,4)dioxin

1,3,7,8-Tetrachlorodibenzodioxin

2,3,6,7-Tetrachlorodibenzo-*para*-dioxin

Chem. Abstr. Services Reg. No.: 34816-53-0

Chem. Abstr. Name: 1,2,7,8-Tetrachlorodibenzo[b,e](1,4)dioxin

1,2,7,8-Tetrachlorodibenzo-1,4-dioxin; 1,2,7,8-tetrachlorodibenzo-*para*-dioxin; 2,3,6,7-tetrachlorodibenzodioxin

2,3,7,8-Tetrachlorodibenzo-*para*-dioxin

Chem. Abstr. Services Reg. No.: 1746-01-6

Chem. Abstr. Name: 2,3,7,8-Tetrachlorodibenzo[b,e](1,4)dioxin

Dioxin; TCDBD; TCDD; 2,3,7,8-tetrachlorodibenzodioxin; 2,3,7,8-tetrachlorodibenzo-1,4-dioxin

1,2,3,4,7-Pentachlorodibenzo-*para*-dioxin

Chem. Abstr. Services Reg. No.: none available

Chem. Abstr. Name: none available

1,2,3,4,7-Pentachlorodibenzodioxin

1,2,3,7,8-Pentachlorodibenzo-*para*-dioxin

Chem. Abstr. Services Reg. No.: 40321-76-4

Chem. Abstr. Name: 1,2,3,7,8-Pentachlorodibenzo[*b,e*](1,4)dioxin

1,2,3,7,8-Pentachlorodibenzodioxin

1,2,4,7,8-Pentachlorodibenzo-*para*-dioxin

Chem. Abstr. Services Reg. No.: none available

Chem. Abstr. Name: none available

1,2,4,7,8-Pentachlorodibenzodioxin

1,2,3,4,7,8-Hexachlorodibenzo-*para*-dioxin

Chem. Abstr. Services Reg. No.: none available

Chem. Abstr. Name: none available

1,2,3,4,7,8-Hexachlorodibenzodioxin

1,2,3,6,7,8-Hexachlorodibenzo-*para*-dioxin

Chem. Abstr. Services Reg. No.: none available

Chem. Abstr. Name: none available

1,2,3,6,7,8-Hexachlorodibenzodioxin

1,2,3,6,7,9-Hexachlorodibenzo-*para*-dioxin

Chem. Abstr. Services Reg. No.: none available

Chem. Abstr. Name: none available

1,2,3,6,7,9-Hexachlorodibenzodioxin

1,2,3,7,8,9-Hexachlorodibenzo-*para*-dioxin

Chem. Abstr. Services Reg. No.: none available

Chem. Abstr. Name: none available

1,2,3,7,8,9-Hexachlorodibenzodioxin

1,2,4,6,7,9-Hexachlorodibenzo-*para*-dioxin

Chem. Abstr. Services Reg. No.: none available

Chem. Abstr. Name: none available

1,2,4,6,7,9-Hexachlorodibenzodioxin

1,2,3,4,6,7,8-Heptachlorodibenzo-*para*-dioxin

Chem. Abstr. Services Reg. No.: 35822-46-9

Chem. Abstr. Name: 1,2,3,4,6,7,8-Heptachlorodibenzo[b,e](1,4)dioxin

1,2,3,4,6,7,8-Heptachlorodibenzodioxin; heptachlorodibenzo-*para*-dioxin

1,2,3,4,6,7,9-Heptachlorodibenzo-*para*-dioxin

Chem. Abstr. Services Reg. No.: none available

Chem. Abstr. Name: none available

1,2,3,4,6,7,9-Heptachlorodibenzodioxin

1,2,3,4,6,7,8,9-Octachlorodibenzo-*para*-dioxin

Chem. Abstr. Services Reg. No.: 3268-87-9

Chem. Abstr. Name: 1,2,3,4,6,7,8,9-Octachlorodibenzo[b,e](1,4)dioxin

1,2,3,4,6,7,8,9-Octachlorodibenzodioxin; octachlorodibenzo-*para*-dioxin; octachloro-*para*-dibenzodioxin; OCDD

1.2 Chemical formulae and molecular weights

Empirical formulae and molecular weights are given only for those chlorodibenzo-*para*-dioxins for which biological data were considered. The structural formula of unsubstituted dibenzo-*para*-dioxin and the numbering of the carbon atoms in the ring are given below. The chlorinated dibenzo-*para*-dioxins contain chlorine atoms at the positions indicated in their names.

Dibenzo-*para*-dioxin

$C_{12}H_8O_2$ Mol. wt: 184.2

2,7-Dichlorodibenzo-*para*-dioxin (DCDD)

$C_{12}H_6Cl_2O_2$ Mol. wt: 253

1,2,3,4-Tetrachlorodibenzo-*para*-dioxin

$C_{12}H_4Cl_4O_2$ Mol. wt: 322

2,3,7,8-Tetrachlorodibenzo-*para*-dioxin (TCDD)

$C_{12}H_4Cl_4O_2$ Mol. wt: 322

1,2,4,6,7,9-Hexachlorodibenzo-*para*-dioxin

$C_{12}H_2Cl_6O_2$ Mol. wt: 390.9

1,2,3,4,7,8-Hexachlorodibenzo-*para*-dioxin

$C_{12}H_2Cl_6O_2$ Mol. wt: 390.9

1,2,3,4,6,7,8,9-Octachlorodibenzo-*para*-dioxin (OCDD)

$C_{12}Cl_8O_2$ Mol. wt: 459.8

1.3 Chemical and physical properties

The physical properties of the chlorinated dibenzo-*para*-dioxins are given, when available, in Table 1. Additional information is given below:

TABLE 1

Physical properties of the chlorinated dioxins[a]

Dibenzo-para-dioxin derivative	Description	Melting point (°C)	λ_{max} (chloroform)	E^1_1	λ_{max} (methanol)	E^1_1	λ_{max} (isooctane)	E^1_1	IR spectra	Mass spectra	Phosphorescence spectra	NMR spectra	Method of synthesis
Unsubstituted	crystals	122-123	248 / 293	53.4 / 199.8	228 / 290	1113 / 200.8	230 / 290	530 / 210	b			e	e
1-chloro-	colourless crystals	104.5-105.5	248 / 294	60.3 / 145.7	232 / 291	1094 / 159.8	236 / 291	479.5 / 139.7	b			e	e
2-chloro-	colourless solid	88-89	248 / 299	52 / 169	231 / 293	106.4 / 183.6	234 / 295	520.5 / 168.5	b			e	e
1,3-dichloro-		113.5-114.6[d]	296[d]	122.5[d]					b	h			h
1,6-dichloro-	colourless needles	184-185[b]							b	f			f
2,3-dichloro-	colourless solid	163-164	247 / 304	72.33 / 126	232 / 306	1067 / 142.3	238 / 298	454.5 / 135.2	b	d	e	e	e
2,7-dichloro-	colourless crystals	209-210	247 / 302	52.96 / 181.4	235 / 298	9842 / 200	236 / 299	466.4 / 169.6	b	f	e	e	see text
2,8-dichloro-	colourless solid	150.5-151	247 / 299	46.6 / 185.4	234 / 297	1079 / 202.4	237 / 299	462.5 / 185	b		e	e	e,i
1,2,4-trichloro-	colourless solid	128-129	253 / 294	183.7 / 78	239 / 295	861 / 76.4	247 / 290	449.6 / 79.5	b		e	e	e
2,3,7-trichloro-		153-158[d] / 162-163[d]	304[d] / 305[d]	120[d] / 180.6					g	d,g	e	g	h
1,2,3,4-tetrachloro-	colourless needles	189	257 / 317	195.3 / 71.1					b	e,f	e	e	see text
1,3,6,8-tetrachloro-	colourless needles	219-219.5	250 / 305	172 / 106.8					b	d	e	e	e
1,3,7,8-tetrachloro-		193.5-195[h]	304[h]	129.2[h]									i
2,3,7,8-tetrachloro-	colourless needles	305-306	248 / 310	92.2 / 173.6					b	d,f	e	e	see text
1,2,3,4,7-pentachloro-	colourless solid	195-196	259 / 306	166.3 / 75.6					b		e	e	g
1,2,3,7,8-pentachloro-		240-241	308	171.4						g	e	g	g
1,2,4,7,8-pentachloro-		205-206	307	103.9						g	e	g	d
1,2,3,4,7,8-hexachloro-	colourless solid	275	259 / 316	137.3 / 93.6					b	g	g		see text
1,2,3,6,7,8-hexachloro-		285-286[o]	316[o]	152[o]					c	o			o,j
1,2,3,7,8,9-hexachloro-		243-244[o]	317[o]	104[o]					b	o			o
1,2,4,6,7,9-hexachloro-	colourless solid	238-240	259 / 310	113.81 / 37.85					b		e	e	see text
1,2,3,4,6,7,8,9-octachloro-		330	261 / 318	285.9 / 52.2					b	f	e		see text

[a] Data from reference in footnote e, unless otherwise specified
[b] Chen, 1973
[c] Gray et al., 1975
[d] Kende & Wade, 1973
[e] Pohland & Yang, 1972
[f] Bau-Hoi et al., 1972a
[g] Gray et al., 1976
[h] Kende et al., 1974
[i] Juillino, 1973
[j] Kende & DeCamp, 1975

(a) Solubility: The solubility of TCDD in various solvents is as follows: (Crummett & Stehl, 1973):

Solvent	Solubility, g/l
ortho-dichlorobenzene	1.4
chlorobenzene	0.72
benzene	0.57
chloroform	0.37
acetone	0.11
n-octanol	0.05
methanol	0.01
water	2×10^{-7}
lard oil	0.04 (Committee on the Effects of Herbicides in Vietnam, 1974)

The solubility of OCDD in various solvents is as follows (Aniline, 1973):

Solvent	Solubility, g/l
acetic acid	0.048
anisole	1.730
chloroform	0.562
ortho-dichlorobenzene	1.832
dioxane	0.384
diphenyl oxide	0.841
pyridine	0.400
xylene	3.575

(b) Stability: These compounds are extremely stable, even on heating to 700°C. DCDD and TCDD were changed chemically when exposed as solutions in isooctane or n-octanol to ultra-violet light. OCDD was stable under such conditions (Stehl *et al.*, 1973). For data on the persistence of these compounds in the environment, see section 2.2.

1.4 Technical products and impurities

The chlorodibenzo-*para*-dioxins are not manufactured commercially, but some of them are present as impurities in certain herbicide and fungicide formulations, such as 2,4,5-T and the pentachlorophenols (see also the following section).

2. Production, Use, Occurrence and Analysis

For background information on this section, see preamble, p. 17.

2.1 Production and use

(a) Production

The herbicide 2,4,5-T produced commercially prior to 1965 contained up to 30 mg/kg or more TCDD (Anon., 1970); 2,4,5-T containing less than 0.05 mg/kg TCDD is now produced in several countries and is available in commercial quantities. Furthermore, techniques have been developed for producing 2,4,5-T that contains levels of TCDD below the limit of detection (0.02 mg/kg) (see Neubert & Dillmann, 1972). Details of its commercial production are given in the monograph on 2,4,5-T, p. 273.

Pentachlorophenol may contain 9-27 mg/kg mixed isomers of hexachlorodibenzo-*para*-dioxin (HCDD) and 575-2510 mg/kg OCDD (Johnson et al., 1973). It was first produced in the US in 1936. Production increased from 18 million kg in 1965 to 24 million kg in 1974; however, in 1975, four US manufacturers reported a total production of only 18 million kg (US International Trade Commission, 1976a,b; US Tariff Commission, 1967). Pentachlorophenol is a fungicide used for slime control in the manufacture of paper pulp and for a variety of other purposes, including processing of oils, leathers, paints, glues and textiles, and has been incorporated into shampoos (Crossland & Shea, 1973). It is currently registered for use in the US as an agricultural seed treatment, for use on wood to provide protection against termites, wood-boring insects and moulds and for other miscellaneous uses (US Environmental Protection Agency, 1973).

Hexachlorophene produced from trichlorophenol is reported to contain less than 15 µg/kg TCDD.

Conventional methods for the laboratory preparation of the chlorinated dibenzo-*para*-dioxins mentioned in the section on biological data involve two types of process: (1) condensation of a polychlorophenol, or (2) direct halogenation of the parent dibenzo-*para*-dioxin or a monochloro derivative. The major drawback of these synthetic methods is the small yield of suitably chlorinated chlorodibenzo-*para*-dioxin. This may be avoided in some cases by carrying out condensation between a catechol dianion and either an appropriate polychlorobenzene in boiling dimethyl sulphoxide (Kende et *al.*, 1974) or an appropriate *ortho*-chloropolychloronitrobenzene (Gray et *al.*, 1976).

Unsubstituted dibenzo-*para*-dioxin has been prepared by heating *ortho*-chlorophenol, anhydrous potassium carbonate and copper powder and refluxing the resultant mixture with aqueous potassium hydroxide (Gilman & Dietrich, 1957).

DCDD has been made by heating the potassium salt of 2,4-dichlorophenol in the presence of copper powder in a vacuum sublimator; the sublimate was recrystallized from methanol (Pohland & Yang, 1972). It can also be made by dissolving 2-bromo-4-chlorophenol and potassium hydroxide in methanol and evaporating to dryness. The residue is mixed with bis(2-ethoxyethyl)ether, ethylene diacetate and a copper catalyst, heated, cooled and eluted from a chromatographic column with chloroform. This residue is evaporated and then sublimed (Aniline, 1973).

1,2,3,4-Tetrachlorodibenzo-*para*-dioxin has been prepared by refluxing a mixture of catechol, potassium carbonate, pentachloronitrobenzene and acetone in nitrogen. The product was recrystallized twice from acetone (Pohland & Yang, 1972).

TCDD has been made by chlorination of dibenzo-*para*-dioxin in chloroform in the presence of iodine and ferric chloride (Sandermann et *al.*, 1957).

1,2,4,6,7,9-HCDD can be made by heating the potassium salt of 2,3,5,6-tetrachlorophenol with powdered copper and potassium carbonate in a vacuum sublimation apparatus (Pohland & Yang, 1972).

1,2,3,4,7,8-HCDD has been prepared by mixing 1,2,3,4-tetrachlorodibenzo-*para*-dioxin, ferric chloride, chloroform and a crystal of iodine and then adding a solution of chlorine in carbon tetrachloride (Pohland & Yang, 1972).

Merz & Weith (1872) obtained OCDD by heating the potassium salt of pentachlorophenol; Sandermann *et al.* (1957) prepared it in poor yield directly from pentachlorophenol by heating. It has been prepared in almost quantitative yield by heating pentachlorophenol in the presence of an initiator, such as chlorine, bromine, iodine or 2,3,4,4,5,6-hexachloro-2,5-cyclohexadienone. Hexachlorocyclohexadienone, when heated in an atmosphere of carbon dioxide for 30 minutes, also yields OCDD (Kulka, 1961).

(b) Use

DCDD has been reported to have some antibacterial action (Tomita & Watanabe, 1951). TCDD has been tested for use in flameproofing polymers, e.g., polyesters (Darsow & Schnell, 1970), and against insects and wood-destroying fungi (Sandermann *et al.*, 1957). It is hoped that these uses have never been exploited commercially.

2.2 Occurrence

The chlorodibenzo-*para*-dioxins found in 2,4,5-T, pentachlorophenol and hexachlorophene are formed during the manufacturing processes used to produce chlorophenols.

TCDD is formed as a by-product during the synthesis of 2,4,5-trichlorophenol, which involves the hydrolysis of 1,2,4,5-tetrachlorobenzene using methanol and caustic soda at elevated pressure or ethylene glycol and caustic soda at atmospheric pressure (Milnes, 1971) (see also Fig. 1). If the reaction is allowed to heat to temperatures higher than the normal $180^{\circ}C$, ethylene glycol is distilled off or polymerized, and an exothermic reaction starts at about $230^{\circ}C$ and proceeds rapidly and uncontrollably to about $410^{\circ}C$. TCDD is formed in the distillate by the condensation of two molecules of sodium trichlorophenate under the influence of the highly exothermic decomposition of sodium-2-hydroxyethanol (Fig. 2A). When the

Figure 1

Schematic representation of the reaction involved in 2,4,5-trichlorophenol production[a]

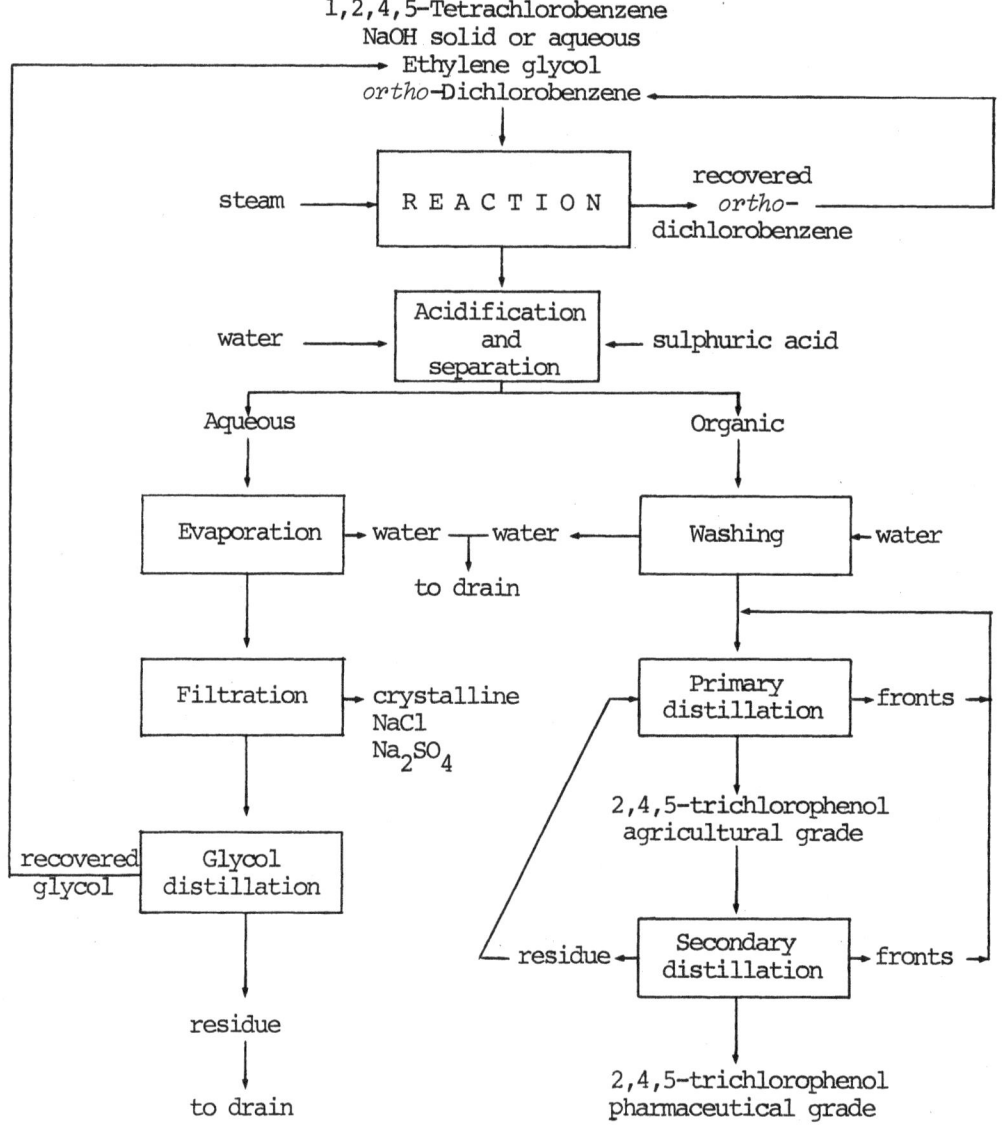

[a]From May, 1973

Figure 2

(A) Formation of TCDD by condensation of sodium trichlorophenate
(Jirásek et al., 1974; Langer et al., 1973; May, 1973; Mercier, 1977; Milnes, 1971).

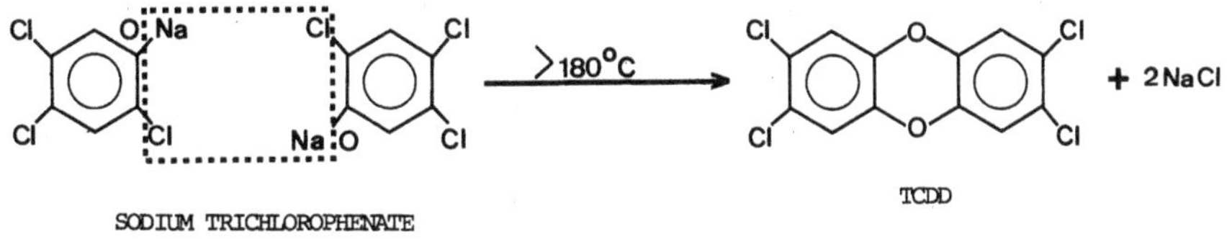

SODIUM TRICHLOROPHENATE $\xrightarrow{>180°C}$ TCDD + 2NaCl

(B) General scheme for production of 2,4,5-T (from Dalderup, 1974; Saint-Ruf, 1977)

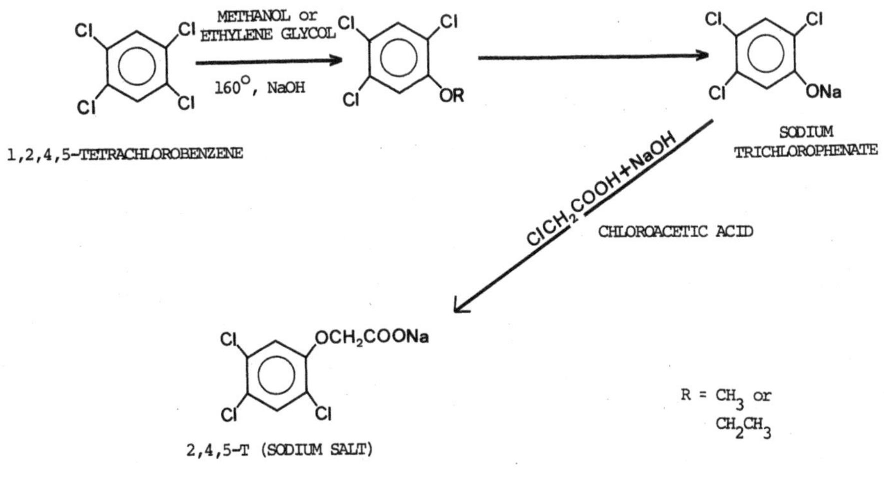

1,2,4,5-TETRACHLOROBENZENE $\xrightarrow[160°, \text{NaOH}]{\text{METHANOL or ETHYLENE GLYCOL}}$ → SODIUM TRICHLOROPHENATE $\xrightarrow{ClCH_2COOH + NaOH \text{ (CHLOROACETIC ACID)}}$ 2,4,5-T (SODIUM SALT)

R = CH_3 or CH_2CH_3

mixture is heated at 180°C, which is the normal reaction temperature, even for long periods, 2,4,5-trichlorophenol contains less than 1 mg/kg TCDD. Much greater amounts of TCDD (e.g., 1600 mg/kg) have been formed when sodium 2,4,5-trichlorophenate was heated at 230-260°C for 2 hours (Mercier, 1977).

2,4,5-Trichlorophenol is also the precursor of 2,4,5-T (Fig. 2B); therefore, another potential source of TCDD is during the manufacture of 2,4,5-T and its esters *per se* (Jirásek *et al.*, 1974; Langer *et al.*, 1973; May, 1973: Mercier, 1977; Milnes, 1971).

In one process, hexachlorobenzenes are subjected to high temperature, high pressure and alkaline conditions, and a reaction between two molecules of pentachlorophenol may occur, resulting in the formation of OCDD. The more highly chlorinated dibenzo-*para*-dioxins may also be formed if too much heat is applied when the chlorophenols are produced by the reaction of chlorine with phenol, especially during the manufacture of tetra- and pentachlorophenols.

2.2.1 Occurrence after accidental contamination

TCDD was a component of the products of an explosion which took place in 1963 at the Philips Duphar 2,4,5-T factory in The Netherlands (Dalderup, 1974). According to Hay (1976), an estimated 30-200 g TCDD were released; the factory was sealed off for 10 years, then dismantled, embedded in concrete and dumped at a deep point into the Atlantic Ocean.

TCDD was identified as a product of an explosion which occurred in the Coalite Company's 2,4,5-trichlorophenol factory in the UK in 1968 (May, 1973; Milnes, 1971), but the quantity of TCDD released was not estimated. The method of manufacture used at this factory involved hydrolysis of 1,2,4,5-tetrachlorobenzene using ethylene glycol and caustic soda at atmospheric pressure.

On 10 July 1976, an accident occurred at the ICMESA 2,4,5-trichlorophenol factory in Italy, in which the ethylene glycol manufacturing process was used (Firestone, 1977; Gruppo PIA *et al.*, 1976; Zedda, 1977). Following a malfunction in thermal regulation, a safety valve blew, and an estimated 2-3 kg TCDD, as well as trichlorophenol and other substances, spread from the factory into a triangular area approximately 3-5 km long and 600-700 m wide. Concentrations of TCDD in samples of soil, including its vegetation, from the more contaminated part of the area within 2 km of the factory (Zone A) were in the range of 1-15 mg/kg; some areas of sampling, however, had the highest concentrations of TCDD ever found in the environment - up to 51.3 mg/kg. In the less contaminated area (Zone B), various levels above 10 µg/kg were found (Hay, 1976; Rawls & O'Sullivan, 1976). In subsequent soil analysis the contamination levels in the soil were expressed in $\mu g/m^2$, as extrapolated from soil samples taken at a depth of 7 cm; the level of sensitivity of the analytical method used was 0.75 $\mu g/m^2$. The highest levels found were over 5000 $\mu g/m^2$ in Zone A and between 15 and 50 $\mu g/m^2$ in Zone B; most of the samples, however, contained levels in the range of 50-500 $\mu g/m^2$ in Zone A and of 0.75-5 $\mu g/m^2$ in Zone B. Most soil samples from a danger area defined around Zones A and B ('Rispetto zone') were negative; about one third of them, however, contained TCDD at levels between 0.75-4.99 $\mu g/m^2$ (Pocchiari, 1977).

Accidental TCDD contamination has occurred in several other factories: in 1953, in Ludwigshafen, Federal Republic of Germany (Goldmann, 1972); in 1954, in Hamburg, Federal Republic of Germany (Bauer et al., 1961); in 1964, in Newark, New Jersey, USA (Poland et al., 1971); in 1965-1968, in Czechoslovakia (Jirásek et al., 1973); and in 1966, in France (Dugois et al., 1968). However, no data on the quantity of TCDD produced or on the concentrations in the working places were available. The only factory which emitted detectable levels into the environment was that described above in Italy.

In Nitro, West Virginia, USA, in 1949 (Firestone, 1977) and in Italy (Hofmann & Meneghini, 1962), symptoms that suggested exposure to TCDD (although the agent was not identified) were observed in workers in 2,4,5-T and trichlorophenol factories after accidental exposures. Similar symptoms were observed in workers in two trichlorophenol factories in the Mittle Rhine in the Federal Republic of Germany in 1952 (W. Hergt, cited by Bauer et al., 1961), in a 2,4,5-T factory in the USSR (Telegina &

Bikbulatova, 1970) and in one in Midland, Michigan, USA in 1964 (Firestone, 1977).

In May and June 1971, waste oil heavily contaminated with TCDD (306-356 mg/kg) was sprayed on the ground of three horse show arenas in rural Missouri in order to control dust. About 7750 litres were sprayed on each of two of the arenas; the concentration of TCDD in the soil from one was 31.8-33 mg/kg (Carter *et al.*, 1975; Commoner & Scott, 1976a).

2.2.2 Residues after herbicide use

Soil: In 1970, analysis for TCDD was begun in experimental sand plots in Lakeland, Florida that had received 2,4-D and 2,4,5-T by aerial application during an 8-year period from 1962-1970. A total of 1060 kg/ha 2,4,5-T had been applied over a 3-year period to these plots (Westing, 1977). This is a massive dose compared to normal application rates for brush control on grazing land, which are 2.24 kg/ha or 6.7 kg/ha over 3 years. No TCDD residues were found in 1 m core samples by analytical methods that had a detection limit of 0.05 mg/kg (Woolson *et al.*, 1973). However, the concentration of TCDD in the applied herbicides is not clearly indicated in the report.

Subsequent to aerial spraying of 2,4,5-T in the Pran Buri region of Vietnam, soil samples were found to contain 1.2-23 µg/kg TCDD (Committee on the Effects of Herbicides in Vietnam, 1974). Westing (1977) has calculated that about 100 kg TCDD were sprayed during 1966-1969 in Vietnam, to give an average concentration in the top cm of soil of about 40 ng/kg.

Animals: Three to four months after spraying of herbicides in Vietnam was stopped, prawns from the Saigon River and fish from the Dong Nai River were found to contain TCDD levels as high as 49 and 1020 ng/kg, respectively, as compared to levels of less than 3 ng/kg in fish obtained in a market in Massachusetts, US. In Vietnam, levels tended to be higher in fish from interior rivers than in those from seacoast locations (Baughman & Meselson, 1973b).

In Florida, aerial spraying of 2,4-D and 2,4,5-T containing an estimated 2-50 g/ha TCDD during a 2-year period (1962-1964) resulted 10 years later in detectable levels of TCDD in tissues of wild mice (1.3 µg/kg), meadow larks (1 µg/kg), reptiles (0.36 µg/kg) and fish (0.08 µg/kg) (Young et al., 1976).

TCDD was found in half of the fat samples taken from cattle grazed on rangeland previously treated with 2,4,5-T (Anon., 1975).

2.2.3 Residues in herbicides and fungicides

In 1970, the US Department of Agriculture analysed 129 samples of 17 herbicides and fungicides derived from chlorophenols for possible contamination by chlorodibenzo-*para*-dioxins; the results are summarized in Table 2, taken from the report (Woolson et al., 1972).

Seven of 8 further samples of technical 2,4,5-T were found to contain 0.1-55 mg/kg TCDD (Storherr et al., 1971).

A total of 21 mono-, di-, tri-, tetra- and pentachlorophenols were analysed for the presence of chlorodibenzo-*para*-dioxins. None were found in samples of 2-chlorophenol, 2,4-dichlorophenol or 2,6-dichlorophenol obtained from laboratory chemical suppliers. From 0.07-6.2 mg/kg TCDD were found in 3/6 samples of 2,4,5-trichlorophenol (or its sodium salt); 49 mg/kg 1,3,6,8-tetrachlorodibenzo-*para*-dioxin were found in a sample of 2,4,6-trichlorophenol. Tetrachlorodibenzo-*para*-dioxins were not found in the tetrachlorophenols, but hexachlorodibenzo-*para*-dioxins were found in 2/3 samples of 2,3,4,6-tetrachlorophenol. One of the tetrachlorophenol samples contained 29, 5.1 and 0.17 mg/kg hexa-, hepta- and octachlorodibenzo-*para*-dioxins, respectively. Analysis for chlorodibenzo-*para*-dioxins in 8 commercial pentachlorophenols (received during the period 1967-1970) showed no tetrachlorodibenzo-*para*-dioxins; heptachlorodibenzo-*para*-dioxins were found in the range of 0.5-39 mg/kg in 7 samples, and 3.3-15 mg/kg were found in 5 samples. The content of hexachlorodibenzo-*para*-dioxins, which are known to be highly toxic, ranged from 0.03 to 38 mg/kg; they were present in all of the 8 pentachlorophenol samples (Firestone et al., 1972).

Commercial samples of 2,3,4,6-tetrachlorophenol (TCP) and of technical pentachlorophenol (PCP), analysed by mass fragmentography for chlorinated

TABLE 2

Number and content of polychlorodibenzo-para-dioxins in selected herbicides

Pesticide	No. of mg/kg of -chlorodibenzo-para-dioxins found[a]												No. of samples contaminated	Total no. of samples tested
	tetra-		hexa-			hepta-			octa-					
	<10	<100	<10	<100	<1000	<10	<100	<1000	<10	<100	<1000			
2,4,5-T	7	13	3	1	0	ND[b]	...	...	ND	...	...		23	42
2-(2,4,5-trichlorophenoxy)propionic acid (Silvex)	1	0	ND	...	...	ND	...	...	ND	...	...		1	7
2,4-D (and its benzoic and propionic acids)	ND	...	1	0	0	ND	...	...	ND	...	...		1	28
3,6-dichloro-2-methoxybenzoic acid (Dicamba)	ND	...	ND	...	...	ND	...	...	ND	...	...		0	8
Chlorophenol tri-	ND	...	4	0	0	1	0	0	2	0	0		4	6
tetra-	ND	...	1	1	0	1	2	0	1	2	0		3	3
penta-	ND	...	0	7	0	0	4	6	0	4	6		10	11
Others	ND	...	1	0	1	3	0	1	3	1	0		7	24

[a] Any sample may contain one or more different dioxins
[b] ND = <0.5 mg/kg of any one chlorodioxin

dibenzo-*para*-dioxins, were found to contain less than 0.2 mg/kg tetra- and pentachlorodibenzo-*para*-dioxins, respectively. The TCP contained 6 mg/kg hexachlorodibenzo-*para*-dioxins, 55 mg/kg heptachlorodibenzo-*para*-dioxins and 39 mg/kg OCDD; the PCP contained 9 mg/kg hexachlorodibenzo-*para*-dioxins, 235 mg/kg heptachlorodibenzo-*para*-dioxins and 250 mg/kg OCDD. The positional isomers of the dioxins were not identified (Buser, 1975).

Hexa-, hepta- and octachlorodibenzo-*para*-dioxins were found in both technical and analytical grades of commercial pentachlorophenol, as determined by gas chromatography coupled with several detection methods. When an electron capture detector was used, the technical grade product was found to contain 42, 24 and 10 mg/kg of the respective dioxins, and the analytical grade product had 0.03, 0.04 and 0.02 mg/kg, respectively. Positional isomers of the various dioxins were not specified (Villanueva *et al.*, 1973).

2.2.4 Generation and persistence in the environment

TCDD can be formed by the pyrolysis at $500^{\circ}C$ for 5 hours of sodium α-(2,4,5-trichlorophenoxy)propionate (Saint-Ruf, 1972).

Irradiation of aqueous solutions of chlorinated dibenzo-*para*-dioxin-free sodium pentachlorophenol with ultra-violet light produced small amounts of OCDD; however, no TCDD could be detected after irradiation of aqueous solutions of 2,4,5-T, 2,4,5-trichlorophenol or sodium 2,4,5-trichlorophenate (Crosby *et al.*, 1973; Helling *et al.*, 1973).

The chlorinated dibenzo-*para*-dioxins, when dissolved in methanol, are degraded by exposure to summer sunlight or irradiation with an ultra-violet lamp (300 nm). Photolysis of OCDD was slower than that of TCDD under similar conditions. 2,3,7-Trichlorodibenzo-*para*-dioxin and small amounts of dichlorodibenzo-*para*-dioxin were produced as breakdown products of TCDD. TCDD was photodecomposed only when dissolved in organic solvents. When 0.1 $\mu g/m^2$ TCDD was applied to a 250 μm layer of soil on glass plates and irradiated for 96 hours, there was no loss due to volatilization or photodecomposition. Irradiation of TCDD in water produced little change after 14 days; however, irradiation of an aqueous suspension dispersed and stabilized by a surfactant reduced the TCDD content (Baughman, 1974; Crosby et al., 1971).

Recent studies involving exposure of ng amounts of TCDD indicated a 50% degradation of TCDD in 5 hours; the total amounts degraded were independent of the amount present (J.R. Plimmer, cited by Isensee, 1977). Application of TCDD combined with formulated 2,4,5-T to soil, glass plates and plant leaves resulted in losses of 15, 60 and 100% of the applied dose after 6 hours' exposure to sunlight (Crosby & Wong, 1977). In contrast to the findings of the earlier study described above, these reports suggest a faster rate of degradation of low than of higher levels of TCDD.

The mobilities of DCDD and TCDD were estimated in five soil samples varying widely in texture and other properties. Both dioxins were immobile in all soils (they were not leached downward into the soil by irrigation or rainfall); however, lateral movement due to surface erosion may occur. These studies revealed that TCDD is not translocated in plants and has a half-life in soil of about one year (Helling et al., 1973).

The persistence of TCDD was determined in silty clay loam in Hagerstown and in sand in Lakeland, Maryland, US, which had received up to 100 mg/kg TCDD. After one year, 71 and 56% of the originally applied TCDD was recovered in the two soil types, respectively (Kearney et al., 1972).

The uptake of ^{14}C-labelled 2,4-dichlorophenol (DCP), DCDD and TCDD from nutrient solutions or soil was measured in oats and soya beans. The solutions contained 0.2 mg/l DCP, 0.26 mg/l DCDD or 0.18 mg/l TCDD; soil samples contained 0.07 mg/kg DCP, 0.1 mg/kg DCDD or 0.06 mg/kg TCDD. After 14 days, the seedling oats and soya beans contained (minus control) 1.84 and 0.13 mg/kg DCP, 0.16 and 0.01 mg/kg DCDD and 0.11 and 0.01 mg/kg TCDD, respectively. At maturity, the oats and soya beans contained (minus control) 0.01 and 0.02 mg/kg DCP, 0.02 and <0.001 mg/kg DCDD and <0.001 and <0.001 mg/kg TCDD, respectively. No translocation of these compounds was observed after their application to foliage (Isensee & Jones, 1971).

Subsurface injections of a herbicide containing an unspecified concentration of TCDD resulted in the occurrence of 15 µg/kg TCDD in soil samples after 282 days and of 2.5 µg/kg TCDD after 3 years (Young et al., 1976). In another part of this study, initiated by the US Air Force in 1962 to investigate the persistence, mobility and effect on various ecosystems of TCDD, levels of up to 1.5 µg/kg TCDD were found in soil 10-12 years after the aerial spraying of herbicides containing TCDD. Under relatively dry conditions (Utah test area) TCDD apparently has a half-life of 330 days; in more moist, warm conditions (Florida test area) TCDD has a half-life of about 190 days (see also Fig. 3). The rate of decay was approximately constant up to 1150 days after initiation of the test (longest period of observation in the Air Force studies). There was no increase in the rate of decay when soil samples were stirred at regular intervals, exposed to more sunlight or received an addition of inorganic nutrients. No appreciable downward migration of TCDD occurred even with a heavy annual rainfall (150 cm). Only about 1% of the TCDD initially deposited at a depth of 0-15 cm was found below 30 cm after 414-557 days (Young et al., 1976).

In the episode in rural Missouri described above, the contaminated soil contained levels of TCDD ranging from 0.12 to 0.85 mg/kg after 3 years, indicating a half-life in soil (in the absence of covering vegetation and of direct sunlight) of 0.5 years; this is consistent with other estimates that range from 0.24 to 1 year (Commoner & Scott, 1976a).

Microbial degradation of TCDD is reported to be relatively rare in nature. Approximately 100 microbial strains that can degrade persistent pesticides were tested: only 5 of them degraded TCDD. It was not possible to change cultural conditions so as to increase the rate of degradation of TCDD by any of the microorganisms (Matsumura & Benezet, 1973).

In two studies, the application of 5000-40,000 mg/kg 2,4-D and 2,4,5-T containing unspecified amounts of TCDD did not sterilize the soil but stimulated the growth of certain microflora. These bacteria, actinomycetes and fungi proliferated in such a way that it seemed probable that they were using the herbicides and TCDD as carbon sources (an exception was the charcoal plots at Eglin); they were thus contributing to the degradation of the herbicides (Young et al., 1976).

Figure 3[a]

Semi-logarithmic plot of TCDD concentrations in Utah, Kansas and Florida degradation test areas

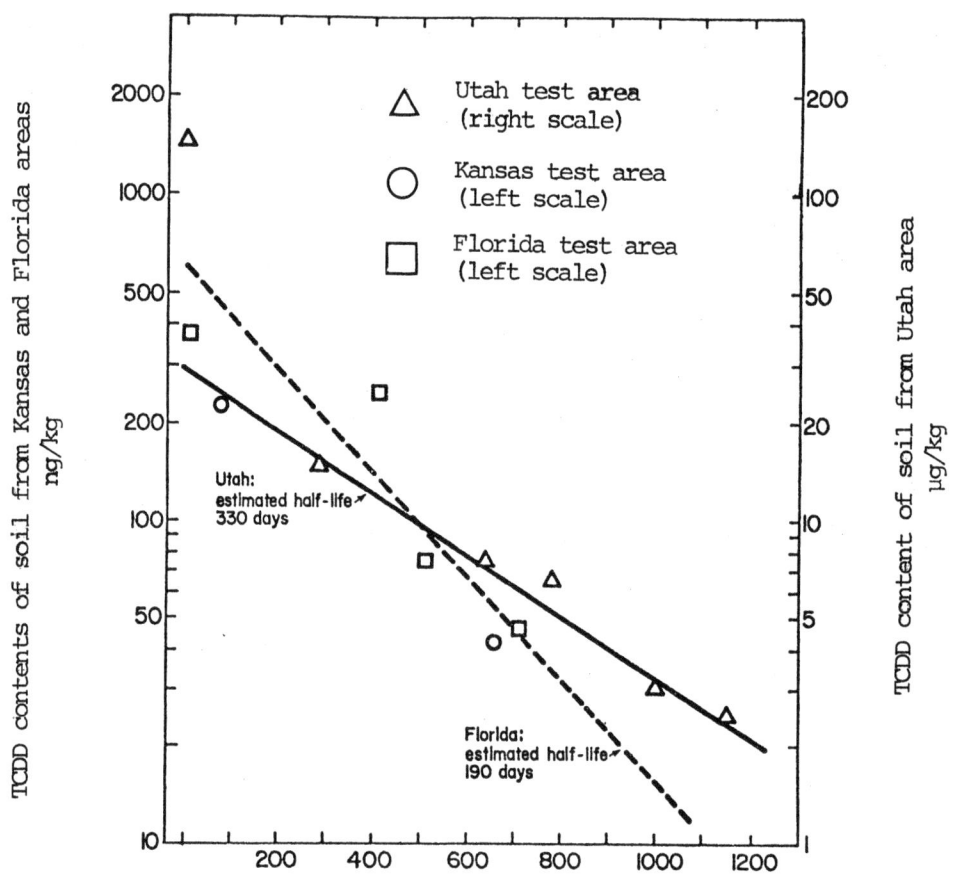

Days after incorporation of TCDD into soil

[a]From Commoner & Scott, 1976b

2.2.5 Accumulation in organisms

Several organisms were exposed in a model ecosystem to ^{14}C-labelled TCDD for up to 31 days to determine its distribution and accumulation in organisms in the aquatic environment (Isensee & Jones, 1975). TCDD accumulation by all organisms was directly related to its concentration in the water (0.05-1330 ng/l); averages were $2.0-2.6 \times 10^4$ (snail, *Gambusia* and daphnid) and $4-9 \times 10^3$ (duckweed, algae and catfish) times the concentration in water, and equilibrium concentrations were reached in tissues in 7-15 days (Isensee, 1977). TCDD accumulation ratios were about the same as those reported for many of the chlorinated hydrocarbon insecticides. No metabolites of TCDD were found in submerged soil, water, snails, *Gambusia* or catfish (Isensee & Jones, 1975).

From the US Air Force studies cited above (Young *et al.*, 1976), it would appear that after aerial spraying of herbicides TCDD accumulated in the livers of rodents, reptiles, birds, fish and insects, although it was calculated that TCDD levels in the livers did not exceed the highest level found in contaminated soil. In reviewing these results, however, Commoner & Scott (1976b) came to different conclusions. Livers of wild mice collected from a zone of the Florida test area contained average levels of 540 ng/kg TCDD in 1973 (males and females together) and 1300 ng/kg (males) and 960 ng/kg (females) in 1974, compared with an average value in the soil of 340 ng/kg (initial concentrations 10 years earlier were about 2 mg/kg); these results point to a concentration effect in the mouse livers. A composite sample of 9 livers from meadow larks contained 1020 ng/kg TCDD, compared with the average value of 46 ng/kg in soil samples in the corresponding area. Pooled samples of whole body and livers of fish taken from a pond in the Florida test field contained concentrations of 150-740 ng/kg; concentrations in the soil samples taken from the region of the pond were 22-85 ng/kg TCDD, again suggesting that accumulation occurrs in various animal species.

Concentrations of 255 ng/g of tissue were found in the livers of rabbits captured in Zone A in Seveso, Italy after the accident at the ICMESA factory (Firestone, 1977).

2.3 Analysis

Two difficult problems are encountered in the analysis of chlorodibenzo-*para*-dioxins: (1) the separation of related compounds, such as the polychlorinated biphenyls and chlorodibenzofurans, among others, which have similar retention times on chromatographic columns, and (2) the difficulty of assigning positions in isomers containing the same number of chlorine atoms during identification by mass spectrometry. Methods of analysis of TCDD in environmental samples have been reviewed by McKinney (1977).

In a method used to monitor commercial chlorinated phenols for the presence of chlorodibenzo-*para*-dioxins, a combination of aluminium oxide column chromatographic cleanup and gas chromatography with mass fragmentographic identification were used. The compounds were determined in isomer groups only, and no attempt was made to separate and determine the isomers (Buser, 1975; Buser & Bosshardt, 1976). In a later study, gas chromatography, using glass capillary columns and a micro-electron capture detector, was used to separate and detect positional isomers. The number of chlorine atoms was determined by mass spectrometry, but no positions were assigned (Buser, 1976).

2,3,4,4,5,6-Hexachloro-2,5-cyclohexadien-1-one, which may be formed during the manufacture of pentachlorophenol, interfered in analysis of the latter for OCDD by gas chromatography (Wilkinson, 1975). An aluminium oxide column has been used to separate chlorodibenzo-*para*-dioxins from polychlorinated biphenyls for determination of the dioxins by gas chromatography with electron capture detection (Porter & Burke, 1971).

Commercial chlorophenols were analysed for chlorodibenzo-*para*-dioxins, chlorodibenzofurans and chlorodiphenyl ethers by fractionation on an aluminium oxide column, followed by gas chromatography with electron capture detection and confirmation by mass spectroscopy. Di-, tri-, tetra-, penta-, hexa-, hepta- and octachlorodibenzo-*para*-dioxins were determined, with a detection limit of 20 µg/kg (Firestone *et al.*, 1972).

A method for analysing samples of unknown origin for chlorodibenzo-*para*-dioxins involves initial use of an ion-exchange resin column to remove chlorophenoxyphenols before determination of the dioxins by gas chromatography and mass spectrometry using multiple-ion detection. Limits of detection were 0.05 mg/kg for TCDD, 0.1 mg/kg for HCDD and 0.5 mg/kg for OCDD in samples of 2,4,5-trichlorophenol, 2,4,5-T and its esters, pentachlorophenol, fats and oils (Crummett & Stehl, 1973). The ion-exchange cleanup technique used in this method was evaluated as the most efficient of four techniques described in the literature (Villanueva et al., 1975).

Solvent extraction with column cleanup followed by gas chromatography and mass fragmentography has been used to analyse samples from the Seveso area in Italy for TCDD. The limit of detection was about 0.1 µg/kg, and recovery, 80% (Cattabeni, 1977).

A method of analysis for TCDD in technical 2,4,5-T which requires minimal cleanup involves gas chromatography with identification by mass fragmentography; recovery was 80-100%, and the detection limit, 50 µg/kg (Buser & Bosshardt, 1974). Time-averaged high-resolution mass spectrometry has been used to detect as little as 0.1 µg/kg TCDD added to human milk. Sample cleanup was accomplished by preparative gas chromatography; recovery, however, was only 25% (Baughman & Meselson, 1973a). An improved cleanup procedure, which eliminates interfering 1,1-dichloro-2,2-bis(*para*-chlorophenyl)ethylene (DDE) and polychlorinated biphenyls, was later developed and applied to the analysis of Vietnamese fish samples; sensitivity of the method was about 15 ng/kg (Baughman & Meselson, 1973b).

Gas chromatography with flame ionization detection and gas chromatography combined with mass spectrometry were used to investigate the formation of chlorodibenzo-*para*-dioxins from the photochemical and thermochemical decomposition of chlorophenoxyphenols (Nilsson et al., 1974).

The Association of Official Analytical Chemists has published an Official First Action for the detection of hexa-, hepta- and octachlorodibenzo-*para*-dioxins in fats, oils, fatty acids or lipid materials by gas chromatography with electron capture detection (Horwitz, 1975).

A method for rapid screening and detection of chlorodibenzo-*para*-dioxins has been suggested, in which compounds are dissolved in strong acids which convert them to their cationic form. Oxidation of these cations produces highly coloured radicals. The chlorodibenzo-*para*-dioxin can then be identified by its visible or electron-spin-resonance spectra, which are less subject to interference than others (Pohland et *al*., 1973).

High-performance, reverse-phase, partition liquid chromatography has been investigated as a means of determining chlorodibenzo-*para*-dioxins in pentachlorophenol. The samples were first subjected to an ion-exchange column cleanup to remove phenoxyphenols. Recoveries of 93-104%, with a relative error of ±10%, and detection limits of 0.2 mg/kg for HCDD and 0.1 mg/kg for OCDD were reported (Pfeiffer, 1976).

The induction of aryl hydrocarbon hydroxylase in embryo chick liver by low levels of TCDD and other toxic dioxins might represent a very valuable screening bioassay for detecting the presence of toxic dioxins in commercial products or environmental samples (Poland & Glover, 1973a).

3. Biological Data Relevant to the Evaluation of Carcinogenic Risk to Man

3.1 Carcinogenicity and related studies in animals

(a) Oral administration

Mouse: According to a preliminary report, 50 10-week old, male random-bred Swiss H/Riop mice received weekly gastric intubations of 7 µg/kg bw TCDD in sunflower oil for 12 months. No tumours were observed in 19 mice autopsied at this time, but 3 had liver cirrhosis and 8 had dermatitis and amyloidosis. Weekly doses of 0.7 µg/kg bw and 0.007 µg/kg bw TCDD were given for 12 months to similar groups of mice, and no pathological changes were observed in 1 and 4 animals killed two months after the end of treatment; the surviving mice are being kept for lifespan. Two groups of 100 male and 100 female, 10-week old, random-bred Swiss H/Riop mice were given weekly oral doses of 70 mg/kg bw 2,4,5-trichlorophenoxyethanol (TCPE) with either 0.7 µg/kg bw or 0.007 µg/kg bw TCDD in 0.5% carboxymethyl cellulose by gastric intubation for 12 months. The TCPE used for the first group contained 10 mg/kg TCDD and that for the second group, 0.1 mg/kg TCDD. The incidences of liver tumours in males after 2 years were reported to be 43% and 54% in the two treated groups, compared with 15-20% in untreated mice of the colony that survived up to 3 years. Three additional groups of mice were given 7 mg/kg bw TCPE with 0.0007 µg/kg bw TCDD, 0.7 mg/kg bw TCPE with 0.00007 µg/kg bw TCDD or 7 mg/kg bw TCPE with 0.07 µg/kg bw TCDD. The incidences of liver tumours in males after 2 years were 15-21% in the three groups, compared with 28% in controls given 0.5% carboxymethyl cellulose alone; this part of the study is still in progress (Tóth et al., 1977) [The Working Group noted that the reporting of these experiments was incomplete].

According to a preliminary report of a study in progress, groups of 50 male and 50 female $B6C3F_1$ mice were fed diets containing 0.5% or 1% unsubstituted dibenzo-para-dioxin or DCDD, or 0.25, 0.5 or 1% OCDD. The numbers of survivors in the various groups at different stages of the experiment are given in Table 3. OCDD induced significant mortality within 20 weeks and pathological changes in the lung and liver. Hyperplasia of the bronchial mucosa occurred in one mouse fed 1% unsubstituted dioxin; another animal fed 0.25% OCDD showed hyperplasia and metaplasia of the bronchial mucosa and a bronchiolar carcinoma. Hepatotoxic changes were also noted, but no hepatic tumours were reported (King et al., 1973).

Rat: In the study by King et al. (1973) described above, groups of 35 male and 35 female Osborne-Mendel rats were fed diets containing the same concentrations of unsubstituted dibenzo-para-dioxin, DCDD and OCDD. The numbers of survivors at different stages of the experiment are shown in Table 3. No tumours were seen in rats treated for up to 42 weeks (time of reporting). Rats fed OCDD had liver changes ranging from early hepatotoxic lesions to cirrhosis.

(b) Skin application

Mouse: In the same study described above, groups of 30 male and 30 female Swiss-Webster mice received thrice weekly skin applications of 0.2 ml acetone containing 0.2, 3 or 80 mg/kg OCDD, DCDD or unsubstituted

TABLE 3

Numbers of animals surviving after various treatment times with various chlorinated dibenzo-*para*-dioxins[a]

Compound	Mice (50 per group)			Rats (35 per group)	
	Sex	Week of test	No. of survivors	Week of test	No. of survivors
Controls	M	31	50	34	35
	F	31	50	34	35
1% unsubstituted dibenzo-*para*-dioxin	M	39	48	42	33
	F	39	29	42	32
0.5% unsubstituted dibenzo-*para*-dioxin	M	34	50	42	31
	F	39	49	42	35
1% DCDD	M	17	49	17	35
	F	17	48	17	35
0.5% DCDD	M	17	50	17	35
	F	17	49	17	35
1% OCDD	M	10	0	32	0
	F	37	5	22	0
0.5% OCDD	M	8	0	37	0
	F	37	45	25	0
0.25% OCDD	M	17	1	17	28
	F	15	0	17	15

[a]From King *et al.*, 1973

dibenzo-*para*-dioxin, respectively. After 60, 64 and 59 weeks, 20 male and 28 female, 17 male and 27 female, and 24 male and 24 female mice, in the three groups, respectively, were still alive. None of the treated mice had skin tumours; 1 male and 1 female treated with OCDD had s.c. tumours (type not specified); 1 female treated with unsubstituted dibenzo-*para*-dioxin had a lymphoma (King et *al.*, 1973).

3.2 Other relevant biological data

(a) Experimental systems

The toxicological and pharmacological effects of the chlorinated dibenzo-*para*-dioxins have been reviewed (Kimbrough, 1974; Moore, 1977; NIEHS, 1973; Schwetz et *al.*, 1973; J.G. Wilson et *al.*, cited by Neubert et *al.*, 1973).

Acute and short-term toxicity

The extremely high acute toxicity of TCDD, the most toxic of the chlorinated dibenzo-*para*-dioxins, has been noted frequently (Carter et *al.*, 1975; Greig et *al.*, 1973; Gupta et *al.*, 1973; Harris et *al.*, 1973; King et *al.*, 1973; Schwetz et *al.*, 1973; Vos et *al.*, 1974; Zinkl et *al.*, 1973). Single oral LD_{50}'s ranged from 0.0006 mg/kg bw in male guinea-pigs to 0.115 mg/kg bw in rabbits of both sexes (Table 4). Lethal doses to rabbits were similar with i.p., oral or skin administration; dogs were less sensitive than rabbits. In mice, single doses of 0.001-0.130 mg/kg bw produced some deaths, with no dose-response relationship.

Death following a lethal dose of TCDD is often delayed for several weeks; approximately half the deaths in mice occurred between 13 and 18 days after treatment (Schwetz et *al.*, 1973). In rats and guinea-pigs, mortality was similar when TCDD was given as a single dose or as divided daily or weekly doses within 4 to 5 weeks, thus demonstrating a cumulative effect (Harris et *al.*, 1973).

Other chlorodibenzo-*para*-dioxins are less toxic than TCDD (Khera & Ruddick, 1973; King et *al.*, 1973; Schwetz et *al.*, 1973). Single oral doses of 1-2 g/kg bw DCDD and OCDD did not kill female rats, and larger

TABLE 4

Acute toxicity of TCDD[a]

Species	Sex	Route	LD_{50} (mg/kg bw)
Rat	M	Oral	0.022
	F	Oral	0.045
Guinea-pig	M	Oral	0.0006
	F	Oral	0.0021
Rabbit	M&F	Oral	0.115
	M&F	Skin	0.275
		I.p.	>0.252

[a]From Schwetz et al., 1973

doses of OCDD (4 g/kg bw) were not lethal to mice. Oral doses of approximately 100 mg/kg bw mixed isomers of hexachlorodibenzo-*para*-dioxin were lethal to male rats (Schwetz et al., 1973). The LD_{50} for mice after i.p. injection of unsubstituted dibenzo-*para*-dioxin was more than 56 mg/kg bw (Vinopal & Casida, 1973).

Hepatic-cell necrosis produced by TCDD is the probable cause of death in rats, while hepatic necrosis and liver insufficiency are minimal in mice and guinea-pigs (Harris et al., 1973; Schwetz et al., 1973; Vos et al., 1973).

In rats, guinea-pigs and mice, changes in the weight of the thymus appeared to be a most sensitive indicator of TCDD exposure, since decreases in thymus weight occurred with doses which had no effect on body weight (Harris et al., 1973).

I.p. injection of 400 µg/kg bw TCDD in monkeys resulted in high concentrations in the skin and produced alopoecia and acne (Van Miller et al., 1976).

Subacute and chronic toxicity

Acute and subacute doses of TCDD produce a variety of toxic effects, including hepatic necrosis, thymic atrophy and lesions of the myocardium in rats (Buu-Hoi et al., 1972b; Gupta et al., 1973), thymic atrophy, depletion of lymphoid organs and haemorrhage and atrophy of adrenal zona glomerulosa in guinea-pigs (Gupta et al., 1973) and hepatic necrosis in rabbits (Schulz, 1968). The main target organs of TCDD in rats, guinea-pigs and mice appear to be the liver and thymus (Gupta et al., 1973; Jones, 1975; Jones & Butler, 1974; Vos et al., 1974). The degree of hepatic involvement appears to be dose-dependent, and the severity of the changes produced varies between species (Gupta et al., 1973).

The most significant findings in both mice and guinea-pigs treated with sublethal doses of TCDD were in the lymphoid system, resulting in suppression of cell-mediated immunity (Vos et al., 1973). Low levels of TCDD that did not produce overt clinical or pathological changes still reduced host defences: 1 µg/kg bw given orally once weekly for 4 weeks to mice before infection with *Salmonella* increased mortality and decreased the time from infection to death (Thigpen et al., 1975). Haematological changes in mice, rats and guinea-pigs treated with TCDD included lymphopenia and thrombocytopenia (Weissberg & Zinkl, 1973; Zinkl et al., 1973).

Oral administration of 25 µg/kg bw TCDD to mice 4 times weekly increased the levels of 8- and 7-carboxyporphyrins in the liver by 2000-fold (Goldstein et al., 1973).

In a 13-week feeding study, Sprague-Dawley rats of both sexes were given 0.01 or 0.001 µg/kg bw TCDD on 5 days per week; a slight increase in relative liver weight occurred in those receiving 0.01 µg/kg bw. Steady state concentrations of TCDD were attained in body tissues by the end of of treatment (Kociba et al., 1976).

In the rabbit ear bioassay for acnegenic activity, solutions of chlorinated dibenzo-*para*-dioxins were applied to the inside of the ear on 5 days per week for 4 weeks. Solutions in benzene that contained more than 0.04 µg/ml TCDD or 10 µg/ml HCDD were active, whereas a chloroform solution of

1,2,3,4-TCDD (50 µg/ml) and chloroform extracts of 10% suspensions of DCDD or OCDD were inactive (Schwetz et al., 1973).

Chick oedema disease, characterized by hydropericardium, subcutaneous oedema, liver necrosis and death, was described in 1957 following the accidental administration of toxic fats in the feed of broiler chickens. The toxic material was later identified in commercial oleic and stearic acids produced from inedible tallow recovered from animal hides; trichlorophenols and pentachlorophenols had been used in curing the hides. TCDD, HCDD and OCDD have also been identified in several commercial fatty acids (Firestone, 1973). Daily doses of 10 or 100 µg/kg bw HCDD or of 1 or 10 µg/kg bw TCDD produced a positive response in the chick oedema bioassay; 0.5% OCDD in the diet had no effect (Schwetz et al., 1973).

Feeding of fat containing unspecified concentrations of chlorinated dibenzo-*para*-dioxins in the diet to *Macaca mulatta* monkeys for 100 days led to alopoecia, s.c. oedema, anaemia, progressive leucopenia and hypoproteinaemia. Enlargement of the liver, hydropericardium, gastric hyperplasia and ulceration and hypoplasia of the lymph tissue and bone marrow were observed at death. A diet containing the same amount of fat was lethal to 50% of chickens fed it for 15 days (Norback & Allen, 1973).

Adult female rhesus monkeys fed a diet containing 500 ng/kg TCDD for 6 months suffered loss of hair, swelling of eyelids, loss of lashes, irregularities in menstrual cycle, poor conception and abortion (Allen et al., 1977).

Absorption, distribution and excretion

Following a single oral administration of 50 µg/kg bw ^{14}C-TCDD to rats, almost 30% was eliminated in the faeces during the first 48 hours; excretion of ^{14}C activity *via* the faeces after this time was from 1-2% per day. After its absorption in the body, most of the activity derived from ^{14}C-TCDD is localized in the liver and fat: the level in these tissues is 10 times that in other tissues. A total of 53.2% of the dose was eliminated *via* the faeces and 13.2% and 3.2% *via* urine and expired air, respectively, within 21 days (Piper et al., 1973a,b).

Following daily oral administration, 5 times a week for 7 weeks, to Sprague-Dawley rats of 0.01, 0.1 or 1.0 µg/kg bw ^{14}C-TCDD, the major route of excretion was *via* the faeces; urine contained 3-18% of the cumulative dose of ^{14}C activity after 7 weeks. The half-life of ^{14}C activity in the rats was 23.7 days (Rose *et al.*, 1976). A half-life of 12-15 days was found when rats were given 7 or 20 µg ^{14}C-TCDD per kg of diet (equivalent to 0.5 or 1.5 µg/kg bw/day) for 42 days (Fries & Marrow, 1975).

^{3}H-TCDD administered by i.p. injection to male mice at the LD_{50} dose (120 µg/kg bw) was not measurably converted to water-soluble products and was eliminated mainly in the faeces and possibly *via* the bile. Traces of tritium activity were detected in the urine. A large proportion of the administered dose persisted in unmetabolized form in the liver, partially concentrated in the microsomal fraction, 11-20 days after treatment (Vinopal & Casida, 1973).

^{3}H-TCDD was not metabolized by liver microsomal fractions from mice, rats and rabbits; however, unsubstituted dibenzo-*para*-dioxin was rapidly metabolized in mice treated intraperitoneally and by liver microsomal systems *in vitro* (Vinopal & Casida, 1973).

Embryotoxicity and teratogenicity

TCDD is embryotoxic and teratogenic in mice (Courtney & Moore, 1971; Neubert & Dillmann, 1972; Neubert *et al.*, 1973; Smith *et al.*, 1976) in repeated or single doses of as little as 1-10 µg/kg bw, causing increased frequencies of cleft palate and kidney abnormalities. In rats, embryo-lethal effects occur under experimental conditions (Sparschu *et al.*, 1970, 1971), and kidney anomalies (Courtney & Moore, 1971), intestinal haemorrhages and general oedema can be produced in the foetuses (Khera & Ruddick, 1973). Few follow-up studies of the effects of prenatal exposure on postnatal functions have been carried out so far.

Table 5 summarizes the teratogenic and embryotoxic effects induced by TCDD in rats and mice that have been reported in the literature. There is a dose-response relationship for the induction of cleft palates in mice by TCDD (Neubert, 1976; Neubert *et al.*, 1973). Other embryotoxic effects

TABLE 5

Evaluation of reported teratogenic and embryotoxic effects
induced by TCDD in rats and mice (From Neubert et al., 1973)

Species	Strain	Embryotoxic/ teratogenic effect	Dose (μg/kg bw)		Period of dosing (days)	Route	Reference
			lowest tested[a]	~ED$_{50}$[b]			
Rat		Intestinal haemorrhage	0.125	0.5?		oral	Sparschu et al., 1971
Mouse	CD	Kidney abnormality	0.5	>1	6-15	s.c.	Courtney & Moore, 1971
	CD-1	Cleft palate	1? 3	>3	6-15	s.c.	" " " "
		Kidney abnormality	1	1-3	6-15	s.c	" " " "
	DBA/2J	Cleft palate	3	>3	6-15	s.c.	" " " "
		Kidney abnormality	3	>3	6-15	s.c.	" " " "
	C57BL/6J	Cleft palate	3	>3	6-15	s.c.	" " " "
		Kidney abnormality	3	<3	6-15	s.c.	" " " "
	NMRI	Cleft palate	3	6.5	6-15	oral	Neubert & Dillmann, 1972
			9	<9	9-13	oral	" " "
			15	40	13	oral	Neubert et al., 1973
			5	15	11	oral	" " " "

[a] The lowest dose with which an embryotoxic or teratogenic effect detectable at birth has been produced is indicated. Since sometimes only one dose level was tested, this does not necessarily represent the lowest dose from which an effect could result.

[b] ED$_{50}$ - dose required to produce an embryotoxic effect in 50% of animals

such as eye abnormalities, reduction of mean foetal weight, gastrointestinal haemorrhages and increased prenatal mortality occurred in hamsters given µg/kg bw doses of TCDD for 5 days (J.G. Wilson et al., cited by Neubert et al., 1973).

In mice, increased incidences in the frequency of cleft palate have been noted in combination experiments involving TCDD and other teratogens such as 2,4,5-T, dexamethasone, cyclophosphamide and 6-aminonicotinamide, administered at 'sub-threshold' and 'threshold' doses during days 6-15 of pregnancy. When 30 mg/kg bw 2,4,5-T, which produced no significant increase in the incidence of cleft palate compared with that in controls, or half this dose, was combined with 2 µg/kg bw TCDD, potentiating effects were observed. However, 1/10 of the TCDD dose (0.2 µg/kg bw) induced no detectable effect with either dose of 2,4,5-T. When the 'minimal effect' dose of 2,4,5-T (60 mg/kg bw) was used, potentiation was observed with 2 µg/kg bw and with 0.2 µg/kg bw TCDD (Neubert et al., 1973).

Postnatal effects of maternal exposure include hydronephrotic kidneys produced in mouse pups nursed by a foster mother treated with TCDD during pregnancy or at the time of parturition. Prenatal and postnatal kidney anomalies had a common aetiology, and the incidence and degree of hydronephrosis was a function of dose and length of target organ exposure (Moore et al., 1973).

Interference with the development of the lymphatic system, including the thymus (Neubert et al., 1973), and fatty infiltration of the foetal liver (Becker, 1973; Neubert et al., 1973) occurred in mice exposed *in utero* to TCDD during the second half of gestation.

A mixture of unspecified isomers of HCDD administered to pregnant rats at a dose of 100 µg/kg bw/day from days 6-15 of pregnancy was teratogenic, producing cleft palate and skeletal abnormalities, while doses of 1 or 10 µg/kg bw/day produced only s.c. oedema. A dose of 0.1 µg/kg bw/day had no toxic effects in embryos or foetuses. OCDD administered to pregnant rats at a dose of 500 mg/kg bw/day from days 6-15 of pregnancy produced s.c. oedema in the foetuses. Doses of 100 mg/kg bw/day DCDD had neither teratogenic nor embryotoxic effects (Schwetz et al., 1973).

In a three-generation reproductive study (B.A. Schwetz, cited by Moore, 1977) with random-bred albino rats, 0.1 µg/kg/day TCDD caused a lowered pregnancy rate and increased mortality of weanling pups. Daily doses of 0.001 µg/kg produced no detectable effects on the parameters studied [The sex of the animals receiving TCDD was not specified].

Enzyme induction

TCDD is a potent inducer of hepatic and renal microsomal drug metabolizing enzymes (Beatty & Neal, 1976; Buu-Hoi et al., 1971, 1972c; Fowler et al., 1975; Greig, 1972; Greig & DeMatteis, 1973; Hook et al., 1975a,b; Lucier et al., 1973, 1975a,b; Woods, 1973). Intoxication with TCDD results in a marked increase in the cellular smooth endoplasmic reticulum content of hepatic and renal cells (Fowler et al., 1973, 1975). TCDD can simultaneously activate and suppress certain microsome-associated foreign-compound- and steroid-hormone-metabolizing enzyme systems (Hook et al., 1975a). It increased the activity of both renal and hepatic glutathione-S transferase, an enzyme that converts several organic compounds to metabolites that are transported by the proximal tubules of the kidney (Kirsch et al., 1975).

TCDD is the most active of the chlorinated dibenzo-*para*-dioxins in inducing hepatic δ-aminolevulinic acid (ALA) synthetase and aryl hydrocarbon hydroxylase (AHH) in chick embryo liver preparations (Poland & Glover, 1973b,c).

All of the chlorinated dibenzo-*para*-dioxins that induce ALA synthetase in chick embryo have two common properties: (1) halogen atoms occupy at least 3 of the 4 ring positions (2,3,7,8), and (2) there is at least one free, non-halogenated carbon atom (Poland & Glover, 1973b). The available toxicological data (Schwetz et al., 1973) indicate that all those chlorodibenzo-*para*-dioxins that are lethal at low doses, teratogenic or produce acne also induce ALA synthetase; those chlorodibenzo-*para*-dioxins that are not toxic do not induce ALA synthetase. The structure-activity relationship of chlorodibenzo-*para*-dioxins in their ability to induce AHH in chick embryos was identical to that in inducing ALA synthetase (Poland & Glover, 1973b).

Mixed function oxidase enzyme systems of mouse strains 'non-responsive' to other aromatic hydrocarbons were induced by single doses of TCDD, as evidenced by increases in hepatic monooxygenase activities and in concentrations of cytochrome P-448 (Chhabra et al., 1974; Kouri & Nebert, 1977; Nebert et al., 1975; Poland et al., 1974). Genetic resistance to induction of AHH by 3-methylcholanthrene in DBA/2J mice was overcome by treatment with TCDD. This result conflicts with the hypothesis that induction of AHH activity is a consequence of the formation of cytochrome P-448 (Chhabra et al., 1976). A component that has a high binding affinity for TCDD was found in mouse liver cytosol (Poland et al., 1976).

TCDD induces AHH even in poorly responsive strains of mice (Niwa et al., 1975a), not only in liver but also in lung, kidney and colon. The DBA/2N strain, which responds only weakly to the sarcomatogenic action of 3-methylcholanthrene, becomes highly susceptible after treatment with TCDD (Kouri, 1976; Kouri & Nebert, 1977).

TCDD is approximately 30,000 times more potent than 3-methylcholanthrene in inducing AHH activity in rat liver (Poland & Glover, 1974).

AHH activity in maternal and foetal livers was increased 14- and 100-fold, but only minimal increases were observed in placentas and adrenal glands following a single administration of 2.5-6.0 µg/kg bw TCDD to Sprague-Dawley rats on day 17 of gestation. Similar results were obtained with regard to rates of 7-, 5-, N-, 3- and 1-hydroxylations of N-2-fluorenyl-acetamide. Benzo(a)pyrene metabolism to diols was also increased in foetal and maternal livers after treatment with TCDD, possibly by an increase in epoxide hydratase activity (Berry et al., 1976).

The kinetics of TCDD induction of AHH in 10 established cell lines, in primary foetal cultures derived from hamsters, rats, rabbits, chicks and 4 inbred strains of mice and in cultured human lymphocytes were similar to those of hydroxylase induction by 3-methylcholanthrene. There was no relationship between the cytotoxicity of TCDD and the level of inducible hydroxylase activity in the cultures (Niwa et al., 1975b).

The concentration of TCDD in growth medium necessary to induce AHH activity in cultured human lymphocytes is 40-60 times less than that of 3-methylcholanthrene needed for maximal hydroxylase induction (Kouri et al., 1974).

Mutagenicity

TCDD increased the reversion frequency to streptomycin independence in *Escherichia coli* Sd-4 at a concentration of 2 µg/ml. In *Salmonella typhimurium*, frameshift mutations in strain TA1532, but not base substitutions in strain TA1530, were induced by toxic concentrations of TCDD (Hussain et al., 1972). In plate assays, the response was positive with *S. typhimurium* TA1532, doubtful with TA1531 and TA1534 and negative with G46 and TA1530 (Seiler, 1973).

OCDD was non-mutagenic to *S. typhimurium* strains G46, TA1530 and TA1531, and doubtful results were obtained with strains TA1532 and TA1534 (Seiler 1973). Metabolic activation systems were not included in any of these microbiological assays.

Inhibition of mitosis and chromosomal abnormalities were observed in endosperm cells of *Haemanthus katherinae* Baker treated with 0.2 or 1.0 µg/l TCDD in the presence or absence of 2,4,5-T (Jackson, 1972).

No chromosomal aberrations were observed in bone-marrow cells of male rats treated with TCDD by i.p. injection (5, 10 and 15 µg/kg bw) or orally (a single dose of 20 µg/kg bw or 5 consecutive daily 10 µg/kg bw doses) (Green & Moreland, 1975). However, when rats of both sexes were treated twice weekly with TCDD (4 µg/kg bw) for 13 weeks, a significant increase in the number of chromosome aberrations was found (Green, 1977).

TCDD did not induce dominant lethal mutations in Wistar rats after its oral administration to males at doses of 4, 8 or 12 µg/kg bw/day for 7 days (Khera & Ruddick, 1973).

(b) Man

Toxic effects in humans due to TCDD have been reported after (i) occupational exposure during the industrial synthesis of 2,4,5-trichlorophenol

(TCP) and 2,4,5-T, (ii) exposure in factories and in the surrounding environment due to accidents occurring during the synthesis of TCP, and (iii) exposure to herbicides and other materials containing TCDD. Exposed subjects have been found to develop a wide variety of lesions and symptoms (Table 6).

Chloracne, one of the most constant and prominent features of TCDD exposure, has been described as a refractory acne characterized by inclusion cysts, comedones and pustules, with eventual scarring of the skin, more frequently originating on the face and sometimes spreading to other parts of the body. Many patients also have blepharoconjunctivitis and irritation of other mucous membranes. Sometimes the chloracne is preceded by erythematous and oedematous skin lesions. The latent period between exposure and the appearance of clear signs of chloracne ranges from a few weeks to several months (May, 1973).

Occupational exposure

Chloracne was observed in 1952 in workers involved in the manufacture of TCP in two factories in the Federal Republic of Germany where some 60 cases were observed (W. Hergt, cited by Bauer *et al.*, 1961).

Two years later, 31 cases of chloracne occurred within a few months at a factory manufacturing 2,4,5-T near Hamburg after a change in the industrial process. On this occasion the investigators were able to show that chloracne was not caused by purified TCP, and it was attributed to TCDD which occurred as a contaminant of technical TCP. Many of the exposed workers showed clinical manifestations of systemic toxicity, mainly muscular weakness, loss of appetite and weight, sleep disturbances, orthostatic hypotension, abdominal pain and liver impairment; most of them had psychopathological changes that were interpreted as a specific syndrome (Bauer *et al.*, 1961; Kimmig & Schulz, 1957; Schulz, 1957).

A similar outbreak of chloracne affected 60 workers at the 2,4,5-T factory of the Dow Chemical Company in Midland, Michigan in 1964 (Firestone, 1977).

TABLE 6

Toxic effects of TCDD in man

EFFECTS	REFERENCES
Dermatological	
chloracne	Bauer et al., 1961; Bert et al., 1976; Bleiberg et al., 1964; Carter et al., 1975; Dugois et al., 1968; Firestone, 1977; Goldmann, 1972, 1973; Jensen & Walker, 1972; Jirásek et al., 1973, 1974; Kimmig & Schulz, 1957; May, 1973; Oliver, 1975; Poland et al., 1971
porphyria cutanea tarda	Bleiberg et al., 1964; Jirásek et al., 1973, 1974
hyperpigmentation and hirsutism	Bleiberg et al., 1964; Oliver, 1975; Poland et al., 1971
Internal	
liver damage[a]	Bauer et al., 1961; Bleiberg et al., 1964; Dugois et al., 1968; Goldmann, 1972, 1973; Jirásek et al., 1973, 1974; May, 1973; Ton That, 1977
raised serum hepatic enzyme levels	Bert et al., 1976; Bleiberg et al., 1964; Jirásek et al., 1973, 1974; May, 1973; Poland et al., 1971; Ton That, 1977
disorders of fat metabolism	Jirásek et al., 1973; Oliver, 1975; Poland et al., 1971
" carbohydrate metabolism	Goldmann, 1972, 1973; Jirásek et al., 1973, 1974; Poland et al., 1971
cardiovascular disorders	Goldmann, 1972, 1973; Jirásek et al., 1973, 1974
urinary tract "	Carter et al., 1975; Goldmann, 1972, 1973
respiratory "	Bauer et al., 1961; Goldmann, 1972, 1973
pancreatic "	Goldmann, 1972, 1973
Neurological	
polyneuropathies	Goldmann, 1972, 1973; Jirásek et al., 1973, 1974
lower extremity weakness	Bauer et al., 1961; Firestone, 1977; Goldmann, 1972, 1973; Jirásek et al., 1973, 1974; Oliver, 1975; Poland et al., 1971
sensorial impairments (sight, hearing, smell, taste)	Goldmann, 1972, 1973; Oliver, 1975; Poland et al., 1971; Ton That, 1977
Psychiatric	
neurasthenic or depressive syndromes	Bauer et al., 1961; Firestone, 1977; Goldmann, 1972, 1973; Jirásek et al., 1973, 1974; Oliver, 1975; Poland et al., 1971

[a] Mild fibrosis, fatty changes, haemofuscin deposition and parenchymal-cell degeneration were observed in a few cases.

Chloracne, as well as hyperlipaemia and hypercholesterolaemia, were reported in 17 workers at a factory producing TCP in France (Dugois & Colomb, 1956, 1957; Dugois et al., 1958).

Of 29 subjects with features of chloracne working in a 2,4-D and 2,4,5-T-producing factory of the Diamond Alkali Co., Newark, New Jersey, US, 11 had increased excretion of uroporphyrins. In 3 cases a diagnosis of porphyria cutanea tarda was unquestionable; 2 of these had raised serum glutamic-oxaloacetic transaminase levels. Many of the workers, whether or not they had uroporphyrinuria, had hirsutism, hyperpigmentation, increased skin fragility and vesicobullous eruptions on exposed areas of skin (Bleiberg et al., 1964; Firestone, 1977).

Poland et al. (1971) re-examined all of the employees of the same factory in 1969, after the level of TCDD in the TCP had been reduced from 10-25 mg/kg to less than 1 mg/kg, and found chloracne in 13/73 workers. A number of subjects had hyperpigmentation or facial hypertrichosis, but no definite diagnosis of porphyria could be made, and only one worker had mild uroporphyrinuria. The authors suggested that chloracne and porphyria cutanea tarda are essentially independent syndromes. About 30% of the workers suffered from gastrointestinal symptoms (nausea, vomiting, diarrhoea, abdominal pains or blood in the stools); about 10% of the workers had other symptoms, such as lower extremity weakness, headache and/or decreased auditory acuity. The severity of chloracne was associated with the degree of hypomania as measured on the Minnesota Multiphasic Personality Inventory hypomanic scale. Serum cholesterol was elevated in 10% of cases and serum lactic dehydrogenase in 29%. Seven persons (10%) had a white blood cell count of less than $5000/mm^3$.

In a report of occupational exposure at a factory in the USSR where production of 2,4,5-T was begun in 1964, 128 workers showed skin lesions, and, among 83 examined, 69 had acne. Many, especially those with severe skin lesions, also had liver impairment; 18 workers had a neurasthenic syndrome (Telegina & Bikbulatova, 1970).

Similar findings were described by Jirásek et al. (1973, 1974), who reported 76 cases of chloracne following exposure to TCDD between 1965-1968 in a factory in Czechoslovakia producing 2,4,5-T and pentachlorophenol. Fifty-five patients were submitted to medical follow-ups for over 5 years; some had symptoms of porphyria cutanea tarda, uroporphyrinuria, abnormal liver tests (bilirubin, serum glutamic-oxaloacetic transaminase, serum glutamic-pyruvic transaminase and bromosulphthalein) and liver enlargement. The majority of patients suffered from severe neurasthenia and depressive syndrome. In 17 subjects, signs of peripheral neuropathy, especially in the lower extremities, were confirmed by electromyographic examinations. More than half of the patients showed raised levels of blood cholesterol and total lipids (see also section 3.3).

Three scientists were poisoned in the course of experimental preparation of TCDD by heating potassium trichlorophenate (Oliver, 1975). Two of them developed typical chloracne 6 and 8 weeks after exposure, respectively. Delayed symptoms, most likely due to TCDD, developed about 2 years after initial exposure in two of the scientists; these symptoms included personality changes, mainly loss of energy and drive, impairments of vision, taste and muscular coordination, sleep disturbances, gastrointestinal symptoms and hirsutism. Hypercholesterolaemia (in excess of 300 mg/100 ml) occurred in all 3 patients.

Exposure due to accidents

The first reported cases of industrial poisoning due to the formation of TCDD in uncontrolled exothermic reactions occurring during the manufacture of TCP were seen in 1949 at a 2,4,5-T-producing factory of the Monsanto Chemical Company in Nitro, West Virginia, US; 228 people were affected. Symptoms included chloracne, melanosis, muscular aches and pain, fatigue, nervousness and intolerance to cold (see Firestone, 1977).

In November 1953, as accident occurred at the Badische Anilin und Soda Fabrik (BASF) factory in Ludwigshafen, Federal Republic of Germany, during the manufacture of TCP (Goldmann, 1972, 1973; Hofmann, 1957); 53 workers were affected by chloracne, 42 in a severe form; 21 of the 42 suffered consequent damage to internal organs or disturbances of the nervous system. The most relevant features were polyneuritis, sensorial impairments and liver damage. The son of one of the workers developed chloracne following contact with his father's clothes. An additional case of poisoning occurred 5 years later in a worker who was involved in repair work at the contaminated site; this worker subsequently died with necrotic pancreatitis.

In a follow-up study of these workers, Thiess & Goldmann (1977) reported that of the 53 workers exposed to TCDD in the 1953 accident, 22 were still working at the factory, 16 had retired, and 15 had died (6 while still employed at the factory and 9 in retirement). Of the 22 workers still employed, 2 still had acne of the face and scrotum, 1 had paralysis of the left leg, and 1 had permanent loss of hearing; the remaining workers were well, except for scars left by the chloracne. Of the 15 deaths, 7 were from cardiovascular diseases, 2 of which were myocardial infarctus and 1, mitral stenosis, 4 from cancer (see also section 3.3), 2 from suicide, 1 from necrotic pancreatitis and 1 from oesophageal haemorrhage. The 16 men who had retired and were still alive were well. No abortions or miscarriages were reported in the wives of exposed workers still employed at the factory.

A similar accident occurred at the 2,4,5-T-producing factory of the Philips Duphar Company in The Netherlands in 1963 (Dalderup, 1974; Hay, 1976). Of 50 people affected, at least 10 still had skin complaints in 1976; 4 workers died within 2 years of the accident.

Five cases of chloracne were reported following an industrial accident in an Italian TCP factory (Hofmann & Meneghini, 1962).

Dugois et al. (1968) observed 21 cases of chloracne after an accident in 1966 in a French factory producing TCP in the Grenoble region. Pain in the right hypochondrium was recorded frequently in affected workers.

A further accident occurred at the TCP-producing factory of Coalite and Chemical Products at Bolsover, Derbyshire, UK, in April 1968 (Jensen & Walker, 1972; May, 1973). Of the 14 men who were in the building during or immediately after the explosion, 10 showed some abnormality in liver function tests (increase in zinc and/or thymol turbidity and/or serum glutamic-pyruvic transaminase); however, all tests were within normal limits 10 days later, and production was started again. Within the next 7 months, 79 workers developed chloracne, with younger men being affected first; most of these workers recovered within 4-6 months. Three years later, chloracne was observed in 2 outside employees who came into contact with a tank that had been contaminated but which had been subject to the most rigorous cleaning after the accident. Although they were exposed for only one or two days, their chloracne was very persistent. In addition, the son of one and the wife of the other developed chloracne some months later.

In July 1976, an accident at the TCP-producing ICMESA factory in Meda, Italy (Bert *et al.*, 1976; Hay, 1976) resulted in the contamination of a large, densely populated area including the towns of Seveso, Meda, Cesano Maderno and Desio. Five days after the accident, animals began to die. Over 700 people have been evacuated from the more heavily contaminated area (evacuation began two-and-a-half weeks after the accident); some 4000-5000 people still live in areas that have been found to be less heavily contaminated. The total population of the four towns involved is about 100,000 people. Hundreds of people complained of acute skin lesions and symptoms of systemic poisoning, and, by the end of October 1976, 37 cases of chloracne had been reported among the evacuated persons, mostly in children and young people. Raised serum transaminase and γ-glutamyl transferase levels were found in about 20% of the people living in or near the affected areas.

TCDD has been identified as the cause of an outbreak of poisoning in humans, horses and other animals in 1971 (Carter *et al.*, 1975; Kimbrough *et al.*, 1977). Exposure was related to the spraying of waste oil contaminated with TCDD on riding arenas for dust control. The most severe effects occurred in a 6-year old girl who played in the arena soil. Her symptoms included headache, epistaxis, diarrhoea, lethargy, haemorrhagic cystitis and focal pyelonephritis. Three other children and one adult who were frequently in the arena complained of skin lesions. In at least 2 of the children, the lesions described were consistent with chloracne. Intermittent arthralgias in two adults have been associated with previous exposure to the arena.

Exposure in Vietnam

Information concerning the effects of herbicides, and especially so-called 'Agent Orange' (a 50:50 mixture of the n-butyl esters of 2,4-D and 2,4,5-T, containing up to 30 mg/kg or more TCDD), on humans is given in a National Academy of Sciences report (Committee on the Adverse Effects of Herbicides in Vietnam, 1974). Interviews with Montagnard people produced remarkably consistent reports of child deaths, diarrhoea, vomiting, skin rashes, fever and abdominal pain following exposure after 'spray missions'. On the other hand, "no consistent pattern of association between rates of congenital malformation and annual amounts of herbicide sprayed" was revealed by a search through the records of two major Saigon hospitals over a 10-year period. It should be noted, however, that people living in the rural areas were more highly exposed than those living in Saigon; an earlier survey (Meselson et al., 1972) reported a higher rate of still-births in 1968-1969 (68 per 1000) in the province of Tay Ninh, which had been heavily sprayed, than in the rest of the country (32 per 1000 in 1966-1969 for the entire country, and 28 per 1000 in 1968-1969 for Saigon). Moreover, this study describes raised frequencies of certain malformations amongst the records of the Saigon children's hospital in 1966-1968, the years of the heaviest herbicide spraying: while total admissions for common birth defects remained relatively constant during the period 1964-1968, there was an increase in the relative frequency of spina bifida (2.1% among 1205 defective livebirths during 1967-1968, the heavy spray period, *versus* a proportion of 0.7% among 2781 defective livebirths during 1959-1966) and of isolated cleft palate (3.0% *versus* 0.8%) (Westing, 1977).

More recent data on the effects of herbicides are available from Ton That (1977), who stresses the high frequency of sight impairments, gastrointestinal haemorrhages and serious hepatitis.

Czeizel & Király (1976) studied the frequency of chromosome aberrations in the peripheral blood lymphocytes of 76 workers at a Budapest chemical factory producing herbicides, and in 33 controls. Thirty-six workers had been exposed to 2,4,5-trichlorophenoxyethanol (TCPE) and 26 to Buvinol, a combination herbicide containing TCPE and 2-chloro-6-ethylamino-4-isopropylamino-1,3,5-triazine (atrazine); 14 had never been engaged in herbicide production or use. The TCDD contamination of the final products was said to be less than 0.1 mg/kg and generally not more than 0.05 mg/kg (Vásárhelyi et al., 1976). The frequency of chromatid-type and unstable chromosome aberrations was found to be statistically significantly higher in the factory workers, whether they had been directly exposed in herbicide production or not. The aberrations were more frequent among workers preparing Buvinol and TCPE than in other factory workers, but the difference was significant only for the chromatid-type effect.

3.3 Case reports and epidemiological studies

A number of reports describe the occurrence of cancer in workers exposed to TCDD. Jirásek et al. (1973, 1974) followed up 55 subjects of a cohort of 78 exposed workers for 5-6 years: 4 deaths were observed, 2 of which were from bronchogenic carcinoma at 47 and 59 years, respectively. Smoking history was not reported and no causal conclusion was drawn [It is worth noting, however, that if 1965 WHO lung cancer mortality rates for Czechoslovakia were applied to the age structure of the whole cohort of 78 workers, the expected number of lung cancer deaths in 5 years would be only 0.12].

Thiess & Goldmann (1977) traced 4 cancer deaths (1 lung carcinoma at 54 years, 2 gastric carcinomas at 64 and 66 years and 1 colonic carcinoma at 70 years) out of 15 deaths occurring in a cohort of 53 workers exposed accidentally to TCDD at the BASF factory in Ludwigshafen, Federal Republic of Germany in 1953 (Goldmann, 1972, 1973); the follow-up study is still in progress.

Ton That et al. (1973) reported an increase in the number of persons with primary liver cancer in proportion to all cancer patients admitted to Hanoi hospitals during the period 1962-1968 (791 liver cancer cases out of 7911 total cancer cases, 10%) as compared to the period 1955-1961 (159 liver cancer cases out of 5492 total cancer cases, 2.9%), which was prior to the start of herbicide spraying. The authors attributed this increase to exposure as a result of the spraying of herbicides containing TCDD in south Vietnam during the 1960's [However, limitations in the reporting of the study make impossible an adequate assessment of the possible relationship between the incidence of liver cancer and herbicide spraying in south Vietnam].

4. Comments on Data Reported and Evaluation[1]

4.1 Animal data

There are data on the toxicity, teratogenicity and mutagenicity of 2,3,7,8-tetrachlorodibenzo-*para*-dioxin (TCDD) and other chlorinated dibenzodioxin derivatives; however, only preliminary reports of a few carcinogenicity studies, not completed at the time of their reporting, were available. In one study, the oral administration of 2,4,5-trichlorophenoxyethanol together with TCDD increased the incidence of liver tumours in male mice.

No evaluation of the carcinogenicity of chlorinated dibenzodioxins can be made on the basis of the available data.

---

[1] Subsequent to the finalization of this evaluation by the Working Group in February 1977, the Secretariat became aware of a preliminary report by Van Miller & Allen (1977). This abstract indicates that among 6 groups of 10 male Sprague-Dawley rats administered 5, 1, 0.5, 0.05, 0.005 or 0.001 µg TCDD/kg of diet for 65 weeks, 12 animals had died: 5 and 4 died in the two higher dose groups, respectively, and 1 in the 0.5 µg/kg group and 2 in the 0.005 µg/kg group. The death of 3 rats in the group receiving 5 µg/kg was attributed to aplastic anaemia; 2 carcinomas of the kidney, 2 carcinomas of the liver, 1 carcinoma of the skin and 1 angiosarcoma were observed in 6 of the 9 remaining animals. In rats that were still alive at the time of reporting, two additional neoplasms (1 bile-duct carcinoma and 1 angiosarcoma) were detected by laparotomy and biopsy.

4.2 Human data

A number of cases of cancer have been reported in workers exposed to TCDD, but no adequate epidemiological studies were available. An increased proportion of liver cancers has been reported in Hanoi, after the spraying of herbicides (2,4-D and 2,4,5-T) containing TCDD in south Vietnam. The significance of these observations cannot be assessed because not enough details were reported. More details of the reported cases and more extensive observation of the exposed people are needed before an evaluation of the carcinogenicity of chlorinated dibenzodioxins to man can be made (see also monograph on 2,4,5-T, p. 273).

5. References

Allen, J.R., Barsotti, D.A. & van Miller, J.P. (1977) Reproductive dysfunction in nonhuman primates exposed to dioxins. Toxicol. appl. Pharmacol. (in press)

Aniline, O. (1973) Preparation of chlorodibenzo-p-dioxins for toxicological evaluation. Advanc. Chem. Ser., 120, 126-135

Anon. (1970) Another herbicide on the blacklist. Nature (Lond.), 226, 309-311

Anon. (1975) EPA has found unsafe level of TCDD in half of beef fat samples. Chem. Eng. News, 53, 10

Bauer, H., Schulz, K.H. & Spiegelberg, U. (1961) Berufliche Vergiftungen bei der Herstellung von Chlorphenol-Verbindungen. Arch. Gewerbepath. Gewerbehyg., 18, 538-555

Baughman, R.W. (1974) Tetrachlorodibenzo-p-dioxins in the Environment. High Resolution Mass Spectrometry at the Picogram Level (Thesis, Harvard University)

Baughman, R.W. & Meselson, M. (1973a) An improved analysis for tetrachlorodibenzo-p-dioxins. Advanc. Chem. Ser., 120, 92-104

Baughman, R.W. & Meselson, M. (1973b) An analytical method for detecting TCDD (dioxin): levels of TCDD in samples from Vietnam. Environm. Hlth Perspect., 5, 27-35

Beatty, P.W. & Neal, R.A. (1976) Induction of DI-diaphorase activity of rat liver by 2,3,7,8-tetrachlorodibenzo-p-dioxin. Toxicol. appl. Pharmacol., 37, 189

Becker, D. (1973) The effect of folate overdose and of 2,3,7,8-tetrachlorodibenzo-p-dioxin (TCDBD) on kidney and liver respectively of rat and mouse embryos. Teratology, 8, 215

Berry, D.L., Zachariah, P.K., Namkung, M.J. & Juchau, M.R. (1976) Transplacental induction of carcinogen-hydroxylating systems with 2,3,7,8-tetrachlorodibenzo-p-dioxin. Toxicol. appl. Pharmacol., 36, 569-584

Bert, G., Manacorda, P.M. & Terracini, B. (1976) I controlli sanitari: la sanità incontrollata. Sapere, 796, 50-60

Bleiberg, J., Wallen, M., Brodkin, R. & Applebaum, I.L. (1964) Industrially acquired porphyria. Arch. Dermatol., 89, 793-797

Buser, H.-R. (1975) Analysis of polychlorinated dibenzo-p-dioxins and dibenzofurans in chlorinated phenols by mass fragmentography. J. Chromat., 107, 295-310

Buser, H.-R. (1976) High-resolution gas chromatography of polychlorinated dibenzo-*p*-dioxins and dibenzofurans. Analyt. Chem., 48, 1553-1557

Buser, H.-R. & Bosshardt, H.-P. (1974) Determination of 2,3,7,8-tetrachlorodibenzo-1,4-dioxin at parts per billion levels in technical-grade 2,4,5-trichlorophenoxyacetic acid, in 2,4,5-T alkyl ester and 2,4,5-T amine salt herbicide formulations by quadrupole mass fragmentography. J. Chromat., 90, 71-77

Buser, H.-R. & Bosshardt, H.-P. (1976) Determination of polychlorinated dibenzo-*p*-dioxins and dibenzofurans in commercial pentachlorophenols by combined gas chromatography-mass spectrometry. J. Ass. off. analyt. Chem., 59, 562-569

Buu-Hoï, N.P., Hien, D.-P., Saint-Ruf, G. & Servoin-Sidoine, J. (1971) Propriétés cancéromimétiques de la tétrachloro-2,3,7,8 dibenzo-*p*-dioxine. C.R. Acad. Sci. (Paris), 272, 1447-1450

Buu-Hoï, N.P., Saint-Ruf, G. & Mangane, M. (1972a) The fragmentation of dibenzo-*p*-dioxin and its derivatives under electron impact. J. het. Chem., 9, 691-693

Buu-Hoï, N.P., Chanh, P.-H., Sesqué, G., Azum-Gelade, M.C. & Saint-Ruf, G. (1972b) Organs as targets of 'dioxin' (2,3,7,8-tetrachlorodibenzo-*p*-dioxin) intoxication. Naturwissenschaften, 59, 174-175

Buu-Hoï, N.P., Chanh, P.-H., Sesqué, G., Azum-Gelade, M.C. & Saint-Ruf, G. (1972c) Enzymatic functions as targets of the toxicity of 'dioxin' (2,3,7,8-tetrachlorodibenzo-*p*-dioxin). Naturwissenschaften, 59, 173-174

Carter, C.D., Kimbrough, R.D., Liddle, J.A., Cline, R.E., Zack, M.M., Jr, Barthel, W.F., Koehler, R.E. & Phillips, P.E. (1975) Tetrachlorodibenzo-dioxin: an accidental poisoning episode in horse arenas. Science, 188, 738-740

Cattabeni, F. (1977) Analysis of 2,3,7,8-tetrachlorodibenzo-*para*-dioxin in the Seveso area. In: Ramel, C., ed., Chlorinated Phenoxy Acids and their Dioxins: Mode of Action, Health Risks and Environmental Effects. Ecol. Bull. (Stockholm), 27 (in press)

Chen, J-Y. T. (1973) Infrared studies of chlorinated dibenzo-*p*-dioxins and structurally related compounds. J. Ass. off. analyt. Chem., 56, 962-975

Chhabra, R.S., Tredger, J.M., Philpot, R.M. & Fouts, J.R. (1974) Selection of inducers: an important factor in characterizing genetic differences to induction of aryl hydrocarbon hydroxylase in strains of mice. Life Sci., 15, 123-130

Chhabra, R.S., Tredger, J.M., Philpot, R.M. & Fouts, J.R. (1976) Relationship between induction of aryl hydrocarbon hydroxylase and *de novo* synthesis of cytochrome P-448 (P_1-450) in mice. Chem.-biol. Interact., 15, 21-31

Committee on the Effects of Herbicides in Vietnam (1974) The Effects of Herbicides in South Vietnam, Part A, Summary and Conclusions, Washington DC, National Academy of Sciences

Commoner, B. & Scott, R.E. (1976a) Accidental Contamination of Soil with Dioxin in Missouri: Effects and Countermeasures, Washington University, Saint Louis, Missouri, Center for the Biology of Natural Systems

Commoner, B. & Scott, R.E. (1976b) US Air Force Studies on the Stability and Ecological Effects of TCDD (Dioxin): An Evaluation Relative to the Accidental Dissemination of TCDD at Seveso, Italy, Washington University, Saint Louis, Missouri, Center for the Biology of Natural Systems

Courtney, K.D. & Moore, J.A. (1971) Teratology studies with 2,4,5-trichlorophenoxyacetic acid and 2,3,7,8-tetrachlorodibenzo-*p*-dioxin. Toxicol. appl. Pharmacol., 20, 396-403

Crosby, D.G. & Wong, A.S. (1977) Environmental degradation of 2,3,7,8-tetrachlorodibenzo-*p*-dioxin (TCDD). Science, 195, 1337-1338

Crosby, D.G., Wong, A.S., Plimmer, J.R. & Woolson, E.A. (1971) Photodecomposition of chlorinated dibenzo-*p*-dioxins. Science, 173, 748-749

Crosby, D.G., Moilanen, K.W. & Wong, A.S. (1973) Environmental generation and degradation of dibenzodioxins and dibenzofurans. Environm. Hlth Perspect., 5, 259-266

Crossland, J. & Shea, K.P. (1973) The hazards of impurities. Environment, 15, 35-38

Crummett, W.B. & Stehl, R.H. (1973) Determination of chlorinated dibenzo-*p*-dioxins and dibenzofurans in various materials. Environm. Hlth Perspect., 5, 15-25

Czeizel, E. & Király, J. (1976) Chromosome examinations in workers producing Klorinol® and Buvinol®. In: Bánki, L., ed., The Development of a Pesticide as a Complex Scientific Task, Budapest, Medicina, pp. 239-256

Dalderup, L.M. (1974) Safety measures for taking down buildings contaminated with toxic material. II. T. soc. Geneesk., 52, 616-623

Darsow, G. & Schnell, H. (1970) Chlorodibenzo-*p*-dioxins. German Offen. 1,930,259, 17 December, to Farbenfabriken Bayer A.-G.

Dugois, P. & Colomb, L. (1956) Acné chlorique au 2-4-5 trichlorophénol. Bull. Soc. franç. Derm. Syph., 63, 262-263

Dugois, P. & Colomb, L. (1957) Remarques sur l'acné chlorique (à propos d'une éclosion de cas provoques par la préparation du 2-4-5-trichlorophénol). J. Méd. Lyon, 38, 899-903

Dugois, P., Maréchal, J. & Colomb, L. (1958) Acné chlorique au 2.4.5. trichlorophénol. Arch. Mal. prof., 19, 626-627

Dugois, P., Amblard, P., Aimard, M. & Deshors, G. (1968) Acné chlorique collective et accidentelle d'un type nouveau. Bull. Soc. franç. Derm. Syph., 75, 260-261

Firestone, D. (1973) Etiology of chick edema disease. Environm. Hlth Perspect., 5, 59-66

Firestone, D. (1977) The 2,3,7,8-tetrachlorodibenzo-*para*-dioxin problem: a review. In: Ramel, C., ed., Chlorinated Phenoxy Acids and their Dioxins: Mode of Action, Health Risks and Environmental Effects. Ecol. Bull. (Stockholm), 27 (in press)

Firestone, D., Ress, J., Brown, N.L., Barron, R.P. & Damico, J.N. (1972) Determination of polychlorodibenzo-*p*-dioxins and related compounds in commercial chlorophenols. J. Ass. off. analyt. Chem., 55, 85-92

Fowler, B.A., Lucier, G.W., Brown, H.W. & McDaniel, O.S. (1973) Ultrastructural changes in rat liver cells following a single oral dose of TCDD. Environm. Hlth Perspect., 5, 141-148

Fowler, B.A., Hook, G.E.R. & Lucier, G.W. (1975) Tetrachlorodibenzo-*p*-dioxin induction of renal microsomal enzyme systems. Toxicol. appl. Pharmacol., 33, 176-177

Fries, G.F. & Marrow, G.S. (1975) Retention and excretion of 2,3,7,8-tetrachlorodibenzo-*p*-dioxin by rats. J. agric. Fd Chem., 23, 265-269

Gilman, H. & Dietrich, J.J. (1957) Halogen derivatives of dibenzo-*p*-dioxin. J. Amer. chem. Soc., 79, 1439-1441

Goldmann, P.J. (1972) Schwerste akute Chlorakne durch Trichlorphenol-Zersetzungsprodukte. Arbeitsmed. Sozialmed. Arbeitshyg., 7, 12-18

Goldmann, P.J. (1973) Schwerste akute Chloracne, eine Massenintoxikation durch 2,3,6,7-Tetrachlordibenzodioxin. Der Hautarzt, 24, 149-152

Goldstein, J.A., Hickman, P., Bergman, H. & Vos, J.G. (1973) Hepatic porphyria induced by 2,3,7,8-tetrachlorodibenzo-*p*-dioxin in the mouse. Res. Commun. chem. Path. Pharmacol., 6, 919-928

Gray, A.P., Cepa, S.P. & Cantrell, J.S. (1975) Intervention of the Smiles rearrangement in syntheses of dibenzo-p-dioxins: 1,2,3,6,7,8- and 1,2,3,7,8,9-hexachlorodibenzo-p-dioxin (HCDD). Tetrahedron. Lett., 33, 2873-2876

Gray, A.P., Cepa, S.P., Solomon, I.J. & Aniline, O. (1976) Synthesis of specific polychlorinated dibenzo-p-dioxins. J. org. Chem., 41, 2435-2437

Green, S. (1977) Cytogenetic effect of 2,3,7,8-tetrachlorodibenzo-p-dioxin on rat bone marrow cells. FDA By-Lines, Washington DC, Food and Drug Administration (in press)

Green, S. & Moreland, F.S. (1975) Cytogenetic evaluation of several dioxins in the rat. Toxicol. appl. Pharmacol., 33, 161

Greig, J.B. (1972) Effect of 2,3,7,8-tetrachlorodibenzo-1,4-dioxin on drug metabolism in the rat. Biochem. Pharmacol., 21, 3196-3198

Greig, J.B. & De Matteis, F. (1973) Effects of 2,3,7,8-tetrachlorodibenzo-p-dioxin on drug metabolism and hepatic microsomes of rats and mice. Environm. Hlth Perspect., 5, 211-219

Greig, J.B., Jones, G., Butler, W.H. & Barnes, J.M. (1973) Toxic effects of 2,3,7,8-tetrachlorodibenzo-p-dioxin. Fd Cosmet. Toxicol., 11, 585-595

Gruppo P.I.A., Mazza, B. & Scatturin, V. (1976) ICMESA: come e perché. Sapere, 796, 10-36

Gupta, B.N., Vos, J.G., Moore, J.A., Zinkl, J.G. & Bullock, B.C. (1973) Pathologic effects of 2,3,7,8-tetrachlorodibenzo-p-dioxin in laboratory animals. Environm. Hlth Perspect., 5, 125-140

Harris, M.W., Moore, J.A., Vos, J.G. & Gupta, B.N. (1973) General biological effects of TCDD in laboratory animals. Environm. Hlth Perspect., 5, 101-109

Hay, A. (1976) Toxic cloud over Seveso. Nature (Lond.), 262, 636-638

Helling, C.S., Isensee, A.R., Woolson, E.A., Ensor, P.D.J., Jones, G.E., Plimmer, J.R. & Kearney, P.C. (1973) Chlorodioxins in pesticides, soils, and plants. J. environm. Qual., 2, 171-178

Hofmann, H.T. (1957) Neuere Erfahrungen mit hoch-toxischen Chlorkohlenwasserstoffen. Naunyn-Schmiedeberg's Arch. exp. Path. Pharmakol., 232, 228-230

Hofmann, M.F. & Meneghini, C.L. (1962) A proposito delle follicolosi da idrocarburi clorosostituiti (acne clorica). G. Ital. Derm., 103, 427-450

Hook, G.E.R., Haseman, J.K. & Lucier, G.W. (1975a) Induction and suppression of hepatic and extrahepatic microsomal foreign-compound-metabolizing enzyme systems by 2,3,7,8-tetrachlorodibenzo-p-dioxin. Chem.-biol. Interact., 10, 199-214

Hook, G.E.R., Orton, T.C., Moore, J.A. & Lucier, G.W. (1975b) 2,3,7,8-Tetrachlorodibenzo-p-dioxin-induced changes in the hydroxylation of biphenyl by rat liver microsomes. Biochem. Pharmacol., 24, 335-340

Horwitz, W., ed. (1975) Official Methods of Analysis of the Association of Official Analytical Chemists, 12th ed., Washington DC, Association of Official Analytical Chemists, pp. 511-512

Hussain, S., Ehrenberg, L., Löfroth, G. & Gejvall, T. (1972) Mutagenic effects of TCDD on bacterial systems. Ambio, 1, 32-33

Isensee, A.R. (1977) Bioaccumulation of 2,3,7,8-tetrachlorodibenzo-*para*-dioxin. In: Ramel, C., ed., Chlorinated Phenoxy Acids and their Dioxins: Mode of Action, Health Risks and Environmental Effects. Ecol. Bull. (Stockholm), 27 (in press)

Isensee, A.R. & Jones, G.E. (1971) Absorption and translocation of root and foliage applied 2,4-dichlorophenol, 2,7-dichlorodibenzo-p-dioxin, and 2,3,7,8-tetrachlorodibenzo-p-dioxin. J. agric. Fd Chem., 19, 1210-1214

Isensee, A.R. & Jones, G.E. (1975) Distribution of 2,3,7,8-tetrachlorodibenzo-p-dioxin (TCDD) in aquatic model ecosystem. Environm. Sci. Technol., 9, 668-672

Jackson, W.T. (1972) Regulation of mitosis. III. Cytological effects of 2,4,5-trichlorophenoxyacetic acid and of dioxin contaminants in 2,4,5-T formulations. J. cell. Sci., 10, 15-25

Jensen, N.E. & Walker, A.E. (1972) Chloracne: three cases. Proc. roy. Soc. Med., 65, 687-688

Jirásek, L., Kalenský, J. & Kubeck, K. (1973) Acne chlorina and porphyria cutanea tarda during the manufacture of herbicides. Cs. Dermatol., 48, 306-317

Jirásek, L., Kalenský, J., Kubeck, K., Pazderová, J. & Lukáš, E. (1974) Acne chlorina, porphyria cutanea tarda and other manifestations of general intoxication during the manufacture of herbicides. II. Cs. Dermatol., 49, 145-157

Johnson, R.L., Gehring, P.J., Kociba, R.J. & Schwetz, B.A. (1973) Chlorinated dibenzodioxins and pentachlorophenol. Environm. Hlth Perspect., 5, 171-175

Jones, G. (1975) A histochemical study of the liver lesion induced by 2,3,7,8-tetrachlorodibenzo-*p*-dioxin (dioxin) in rats. J. Pathol., 116, 101-105

Jones, G. & Butler, W.H. (1974) A morphological study of the liver lesion induced by 2,3,7,8-tetrachlorodibenzo-*p*-dioxin in rats. J. Pathol., 112, 93-97

Kearney, P.C., Woolson, E.A. & Ellington C.P., Jr (1972) Persistence and metabolism of chlorodioxins in soils. Environm. Sci. Technol., 6, 1017-1019

Kende, A.S. & DeCamp, M.R. (1975) Smiles rearrangements in the synthesis of hexachlorodibenzo-*p*-dioxins. Tetrahedron Lett., 33, 2877-2880

Kende, A.S. & Wade, J.J. (1973) Synthesis of new steric and electronic analogs of 2,3,7,8-tetrachlorodibenzo-*p*-dioxin. Environm. Hlth Perspect., 5, 49-57

Kende, A.S., Wade, J.J., Ridge, D. & Poland, A. (1974) Synthesis and Fourier transform carbon-13 nuclear magnetic resonance spectroscopy of new toxic polyhalodibenzo-*p*-dioxins. J. org. Chem., 39, 931-937

Khera, K.S. & Ruddick, J.A. (1973) Polychlorodibenzo-*p*-dioxins: perinatal effects and the dominant lethal test in Wistar rats. Advanc. Chem. Ser., 120, 70-84

Kimbrough, R.D. (1974) The toxicity of polychlorinated polycyclic compounds and related chemicals. Crit. Rev. Toxicol., 2, 445-498

Kimbrough, R.D., Carter, C.D., Liddle, J.A., Cline, R.E. & Phillips, P.E. (1977) Epidemiology and pathology of a tetrachlorodibenzodioxin poisoning episode. Arch. environm. Hlth, 32, 77-86

Kimmig, J. & Schulz, K.H. (1957) Berufliche Akne (sog. Chlorakne) durch chlorierte aromatische zyklische Äther. Dermatologia, 115, 540-546

King, M.E., Shefner, A.M. & Bates, R.R. (1973) Carcinogenesis bioassay of chlorinated dibenzodioxins and related chemicals. Environm. Hlth Perspect., 5, 163-170

Kirsch, R., Fleischner, G., Kamisaka, K. & Arias, I.M. (1975) Structural and functional studies of ligandin, a major renal organic anion-binding protein. J. clin. Invest., 55, 1009-1019

Kociba, R.J., Keeler, P.A., Park, C.N. & Gehring, P.J. (1976) 2,3,7,8-Tetrachlorodibenzo-*p*-dioxin (TCDD): results of a 13-week oral toxicity study in rats. Toxicol. appl. Pharmacol., 35, 553-574

Kouri, R.E. (1976) Relationship between levels of aryl hydrocarbon hydroxylase activity and susceptibility to 3-methylcholanthrene and benzo(a)-pyrene induced cancers in inbred strains of mice. In: Freudenthal, R.I. & Jones, P.W., eds, Polynuclear Aromatic Hydrocarbons: Chemistry, Metabolism and Carcinogenesis, Vol. 1, New York, Raven Press, pp. 139-151

Kouri, R.E. & Nebert, D.W. (1977) Genetic regulation of susceptibility to polycyclic hydrocarbon-induced tumors in the mouse. In: Proceedings of a Symposium on Origins of Human Cancer, Cold Spring Harbour, 1976 (in press)

Kouri, R.E., Ratrie, H., III, Atlas, S.A., Niwa, A. & Nebert, D.W. (1974) Aryl hydrocarbon hydroylase induction in human lymphocyte cultures by 2,3,7,8-tetrachloro dibenzo-p-dioxin. Life Sci., 15, 1585-1595

Kulka, M. (1961) Octahalogenodibenzo-p-dioxins. Canad. J. Chem., 39, 1973-1976

Langer, H.G., Brady, T.P. & Briggs, P.R. (1973) Formation of dibenzodioxins and other condensation products from chlorinated phenols and derivatives. Environm. Hlth Perspect., 5, 3-7

Lucier, G.W., McDaniel, O.S., Hook, G.E.R., Fowler, B.A., Sonawane, B.R. & Faeder, E. (1973) TCDD-induced changes in rat liver microsomal enzymes. Environm. Hlth Perspect., 5, 199-209

Lucier, G.W., McDaniel, O.S. & Hook, G.E.R. (1975a) Nature of the enhancement of hepatic uridine diphosphate glucuronyltransferase activity by 2,3,7,8-tetrachlorodibenzo-p-dioxin in rats. Biochem. Pharmacol., 24, 325-334

Lucier, G.W., Sonawane, B.R., McDaniel, O.S. & Hook, G.E.R. (1975b) Postnatal stimulation of hepatic microsomal enzymes following administration of TCDD to pregnant rats. Chem.-biol. Interact., 11, 15-26

Matsumura, F. & Benezet, H.J. (1973) Studies on the bioaccumulation and microbial degradation of 2,3,7,8-tetrachlorodibenzo-p-dioxin. Environm. Hlth Perspect., 5, 253-258

May, G. (1973) Chloracne from the accidental production of tetrachlorodibenzodioxin. Brit. J. industr. Med., 30, 276-283

McKinney, J.D. (1977) Analysis of 2,3,7,8-tetrachlorodibenzo-$para$-dioxin in environmental samples. In: Ramel, C., ed., Chlorinated Phenoxy Acids and their Dioxins: Mode of Action, Health Risks and Environmental Effects. Ecol. Bull. (Stockholm), 27 (in press)

Mercier, M.J. (1977) 2,3,7,8-Tetrachlorodibenzo-p-dioxin: an overview. In: Berlin, A., Buratta, A. & Van der Venne, M.-T., eds, Proceedings of the Expert Meeting on the Problems Raised By TCDD Pollution, Milan, 1976 (in press)

Merz, V. & Weith, W. (1872) Zur Kenntmiss des Perchlorphenols. Ber. dtsch. chem. Ges., 5, 458-463

Meselson, M.S., Westing, A.H. & Constable, J.D. (1972) Background material relevant to presentations at the 1970 Annual Meeting of the AAAS. American Association for the Advancement of Science, Herbicide Assessment Commission, 92nd Congress, 2nd Session, US Congressional Record, 118, S3227-S3233

Milnes, M.H. (1971) Formation of 2,3,7,8-tetrachlorodibenzodioxin by thermal decomposition of sodium 2,4,5-trichlorophenate. Nature (Lond.), 232, 395-396

Moore, J.A. (1977) Toxicity of 2,3,7,8-tetrachlorodibenzo-*para*-dioxin. In: Ramel, C., ed., Chlorinated Phenoxy Acids and their Dioxins: Mode of Action, Health Risks and Environmental Effects. Ecol. Bull. (Stockholm), 27 (in press)

Moore, J.A., Gupta, B.N., Zinkl, J.G. & Vos, J.G. (1973) Postnatal effects of maternal exposure to 2,3,7,8-tetrachlorodibenzo-*p*-dioxin (TCDD). Environm. Hlth Perspect., 5, 81-85

Nebert, D.W., Robinson, J.R., Niwa, A., Kumaki, K. & Poland, A.P. (1975) Genetic expression of aryl hydrocarbon hydroxylase activity in the mouse. J. cell. Physiol., 85, 393-414

Neubert, D. (1976) Some remarks to the toxicity of polychlorinated dibenzodioxins. In: Proceedings of the Congress of the European Teratology Society, Gaspiano, 1976 (in press)

Neubert, D. & Dillmann, I. (1972) Embryotoxic effects in mice treated with 2,4,5-trichlorophenoxyacetic acid and 2,3,7,8-tetrachlorodibenzo-*p*-dioxin. Naunyn-Schmiedeberg's Arch. exp. Path. Pharmakol., 272, 243-264

Neubert, D., Zens, P., Rothenwallner, A. & Merker, H.-J. (1973) A survey of the embryotoxic effects of TCDD in mammalian species. Environm. Hlth Perspect., 5, 67-79

NIEHS (National Institute of Environmental Health Sciences) (1973) Conference on Chlorinated Dibenzodioxins and Dibenzofurans, Research Triangle Park, North Carolina, 2-3 April 1973. Environm. Hlth Perspect., 5, 59-251

Nilsson, C.-A., Andersson, K., Rappe, C. & Westermark, S.-O. (1974) Chromatographic evidence for the formation of chlorodioxins from chloro-2-phenoxyphenols. J. Chromat., 96, 137-147

Niwa, A., Kumaki, K., Nebert, D.W. & Poland, A. (1975a) Genetic expression of aryl hydrocarbon hydroxylase activity in the mouse. Arch. Biochem. Biophys., 166, 559-564

Niwa, A., Kumaki, K. & Nebert, D.W. (1975b) Induction of aryl hydrocarbon hydroxylase activity in various cell cultures by 2,3,7,8-tetrachlorodibenzo-p-dioxin. Mol. Pharmacol., 11, 399-408

Norback, D.H. & Allen, J.R. (1973) Biological responses of the nonhuman primate, chicken and rat to chlorinated dibenzo-p-dioxin ingestion. Environm. Hlth Perspect., 5, 233-240

Oliver, R.M. (1975) Toxic effects of 2,3,7,8-tetrachlorodibenzo 1,4-dioxin in laboratory workers. Brit. J. industr. Med., 32, 49-53

Pfeiffer, C.D. (1976) Determination of chlorinated dibenzo-p-dioxins in pentachlorophenol by liquid chromatography. J. chromat. Sci., 14, 386-391

Piper, W.N., Rose, J.Q. & Gehring, P.J. (1973a) Excretion and tissue distribution of 2,3,7,8-tetrachlorodibenzo-p-dioxin in the rat. Environm. Hlth Perspect., 5, 241-244

Piper, W.N., Rose, J.Q. & Gehring, P.J. (1973b) Excretion and tissue distribution of 2,3,7,8-tetrachlorodibenzo-p-dioxin in the rat. Advanc. Chem. Ser., 120, 85-91

Pocchiari, F. (1977) Decontamination of 2,3,7,8-tetrachlorodibenzo-$para$-dioxin. In: Ramel, C., ed., Chlorinated Phenoxy Acids and their Dioxins: Mode of Action, Health Risks and Environmental Effects. Ecol. Bull. (Stockholm), 27 (in press)

Pohland, A.E. & Yang, G.C. (1972) Preparation and characterization of chlorinated dibenzo-p-dioxins. J. agric. Fd Chem., 20, 1093-1099

Pohland, A.E., Yang, G.C. & Brown, N. (1973) Analytical and confirmative techniques for dibenzo-p-dioxins based upon their cation radicals. Environm. Hlth Perspect., 5, 9-14

Poland, A. & Glover, E. (1973a) Studies on the mechanism of toxicity of the chlorinated dibenzo-p-dioxins. Environm. Hlth Perspect., 5, 245-251

Poland, A. & Glover, E. (1973b) Chlorinated dibenzo-p-dioxins: potent inducers of δ-aminolevulinic acid synthetase and aryl hydrocarbon hydroxylase. II. A study of the structure-activity relationship. Mol. Pharmacol., 9, 736-747

Poland, A. & Glover, E. (1973c) 2,3,7,8-Tetrachlorodibenzo-p-dioxin: a potent inducer of δ-aminolevulinic acid synthetase. Science, 179, 476-477

Pohland, A. & Glover, E. (1974) Comparison of 2,3,7,8-tetrachlorodibenzo-p-dioxin, a potent inducer of aryl hydrocarbon hydroxylase, with 3-methylcholanthrene. Mol. Pharmacol., 10, 349-359

Poland, A.P., Smith, D., Metter, G. & Possick, P. (1971) A health survey of workers in a 2,4-D and 2,4,5-T plant with special attention to chloracne, porphyria cutanea tarda, and psychologic parameters. Arch. environm. Hlth, 22, 316-327

Poland, A.P., Glover, E., Robinson, J.R. & Nebert, D.W. (1974) Genetic expression of aryl hydrocarbon hydroxylase activity. Induction of mono-oxygenase activities and cytochrome P_1-450 formation by 2,3,7,8-tetrachlorodibenzo-p-dioxin in mice genetically 'non-responsive' to other aromatic hydrocarbons. J. biol. Chem., 249, 5599-5606

Poland, A.P., Glover, E. & Kende, A.S. (1976) Stereospecific, high affinity binding of 2,3,7,8-tetrachlorodibenzo-p-dioxin by hepatic cytosol. J. biol. Chem., 251, 4936-4946

Porter, M.L. & Burke, J.A. (1971) Separation of three chlorodibenzo-p-dioxins from some polychlorinated biphenyls by chromatography on an aluminum oxide column. J. Ass. off. analyt. Chem., 54, 1426-1428

Rawls, R.L. & O'Sullivan, D.A. (1976) Italy seeks answers following toxic release. Chem. Eng. News, 54, 27-28, 33, 35

Rose, J.Q., Ramsey, J.C., Wentzler, T.H., Hummel, R.A. & Gehring, P.J. (1976) The fate of 2,3,7,8-tetrachlorodibenzo-p-dioxin following single and repeated oral doses to the rat. Toxicol. appl. Pharmacol., 36, 209-226

Saint-Ruf, G. (1972) Formation of 'dioxin' in the pyrolysis of sodium α-(2,4,5-trichlorophenoxy)-propionate. Naturwissenschaften, 59, 648

Saint-Ruf, G. (1977) La dioxine. In: Berlin, A., Buratta, A. & Van der Venne, M.-T., eds, Proceedings of the Expert Meeting on the Problems Raised by TCDD Pollution, Milan, 1976 (in press)

Sandermann, W., Stockmann, H. & Casten, R. (1957) Über die Pyrolyse des Pentachlorphenols. Chem. Ber., 90, 690-692

Schulz, K.H. (1957) Klinische und experimentelle Untersuchungen zur Ätiologie der Chloracne. Arch. Klin. exp. Dermatol., 206, 589-596

Schulz, K.H. (1968) Zur Klinik und Ätiologie der Chlorakne. Arbeitsmed. Sozialmed. Arbeitshyg., 3, 25-29

Schwetz, B.A., Norris, J.M., Sparschu, G.L., Rowe, V.K., Gehring, P.J., Emerson, J.L. & Gerbig, C.G. (1973) Toxicity of chlorinated dibenzo-p-dioxins. Environm. Hlth Perspect., 5, 87-99

Seiler, J.P. (1973) A survey on the mutagenicity of various pesticides. Experientia, 29, 622-623

Smith, F.A., Schwetz, B.A. & Nitschke, K.D. (1976) Teratogenicity of 2,3,7,8-tetrachlorodibenzo-p-dioxin in CF-1 mice. Toxicol. appl. Pharmacol., 38, 517-523

Sparschu, G.L., Dunn, F.L. & Rowe, V.K. (1970) Teratogenic study of 2,3,7,8-tetrachlorodibenzo-p-dioxin in the rat. Toxicol. appl. Pharmacol., 17, 317

Sparschu, G.L., Dunn, F.L. & Rowe, V.K. (1971) Study of the teratogenicity of 2,3,7,8-tetrachlorodibenzo-p-dioxin in the rat. Fd Cosmet. Toxicol., 9, 405-412

Stehl, R.H., Papenfuss, R.R., Bredeweg, R.A. & Roberts, R.W. (1973) The stability of pentachlorophenol and chlorinated dioxins to sunlight, heat, and combustion. Advanc. Chem. Ser., 120, 119-125

Storherr, R.W., Watts, R.R., Gardner, A.M. & Osgood, T. (1971) Steam distillation technique for the analysis of 2,3,7,8-tetrachlorodibenzo-p-dioxin in technical 2,4,5-T. J. Ass. off. analyt. Chem., 54, 218-219

Telegina, K.A. & Bikbulatova, L.I. (1970) Affection of the follicular apparatus of the skin in workers occupied in production of butyl ether of 2,4,5-trichlorphenoxyacetic acid. Vestn. Dermatol. Venerol., 44, 35-39

Thiess, A.M. & Goldmann, P. (1977) Über das Trichlorphenol-Dioxin-Unfallgeschehen in der BASF AG vom 13. November 1953. In: Vortrag. auf dem IV. Medichem-Kongress, Haifa, 1976 (in press)

Thigpen, J.E., Faith, R.E., McConnell, E.E. & Moore, J.A. (1975) Increased susceptibility to bacterial infection as a sequela of exposure to 2,3,7,8-tetrachlorodibenzo-p-dioxin. Infect. Immun., 12, 1319-1324

Tomita, M. & Watanabe, W. (1951) Antibacterial activity of some organic compounds *in vitro*. II. Antibacterial activity of dibenzo-p-dioxin, phenoxathiin, and 1,4-benzodioxan derivatives on *Mycobacterium tuberculosis, Staphylococcus aureus,* and *Escherichia coli*. J. pharm. Soc. Japan, 71, 1204-1206

Ton That, T. (1977) Pathologie humaine et animale de la dioxine. Rev. Méd. (Paris) (in press)

Ton That, T., Tran Thi, A., Nguyen Dang, T., Pham Hoang, P., Nguyen Nhu, B., Ton That, B., Hoang Van, S. & Do Kim, S. (1973) Le cancer primaire du foie au Viêt-nam. Chirurgie, 99, 427-436

Tóth, K., Sugár, J., Somfai-Relle, S. & Bence, J. (1977) Carcinogenic bioassay of the herbicide, 2,4,5-trichlorophenoxy-ethanol (TCPE) with different 2,3,7,8-tetrachlorodibenzo-p-dioxin (dioxin) content in Swiss mice. In: International Conference on Ecological Perspectives on Carcinogens and Cancer Control, Cremona, 1976, Basel, Karger AG (in press)

US Environmental Protection Agency (1973) EPA Compendium of Registered Pesticides, Vol. II, Fungicides and Nematicides, Part I, Washington DC, US Government Printing Office, pp. P-11-00.01-P-11-00.05

US International Trade Commission (1976a) Synthetic Organic Chemicals, US Production and Sales, 1974, ITC Publication 776, Washington DC, US Government Printing Office, p. 185

US International Trade Commission (1976b) Synthetic Organic Chemicals, US Production and Sales of Pesticides and Related Products, 1975 Preliminary, Washington DC, US Government Printing Office, pp. 2,4

US Tariff Commission (1967) Synthetic Organic Chemicals, US Production and Sales, 1965, TC Publication 206, Washington DC, US Government Printing Office, p. 53

Van Miller, J.P. & Allen, J.R. (1977) Chronic toxicity of 2,3,7,8-tetrachlorodibenzo-p-dioxin in rats. Fed. Proc., 36, 396

Van Miller, J.P., Marlar, R.J. & Allen, J.R. (1976) Tissue distribution and excretion of tritiated tetrachlorodibenzo-p-dioxin in non-human primates and rats. Fd Cosmet. Toxicol., 14, 31-34

Vásárhelyi, E., Hegedüs, I. & Szöke, S. (1976) Production and analytics of Klorinol® (TCPE) and some of its related compounds. In: Banki, L., ed., The Development of a Pesticide as a Complex Scientific Task, Budapest, Medicina, pp. 39-51

Villanueva, E.C., Burse, V.W. & Jennings, R.W. (1973) Chlorodibenzo-p-dioxin contamination of two commercially available pentachlorophenols. J. agric. Fd Chem., 21, 739-740

Villanueva, E.C., Jennings, R.W., Burse, V.W. & Kimbrough, R.D. (1975) A comparison of analytical methods for chlorodibenzo-p-dioxins in pentachlorophenol. J. agric. Fd Chem., 23, 1089-1091

Vinopal, J.H. & Casida, J.E. (1973) Metabolic stability of 2,3,7,8-tetrachlorodibenzo-p-dioxin in mammalian liver microsomal systems and in living mice. Arch. environm. Contam. Toxicol., 1, 122-132

Vos, J.G., Moore, J.A. & Zinkl, J.G. (1973) Effect of 2,3,7,8-tetrachlorodibenzo-p-dioxin on the immune system of laboratory animals. Environm. Hlth Perspect., 5, 149-162

Vos, J.G., Moore, J.A. & Zinkl, J.G. (1974) Toxicity of 2,3,7,8-tetrachlorodibenzo-p-dioxin (TCDD) in C57Bl/6 mice. Toxicol. appl. Pharmacol., 29, 229-241

Weissberg, J.B. & Zinkl, J.G. (1973) Effects of 2,3,7,8-tetrachlorodibenzo-p-dioxin upon hemostasis and hematologic function in the rat. Environm. Hlth Perspect., 5, 119-123

Westing, A.H. (1977) Ecological considerations regarding environmental dioxin contamination. In: Ramel, C., ed., Chlorinated Phenoxy Acids and their Dioxins: Mode of Action, Health Risks and Environmental Effects. Ecol. Bull. (Stockholm) (in press)

Wilkinson, J.E. (1975) Interference of 2,3,4,4,5,6-hexachloro-2,5-cyclohexadien-1-one in the gas-liquid chromatographic analysis of octachlorodibenzo-p-dioxin in commercial pentachlorophenol. J. Ass. off. analyt. Chem., 58, 974-977

Woods, J.S. (1973) Studies of the effects of 2,3,7,8-tetrachlorodibenzo-p-dioxin on mammalian hepatic δ-aminolevulinic acid synthetase. Environm. Hlth Perspect., 5, 221-225

Woolson, E.A., Thomas, R.F. & Ensor, P.D.J. (1972) Survey of polychlorodibenzo-p-dioxin content in selected pesticides. J. agric. Fd Chem., 20, 351-354

Woolson, E.A., Ensor, P.D.J., Reichel, W.L. & Young, A.L. (1973) Dioxin residues in Lakeland sand and bald eagle samples. Advanc. Chem. Ser., 120, 112-118

Young, A.L., Thalken, C.E., Arnold, E.L., Cupello, J.M. & Cockerham, L.G. (1976) Fate of 2,3,7,8-tetrachlorodibenzo-p-dioxin (TCDD) in the environment: summary and decontamination recommendations. USAFA-TR-76-18, Colorado, US Air Force Academy

Zedda, S. (1977) La lezione della chloracne. In: Cerruti, G. *et al.*, eds., ICMESA, Una Rapina di Saluti, di Lavoro e di Territorio, Milan, Mazzotta, pp. 17-43

Zinkl, J.G., Vos, J.G., Moore, J.A. & Gupta, B.N. (1973) Hematologic and clinical chemistry effects of 2,3,7,8-tetrachlorodibenzo-p-dioxin in laboratory animals. Environm. Hlth Perspect., 5, 111-118

COPPER 8-HYDROXYQUINOLINE

1. Chemical and Physical Data

1.1 Synonyms and trade names

Chem. Abstr. Services Reg. No.: 10380-28-6

Chem. Abstr. Name: Bis(8-quinolinolato-N^1,O^8)copper

Bis(8-oxyquinoline)copper; bis(8-quinolinato)copper; bis(8-quinolinolato)copper; copper hydroxyquinolate; copper 8-hydroxyquinolate; copper hydroxyquinolinate; copper 8-hydroxyquinolinate; copper oxinate; copper(2+) oxinate; copper oxine; copper oxyquinolate; copper oxyquinoline; copper quinolate; copper 8-quinolate; copper 8-quinolinol; copper quinolinolate; copper 8-quinolinolate; cupric 8-hydroxyquinolate; cupric 8-quinolinolate; oxine copper

Bioquin; Cunilate 2472; Cuproquin; Dormycin; Milmer 1; Quinolate; Quinolate 15; Quinolate 20; Tomo-oxiran

1.2 Chemical formula and molecular weight

$C_{18}H_{12}CuN_2O_2$ Mol. wt: 351.9

1.3 Chemical and physical properties of the pure substance

(a) Description: Greenish-yellow crystalline powder (Turner, 1966)

(b) Spectroscopy data: Infra-red absorption spectra are given by Shevchenko & Bidulya (1967) and mass spectra by Kidani *et al.* (1972).

(c) **Solubility**: Insoluble in water, ethanol and common organic solvents; slightly soluble in pyridine and quinoline (Turner 1966)

(d) **Volatility**: Non-volatile

1.4 Technical products and impurities

Copper 8-hydroxyquinoline is available in the US in liquid concentrates containing 0.25 to 10.0%, as pastes containing 5.0 to 30.0%, as solids containing 5.0 to 10.0% and as ready-to-use liquids containing 0.25 to 1.5% of the pure chemical, and as a 5.0% liquid concentrate in combination with 17.6% pentachlorophenol and 2.5% tetrachlorophenol. It is also used in combination with zinc petroleum sulphonate (US Environmental Protection Agency, 1973).

A technical grade of this chemical is also available in the US and Japan. Typical specifications are for 99% purity, a maximum of 10 mg/kg free copper and a maximum particle size of 5 microns for the granular form. Free copper and free 8-hydroxyquinoline are impurities.

Combination products with streptomycin and with captan are available for use as agricultural fungicides in Japan (Japan Plant Protection Association, 1973).

2. Production, Use, Occurrence and Analysis

For background information on this section, see preamble, p. 17.

2.1 Production and use

(a) **Production**

Copper 8-hydroxyquinoline can be prepared by mixing solutions of copper salts such as copper acetate with 8-hydroxyquinoline[1] (Spencer, 1973).

---

[1] See IARC, 1977

Production or sale of copper 8-hydroxyquinoline was first reported in the US in 1949 (US Tariff Commission, 1950). The company that first reported production is currently the only US producer of the chemical (US International Trade Commission, 1976a) and produces about 45 thousand kg annually. Imports of the chemical through the principal US custom districts in 1974 amounted to 15 thousand kg (US International Trade Commission, 1976b).

Copper 8-hydroxyquinoline is produced in France.

It was first produced in Japan in 1965. In 1975, about 300 thousand kg were produced by the only manufacturer; minor quantities were exported from Japan in 1972-1974.

About 70,000 kg were imported into Australia in 1975-1976.

(b) Use

Copper 8-hydroxyquinoline is a fungicide used in the treatment of textiles, as an ingredient of paints, in wood and paper preservation and in agriculture (Turner, 1966).

In the US, about 75% of the copper 8-hydroxyquinoline used is in the treatment of textiles (fabric, rope, thread, webbing and cordage, including fishing nets). It is also used in the US for protection against fungal attack on interior paints where mercurial compounds cannot be used because of their toxicity. Its use is limited to green paints (Turner, 1966). It is approved in the US for use as a fungicide on wooden containers which are in contact with food products, such as beverage boxes, field crates, hampers, pallets, and other wooden containers for fruits and vegetables. It is sometimes used in combination with zinc sulphonates for these purposes (US Environmental Protection Agency, 1973; US Food and Drug Administration, 1976). Minor uses in the US include its incorporation into plastics and paper (Turner, 1966) and its application on ornamental crops (US Environmental Protection Agency, 1973).

Less than 5 thousand kg copper 8-hydroxyquinoline are used annually in the UK, mostly in the treatment of textiles. In Japan, all of the copper 8-hydroxyquinoline produced is used as fungicide.

2.2 Occurrence

Copper 8-hydroxyquinoline is not known to occur as a natural product.

A significant but undetermined quantity of the chemical is believed to be widely dispersed in households in which interior paints containing it have been applied. A minor quantity may reach food products through the use of the chemical on fishing nets and fruit and vegetable containers.

2.3 Analysis

Spencer (1973) summarized two methods of analysis for copper 8-hydroxyquinoline; in both of these the copper is determined after its conversion to copper sulphate, and the 8-hydroxyquinoline moiety is determined spectrophotometrically after extraction in an organic solvent.

Copper 8-hydroxyquinoline can be analysed in samples of organic material by ashing in an atmosphere of oxygen and measuring the copper content in the ash by spectrophotometry of the rubeanic acid complex (Desai & Chapin, 1967). The copper has also been determined spectrophotometrically by measuring the absorbance at 610 nm of a copper-dithizone complex formed by adding dithizone to a solution of copper 8-hydroxyquinoline (Sasaki, 1972).

3. Biological Data Relevant to the Evaluation of Carcinogenic Risk to Man

3.1 Carcinogenicity and related studies in animals

(a) Oral administration

Mouse: Groups of 18 male and 18 female (C57BL/6xC3H/Anf)F_1 mice and 18 male and 18 female (C57BL/6xAKR)F_1 mice received copper 8-hydroxyquinoline according to the following dose schedule: 1000 mg/kg bw in 0.5% gelatine by stomach tube at 7 days of age and the same absolute amount (not adjusted for increasing body weight) daily up to 4 weeks of age; subsequently, the mice were given 2800 mg/kg of diet. The dose given was the maximum tolerated dose for infant and young mice. The experiment was terminated when the animals were about 78 weeks of age, at which time 11,

17, 17 and 18 mice in the four groups, respectively, were still alive. The tumour incidences in treated mice were not increased (P>0.05) for any type of tumour in any group or combination of groups compared with those in groups of 79, 87, 90 and 82 mice of each sex and strain which were either untreated or had received gelatine only (Innes et al., 1969; NTIS, 1968).

(b) Subcutaneous and/or intramuscular administration

Mouse: Groups of 18 male and 18 female (C57BL/6xC3H/Anf)F_1 mice and 18 male and 18 female (C57BL/6xAKR)F_1 mice were given single s.c. injections of 1000 mg/kg bw copper 8-hydroxyquinoline in 0.5% gelatine on the 28th day of life and were observed until they were about 78 weeks of age, at which time 14, 16, 18 and 17 mice in the four groups, respectively, were still alive. Of 17 necropsied male (C57BL/6xC3H/Anf)F_1 mice, 6 had generalized reticulum-cell sarcomas, compared with 8/141 control males of that strain [P<0.001]; such tumours were not observed in treated or untreated males of the second strain. In females, 1/18 and 3/18 mice of the first and second strains developed such tumours, compared with 1/154 and 5/157 controls (NTIS, 1968).

3.2 Other relevant biological data

No data were available to the Working Group.

3.3 Case reports and epidemiological studies

No data were available to the Working Group.

4. Comments on Data Reported and Evaluation

4.1 Animal data

Copper 8-hydroxyquinoline has been tested in two strains of mice by oral and by single subcutaneous administration. Although a significantly increased incidence of reticulum-cell sarcomas was observed only in males of one strain following single subcutaneous injection, no evaluation of the carcinogenicity of this compound can be made on the basis of the available data.

4.2 _Human data_

No case reports or epidemiological studies were available to the Working Group.

5. References

Desai, A.G. & Chapin, J.C. (1967) Copper determinations by use of the oxygen combustion flask technique. Int. Biodetn Bull., 3, 13-14

IARC (1977) IARC Monographs on the Evaluation of Carcinogenic Risk of Chemicals to Man, 13, Some Miscellaneous Pharmaceutical Substances, Lyon, pp. 101-112

Innes, J.R.M., Ulland, B.M., Valerio, M.G., Petrucelli, L., Fishbein, L., Hart, E.R., Pallotta, A.J., Bates, R.R., Falk, H.L., Gart, J.J., Klein, M., Mitchell, I. & Peters, J. (1969) Bioassay of pesticides and industrial chemicals for tumorigenicity in mice: a preliminary note. J. nat. Cancer Inst., 42, 1101-1114

Japan Plant Protection Association (1973) 1972 Evaluation of candidate pesticides. Japan Pesticide Information, No. 16, Tokyo, pp. 21-22

Kidani, Y., Naga, S. & Koike, H. (1972) Mass spectrometry of divalent metal oxinates. Chem. Lett., 7, 507-510

NTIS (National Technical Information Service) (1968) Evaluation of Carcinogenic, Teratogenic and Mutagenic Activities of Selected Pesticides and Industrial Chemicals, Vol. 1, Carcinogenic Study, Washington DC, US Department of Commerce

Sasaki, Y. (1972) Extraction and spectrometric determination of copper by the ligand-exchange of copper oxinate with dithizone in chloroform. Bunseki Kagaku, 21, 1037-1042

Shevchenko, L.L. & Bidulya, L.P. (1967) Infrared absorption spectra of thiooxinates and oxinates of some metals. Ukr. Khim. Zh., 33, 1229-1235

Spencer, E.Y. (1973) Guide to the Chemicals Used in Crop Protection, Publication 1093, 6th ed., London, Ontario, University of Western Ontario, Research Branch, Agriculture Canada, p. 383

Turner, N.J. (1966) Fungicides. In: Kirk, R.E. & Othmer, D.F., eds, Encyclopedia of Chemical Technology, 2nd ed., Vol. 10, New York, John Wiley and Sons, pp. 231-236

US Environmental Protection Agency (1973) EPA Compendium of Registered Pesticides, Vol. II, Fungicides and Nematicides, Part I, Washington DC, US Government Printing Office, pp. C-54-00.01-C.54-00.03, Z-07-00.01

US Food and Drug Administration (1976) Preservatives for wood. US Code of Federal Regulations, Title 21, part 121.2556, p. 522

US International Trade Commission (1976a) *Synthetic Organic Chemicals, US Production and Sales of Pesticides and Related Products, 1975 Preliminary*, Washington DC, US Government Printing Office, p. 4

US International Trade Commission (1976b) *Imports of Benzenoid Chemicals and Products, 1974*, ITC Publication 762, Washington DC, US Government Printing Office, p. 97

US Tariff Commission (1950) *Synthetic Organic Chemicals, US Production and Sales, 1949*, Report No. 169, Second Series, Washington DC, US Government Printing Office, p. 125

2,4-D AND ESTERS

1. Chemical and Physical Data

1.1 Synonyms and trade names

Chem. Abstr. Services Reg. No.: 94-75-7

Chem. Abstr. Name: (2,4-Dichlorophenoxy)acetic acid

Dichlorophenoxyacetic acid; 2,4-dichlorophenoxyacetic acid

For a representative list of other synonyms and trade names of products containing 2,4-D, its salts or esters, either as the sole active ingredient or as mixtures with other compounds, see Appendix A.

1.2 Chemical formula and molecular weight

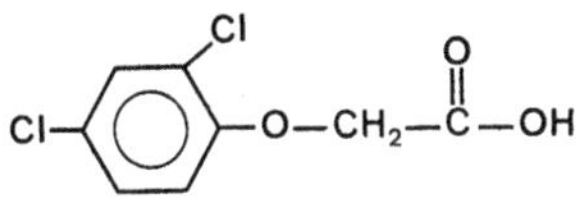

$C_8H_6Cl_2O_3$ Mol. wt: 221.0

1.3 Chemical and physical properties of the pure substance

From Weed Science Society of America (1974), unless otherwise specified

(a) Description: Odourless white crystals

(b) Boiling-point: 160°C at 0.4 mm

(c) Melting-point: 140-141°C

(d) Spectroscopy data: Infra-red and ultra-violet spectra are given by Gore et al. (1971).

(e) Solubility: Soluble in 95% ethanol and in acetone, dioxane and isopropyl alcohol

(f) Stability: Stable up to and including its melting-point

(g) Reactivity: Forms salts that are soluble in water

1.4 Technical products and impurities

Technical grade 2,4-D is available in the US as the free acid (98% purity), as salts (dimethylamine, mixed ethanolamine and isopropanolamine, lithium and sodium) and as esters of the following alcohols: isopropyl, *n*-butyl, sec-butyl, iso-octyl, 2-butoxyethyl and butoxypolypropylene glycol (US International Trade Commission, 1976a).

Of 28 samples of 2,4-D tested for content of chlorodibenzo-*para*-dioxins, one was found to contain <10 mg/kg hexachlorodibenzo-*para*-dioxin (Woolson *et al.*, 1972). Bis(2,4-dichlorophenoxy)methane has been identified as the major contaminant of 2,4-D, and bis(2,6-dichlorophenoxy)methane and 2,2',4,6'-tetrachlorodiphenoxymethane as minor contaminants (Huston, 1972).

N-Nitrosodimethylamine[1] has been detected at a level of 300 µg/l in dimethylamine salt of 2,4-D which was stored in metal containers the interiors of which had been presprayed with sodium nitrite as an antioxidant (Fine *et al.*, 1977).

Technical 2,4-D produced in Japan is more than 99% pure.

2. Production, Use, Occurrence and Analysis

For background information on this section, see preamble, p. 17.

2.1 Production and use

(a) Production

2,4-D was prepared in 1941 by the interaction of 2,4-dichlorophenol, monochloracetic acid and sodium hydroxide (Pokorny, 1941), and a similar process is believed to be used in its commercial production.

Production was first reported in the US in 1944 (US Tariff Commission, 1946). The quantity of 2,4-D produced increased steadily between 1963 and 1968, when it reached a maximum of 36 million kg; production decreased to about 20 million kg in 1970 (US Department of Agriculture, 1973) and

---

[1] See IARC, 1972

gradually increased again to an estimated 27 million kg in 1974. In 1975, three US companies reported production of 2,4-D acid; three others reported the production of esters or salts of 2,4-D, presumably from purchased acid. Separate production data for 1975 are available only for the dimethylamine salt of 2,4-D, 11.6 million kg of which were produced, and for the iso-octyl ester, 4.5 million kg of which were produced (US International Trade Commission, 1976a). In 1973, 115 thousand kg of 2,4-D acid and 57 thousand kg of mixed butyl esters were imported through the principal US customs districts (US Tariff Commission, 1974). In 1974, 365 kg of the mixed butyl esters were imported (US International Trade Commission, 1976b). Combined US exports of 2,4-D and 2,4,5-T amounted to 5.7 million kg in 1975 (US Department of Commerce, 1975).

The Federal Republic of Germany and the UK are the major producing countries in western Europe, where annual production is estimated to be 3-30 million kg; in eastern Europe it is estimated to be less than 10 million kg.

2,4-D was first produced commercially in Japan before 1945 by a process similar to that used in the US. Production in 1975 by two producers amounted to 511 thousand kg, and 176 thousand kg were exported.

About 90,000 kg were imported into Australia in 1975-76.

(b) Use

2,4-D is a systemic herbicide widely used for control of broadleaf weeds in cereal crops and sugar cane and on turf, pastures and non-cropland (Weed Science Society of America, 1974). It is also used to control the ripening of bananas and citrus fruits, to delay preharvest dropping of some fruits and in some countries as a fungicide for the control of *Alternaria* rots when lemons are to be held for storage (WHO, 1975).

An estimated 27 million kg of 2,4-D acid equivalent, largely in the form of esters and salts, were used in the US in 1975, as follows: wheat and other small grains, 31%; corn and grain sorghum, 26%; pasture and rangeland, 25%; industrial and commercial uses, 9%; lawns and turf, 5%; aquatic weed control, 3%; rice and fruit, 1%.

2,4-D was used to defoliate jungle areas in south Vietnam, where it was a component of 'Agent Orange' (a 50:50 mixture of the n-butyl esters of 2,4-D and 2,4,5-T, containing up to 30 mg/kg or more TCDD) (Davis, 1974). About 40 million litres of 'Agent Orange' were sprayed in south Vietnam between 1965-1971 for defoliation or crop destruction (Committee on the Effects of Herbicides in Vietnam, 1974).

National tolerances are in effect in several countries. Examples were reported to the Joint Meeting of the FAO Working Party of Experts on Pesticide Residues and the WHO Expert Committee on Pesticide Residues in 1975. The previously established acceptable daily intake for man of 0-0.3 mg/kg bw was considered and confirmed at this meeting (WHO, 1977).

The US Occupational Safety and Health Administration health standards for exposure to air contaminants require that an employee's exposure to 2,4-D does not exceed an eight-hour time-weighted average of 10 mg/m^3 in the working atmosphere during any eight-hour work shift of a forty-hour work week. The corresponding standard in the Federal Republic of Germany is also 10 mg/m^3, and the acceptable ceiling concentration in the USSR is 1 mg/m^3 (Winell, 1975).

2.2 Occurrence

2,4-D is not known to occur as a natural product.

It is broken down by soil microorganisms, and there is reportedly no accumulation in the soil as a result of normal agricultural use (Weed Science Society of America, 1974).

In a continuing programme involving the monitoring of pesticide residues in food, the US Department of Health, Education and Welfare found a decreasing level of 2,4-D in food samples collected at retail outlets during the period 1965-1973. Between June 1964 and April 1965, 2,4-D was found in 10 of 216 composite food samples examined, including leafy vegetables, oils, fat and shortening, sugar and adjuvants (Duggan et al., 1966). In 1973, an insignificant amount of 2,4-D was found during this programme: a trace was found in one of 360 composite potato samples (US Bureau of Foods, 1975).

Air samples were collected near wheat-growing areas around Pullman and Kennewick Highlands, Washington, USA between April and August 1964 after applications of 2,4-D. Although data were given for several products containing 2,4-D, those for the isopropyl ester were the highest: an average concentration of 0.116 $\mu g/m^3$ and a maximum concentration of 1.96 $\mu g/m^3$ of an aerosol form of the ester and an average concentration of 0.007 $\mu g/m^3$ and a maximum concentration of 0.69 $\mu g/m^3$ of the vaporized ester were found in 24-hour samples near Pullman (Finkelstein, 1969).

Residues of 2,4-D in pond waters declined from maximums of 0.345 and 0.692 mg/l in Florida and Georgia, respectively, to less than 0.005 mg/l 28 days after treatment and from 0.630 mg/l in Missouri pond waters to less than 0.005 mg/l 56 days after treatment. Residues in mud from the Florida and Georgia ponds never exceeded 0.05 mg/kg and had declined to trace or nondetectable levels 56 days after treatment. The highest residue found was 0.170 mg/kg in samples of mud taken on the first and third days in the most heavily treated Missouri pond. In mud from one Missouri pond, residues were detected as late as 28 days after treatment; no residues occurred in any ponds after that time (Schultz & Harman, 1974).

In September 1971, soil samples were obtained from an area in Thailand that had been used for calibrating aerial herbicide spray equipment and that had received about 940 kg/ha 2,4-D and large amounts of other herbicides in 1964-65. Two of 6 samples contained 0.18 and 0.21 kg/ha 2,4-D (Committee on the Effects of Herbicides in Vietnam, 1974).

2.3 Analysis

The Association of Official Analytical Chemists (AOAC) has published three Official Final Actions for the determination of 2,4-D in formulations: (1) titration, for formulations of the free acid; (2) determination of total chlorine after calorimetric destruction for formulations of 2,4-D compounds; and (3) infra-red spectroscopy for 3,6-dichloro-2-methoxybenzoic acid (Dicamba)/2,4-D formulations. Official First Actions have been published for determination of the free acid in formulations of 2,4-D esters by titration to pH 7, and for determination in formulations with 4-amino-3,5,6-trichloropicolonic acid (picloram) by high-pressure liquid chromatography (Beroza, 1976; Horwitz, 1975). Results of collaborative studies of several of these methods have been published (Hammond, 1973; Malina, 1971; Skelly et al., 1976).

Another method for determining 2,4-D in formulations involves gas chromatography of its trimethylsilyl derivative (Zweig, 1972). With a similar method, recoveries of 100.5 ± 1% compare favourably with those obtained using the AOAC infra-red spectroscopy method (Collier & Grimes, 1974).

Methods of analysis for 2,4-D residues in various commodities using gas chromatography have been summarized and tabulated in a recent review (WHO, 1975). In a more recent publication (WHO, 1977) attention was drawn to the low recoveries frequently encountered due to conjugation of 2,4-D with plant constituents. The <u>Pesticide Analytical Manual</u> (US Food & Drug Administration, 1975a,b) summarizes several methods for determining 2,4-D residues, using gas, thin-layer and paper chromatography; a general method for extraction and clean-up of chlorophenoxy acids in a variety of foods provides more than 80% recovery. Limits of detection for gas chromatography are in the order of 10 µg/kg when microcoulometric detection is used and 0.2 µg/kg with electron capture.

A gas chromatographic procedure has been used to separate mixtures of herbicidal acids as their pentafluorobenzyl derivatives, which generally provide better separation and better responses in the electron capture detector than do the methyl or silyl derivatives; the method has a sensitivity of 0.4 µg/kg for 2,4-D (Chau & Terry, 1976). An automated, gel-permeation chromatographic procedure permits clean-up of pesticide residues in lipid-containing plant and animal extracts prior to their determination by gas chromatography with electron-capture detection, and provides recovery of more than 80% 2,4-D esters (Johnson et al., 1976).

A low-temperature extraction and clean-up method is used to separate multiple residues of 2,4-D and other pesticides for eventual gas chromatographic analysis with electron capture and flame photometric detectors; 82-108% of added 4 mg/kg 2,4-D could be recovered (McLeod & Wales, 1972).

Gas chromatography combined with electron-capture detection has been used to determine 0.5 mg/kg 2,4-D residues in oysters (Duffy & Shelfoon, 1967) and 0.05 mg/kg in soil, wheat and barley (Khan, 1975).

3. Biological Data Relevant to the Evaluation of Carcinogenic Risk to Man

3.1 Carcinogenicity and related studies in animals

(a) Oral administration

Mouse: Groups of 18 male and 18 female (C57BL/6xC3H/Anf)F_1 mice and 18 male and 18 female (C57BL/6xAKR)F_1 mice received commercial 2,4-D (90%, m.p. 136-140°C) according to the following dose schedule: 46.4 mg/kg bw in 0.5% gelatine by stomach tube at 7 days of age and the same amount (not adjusted for increasing body weight) daily up to 28 days of age; subsequently, the mice were given 149 mg/kg of diet. A further group of 18 male and 18 female (C57BL/6xAKR)F_1 mice were given oral doses of 100 mg/kg bw/day from 7-28 days of age and subsequently fed 323 mg/kg of diet. The experiment was terminated when the mice were about 78 weeks of age, at which time 15, 16, 16 and 16 given the lower dose level and 11 and 13 given the higher dose level were still alive in the respective groups. Tumour incidences were compared with those observed among groups of 79, 87, 90 and 82 control mice, which had either been untreated or had received gelatine only: the incidences were not significantly greater ($P>0.05$) when any group or combination of groups was considered. Similar results were obtained in groups of mice given 2,4-D isopropyl, butyl or isooctyl esters (99%, 99% and 97% pure) at doses of 46.4 mg/kg bw from 7-28 days of age and, subsequently, 111, 149 and 130 mg/kg of diet, respectively, up to 78 weeks of age (Innes *et al.*, 1969; NTIS, 1968a).

Rat: Groups of 25 male and 25 female 3-week old Osborne-Mendel rats were fed for two years on diets containing 0, 5, 25, 125, 625 or 1250 mg/kg of diet 2,4-D. The 2,4-D was 96.7% pure and contained no detectable levels of 2,7-dichloro- or 2,3,7,8-tetrachlorodibenzo-*para*-dioxin; the limit of sensitivity of the method of analysis was 1 mg/kg . The numbers of male and female rats with malignant tumours were 6 in controls and 8, 7, 7, 8 and 14 in the treated groups, respectively. Tumours were randomly distributed and were also found in ageing rats of this strain. According to the authors, a statistical increase ($P<0.05$) in the number of treated rats with malignant tumours over controls was found only in males receiving the highest dose level (Hansen et al., 1971).

Groups of 120 male and 45 female random-bred rats, weighing 80-100 g at the start of the test, were given 2,4-D as the amine salt (amount not specified) mixed in the food at a concentration which corresponded to a daily intake of one-tenth of the LD_{50} (not specified, but see Table 1, section 3.2). Two treated rats developed tumours (a mammary fibroadenoma and a haemangioma of the mesenterium) after 23 months, and one untreated rat had a mammary fibroadenoma after 27 months (Arkhipov & Koslova, 1974).

(b) Subcutaneous and/or intramuscular administration

Mouse: Groups of 18 male and 18 female (C57BL/6xC3H/Anf)F_1 mice and 18 male and 18 female (C57BL/6xAKR)F_1 mice were given single s.c. injections of 215 mg/kg bw 2,4-D (90% pure, m.p. 136-140°C) in dimethyl sulphoxide on the 28th day of life and observed up to 78 weeks of age, at which time 16, 17, 18 and 18 mice in the four groups, respectively, were still alive. Tumour incidences were compared with those in groups of 141, 154, 161 and 157 controls that were either untreated or were injected with dimethyl sulphoxide, 0.5% aqueous gelatin or corn oil. The tumour incidence in any group or combination of groups was not significantly different from that in controls ($P>0.05$). No increase in the incidence of tumours was observed in similar groups of mice treated with single s.c. injections of 21.5 mg/kg bw butyl or 100 mg/kg bw isopropyl esters of 2,4-D (both 99% pure). Of mice treated with 21.5 mg/kg bw isooctyl ester of 2,4-D (97% pure), 5/17 females of the second strain developed reticulum-cell sarcomas ($P=0.01$) (NTIS, 1968a).

3.2 Other relevant biological data

(a) Experimental systems

The toxicity of 2,4-D was reviewed by Dalgaard-Mikkelsen & Poulsen (1962).

Acute and short-term toxicity

There are species differences in the acute oral toxicity of 2,4-D and of its derivatives (Table 1). The symptoms of acute toxicity in mice, rabbits, guinea-pigs and rats are essentially similar (Bucher, 1946; Hill & Carlisle, 1947). Some animals died suddenly, apparently from ventricular fibrillation; those that did not die immediately developed stiffness of the extremities, incoordination, lethargy, stupor and coma prior to death (Hill & Carlisle, 1947). Symptoms of myotonia were evident in mice after the parenteral administration of 150-200 mg/kg bw; and in mice acutely intoxicated with 2,4-D, dilatation of the blood vessels of lungs, liver and kidneys was observed (Bucher, 1946). Rats and guinea-pigs administered lethal doses of 2,4-D exhibited congestion of the viscera and enlarged, swollen kidneys; microscopically, there was massive cloudy swelling of the proximal convoluted tubules with cast formation (Hill & Carlisle, 1947). S.c. injections of 100 mg/kg bw 2,4-D resulted in a decrease of both thyroid and body weights in male rats (Florsheim & Velcoff, 1962).

Oral administration of 625 mg/kg bw to rats resulted in changes in the levels of several serum enzymes and globulins (Szöcs et al., 1970). 2,4-D was found to be a potent uncoupling agent for oxidative phosphorylation and to stimulate the respiration of rat liver mitochondria in a phosphate-deficient medium (Brody, 1952).

In dogs, toxic symptoms were often not present until 6 hours after oral administration of a lethal dose of 2,4-D; the animals became ataxic, with progressive increase in spasm. Death appeared to be due in most cases to hepatic congestion or to pneumonia. Pathological changes, limited to the gastrointestinal tract, lung and liver, followed the development of anorexia, weight loss and myotonia (Drill & Hiratzka, 1953). Dogs exhibited evidence of liver damage more frequently than other animals studied (Bucher, 1946; Drill & Hiratzka, 1953).

No toxic symptoms were noted in monkeys given 214 mg/kg bw orally, or 428 mg/kg bw intraperitoneally; however, oral plus i.p. injection of a total of 500 mg/kg bw 2,4-D caused nausea, vomiting, lethargy, muscular incoordination and head drop (Hill & Carlisle, 1947). Acute toxic doses

TABLE 1

Acute oral toxicity of 2,4-D and esters

Compound of 2,4-D	Species	Sex	LD_{50} (mg/kg bw)	Reference
Acid	Mice	M	375	Hill & Carlisle (1947)
	Mice	M	368	Rowe & Hymas (1954)
	Rats	M	375	" " "
	Rats		666	Hill & Carlisle (1947)
	Guinea-pigs	M&F	469	Rowe & Hymas (1954)
	Guinea-pigs		1000	Hill & Carlisle (1947)
	Rabbits		800	" " "
	Dogs		100	Drill & Hiratzka (1953)
	Chicks	M&F	541	Rowe & Hymas (1954)
Butyl ester	Mice		380	Konstantinova (1970)
	Rats		1500	Schillinger (1960)
	Rats		920	Konstantinova (1970)
	Cats		820	" "
Esters of mono-, di- and tripropylene glycol butyl ethers	Rats	F	570	Rowe & Hymas (1954)
Isopropyl ester	Mice	M	541	Rowe & Hymas (1954)
	Rats	M&F	700	" " "
	Guinea-pigs	M	550	" " "
	Chicks	M&F	1420	" " "
Mixed butyl esters	Mice	F	713	Rowe & Hymas (1954)
	Rats	F	620	" " "
	Guinea-pigs	F	848	" " "
	Rabbits	M&F	1420	" " "
	Chicks	M&F	2000	" " "
Sodium salt	Mice		375	Rowe & Hymas (1954)
	Rats	F	805	" " "
	Rats		2000	Schillinger (1960)
	Guinea-pigs	M	551	Rowe & Hymas (1954)
	Rabbits		800	" " "
Alkanolamine salt	Chicks		380-765	Rowe & Hymas (1954)

of 2,4-D (765 mg/kg bw) produce fatty degeneration of the liver, spleen, kidneys and heart and haemorrhagic gastroenteritis in chickens (Bjorn & Northen, 1948), and acute toxic doses have similar effects in sheep and cattle (Palmer & Radeleff, 1964).

Subacute and chronic toxicity

2,4-D administered subcutaneously to mice at doses of 50-90 mg/kg bw once or twice daily for 3 weeks to 3 months produced no clear-cut chronic symptoms. Levels of 70 mg/kg bw and more retarded growth, probably by reducing food intake (Bucher, 1946).

Rats fed 1000 mg/kg of diet 2,4-D for one month showed no signs of toxic effects (Hill & Carlisle, 1947). No adverse effects were noted in young female rats fed 100 and 300 mg/kg of diet 2,4-D (purity unspecified) for periods of up to 113 days, while those given 1000 mg/kg of diet over the same period had increased mortality, depressed growth rate, slightly increased liver weight and slight cloudy swelling of the liver. Animals fed 3000 or 10,000 mg/kg of diet were sacrificed after 12 days because of food refusal and rapid weight loss. Increased liver and kidney weights and unstated slight pathological changes were noted in these organs (Rowe & Hymas, 1954).

No significant adverse effects were noted when 15 ml of each of 3 commercially available formulations of 2,4-D (the dimethylamine salt and the isooctyl and butyl esters) were administered 5 times weekly for 3 weeks to the intact and abraded skin of rabbits at two concentrations, 0.626% and 3.13% (the dimethylamine salt was diluted in water and the ester in either oil or water) (Kay *et al.*, 1965).

Groups of 3 male and 3 female beagle dogs were fed 10, 50, 100 or 500 mg/kg of diet 2,4-D (96.7% pure, with no detectable chlorodibenzo-*para*-dioxin content) for 2 years, starting at 6-8 months of age. Twenty-eight dogs that survived the 2-year period were clinically normal. No adverse effects related to 2,4-D administration were observed (Hansen *et al.*, 1971).

Dogs of both sexes were given 2, 5 or 10 mg/kg bw commercial 2,4-D (98.5% pure) orally by capsule for 5 days per week for 13 weeks; no signs of toxicity were observed. Dogs given 20 mg/kg bw survived for periods ranging from 18-49 days, with loss of weight occurring after 7-12 days and with ataxia, increased muscle tonus and a terminal fall in lymphocyte count prior to death (Drill & Hiratzka, 1953).

Young pigs treated at varying intervals up to 103 days with 50, 100 or 300 mg/kg bw of the commercial triethanolamine salt or butyl ester of 2,4-D exhibited symptoms of intoxication and pathology analagous to those seen in laboratory animals. Clinical signs of anorexia and retarded growth were found in one animal given 51 doses of 50 mg/kg bw triethanolamine salt over 103 days. Pigs fed 500 mg/kg of diet triethanolamine salt of 2,4-D for up to 12 months developed locomotor disturbances of increasing severity after about one month. Animals sacrificed after 2-12 months had normal organ weights and no gross pathological changes. Clinico-chemical observations included lowered haemoglobin and haematocrit values, elevation of glutamic-oxaloacetic transaminase and reduced albumin and albumin: globulin ratios in the treated animals (Björklund & Erne, 1966).

Absorption, distribution and excretion

In rats, pigs, calves and chickens, 2,4-D administered in doses of 50-100 mg/kg bw orally as salts was readily absorbed and eliminated, mainly in the urine, with plasma half-lives varying from 3-12 hours (Erne, 1966a,b). The rate of 2,4-D elimination in rats was dosage dependent. Following administration of ^{14}C-2,4-D, radioactivity was found in all organs and tissues examined (Khanna & Fang, 1966).

2,4-D esters are hydrolysed in animals. The phenoxy acids are excreted predominantly as such in the urine of rats after their oral administration, although a minor portion is conjugated with the amino acids glycine and taurine and with glucuronic acid (Grunow & Böhme, 1974). No 2,4-dichlorophenol was, however, detected in the urine of C57BL/6 mice treated subcutaneously with 2,4-D or its butyl or isooctyl esters. The rates of disappearance from the plasma of 2,4-D and its butyl and isooctyl esters following single s.c. injections of 100 mg/kg bw of the compounds to female C57BL/6 mice were: butyl ester>isooctyl ester>2,4-D (Zielinski & Fishbein, 1967).

After oral administration of 0.05 mg/kg bw 2,4-D to rats, traces were detected in the milk of lactating animals for 6 days. Within 24 hours after administration of 2,4-D to pregnant rats, 16.8% of the dose was detected in the uterus, placenta, foetus and amniotic fluid (Fedorova & Belova, 1974). 2,4-D was also found to pass the placental barrier in pigs (Björklund & Erne, 1966).

Embryotoxicity and teratogenicity

Results of teratological studies with 2,4-D were variable; teratogenic effects are observed with doses close to those which cause maternal toxicity.

Administration of 2,4-D or its isopropyl, butyl or isooctyl esters orally or subcutaneously during days 6-14 of pregnancy increased the incidence of foetal anomalies among BL6, AKR and/or C3H strains of mice but not among B6AK and A/Ha strains. The purity of the compounds was: 2,4-D, 90%, m.p. 136-140°C; isopropyl and butyl esters, 99%; isooctyl ester, 97% (NTIS, 1968a,b).

Sprague-Dawley rats were given 1000 mg/l 2,4-D in the drinking-water during pregnancy and for a further 10 months, and 2,4-D was administered to the second generation for up to 2 years. Pregnancy and parturition were normal; litter size was not significantly reduced, and no malformations were noted in the young. Except for retarded growth and increased mortality in the second generation, no unequivocal clinical or morphological changes were seen. When 2,4-D was administered at a concentration of 500 mg/kg of diet during the entire pregnancy of a sow, anorexia was noted; the newborn piglets were underdeveloped and apathetic, and 10/15 died within 24 hours. Continued feeding of 500 mg/kg of diet to the survivors until they were 8 months of age caused marked growth depression, persistent anaemia and moderate degenerative changes of liver and kidneys (Björklund & Erne, 1966).

Female rats (10 per group) were fed 2,4-D (purity unspecified) at levels of 0, 1000 and 2000 mg/kg of diet for 95 days and then mated with untreated males and continued on their respective diets through gestation and lactation. Pups born to females fed the highest level were small at birth; 94% died before weaning; some deaths also occurred in pups of rats fed the lower level (T.B. Gaines & R.D. Kimbrough, cited by Hansen et al., 1971).

The maximum tolerated oral dose of 2,4-D (98.7% purity, no chlorinated dibenzo-*para*-dioxins found with the limit of detection of 0.2 mg/kg) or an equimolar dose of 2,4-D propylene glycol butyl ether ester or of the iso-octyl ester of 2,4-D had embryolethal and growth retarding effects but no teratogenicity when given to pregnant Sprague-Dawley (Spartan strain) rats on days 6-15 of gestation. Other signs of foetotoxicity were s.c. oedema, delayed ossification and wavy ribs. 2,4-D did not affect fertility, gestation, lactation or viability of the newborn; the propylene glycol butyl ether and isooctyl esters decreased viability of the newborn and lactation indices[1] (Schwetz et al., 1971). Similar effects were observed in Wistar rats given single daily oral doses of 100-150 mg/kg bw 2,4-D or the butyl, isooctyl, butoxyethanol dimethylamine derivatives of 2,4-D on days 6-15 of pregnancy (Khera & McKinley, 1972).

No consistent embryotoxic effects were noted when 2,4-D was administered orally to hamsters at doses up to 100 mg/kg on days 6-10 of gestation (Collins & Williams, 1971).

Lutz-Ostertag & Lutz (1970) tried to simulate field conditions for spraying with 2,4-D and to evaluate the effect on pheasant eggs and development of chicks. A high mortality rate and morphological alterations were observed in the embryos and chicks, the toxicity apparently being higher than for mammalian species. Total or partial paralysis was observed in most of the surviving embryos, and 50% of the surviving chicks were sterile.

In a 3-generation reproduction study, Osborne-Mendel rats were fed 100 or 500 mg/kg of diet 2,4-D that was 96.7% pure, with no detectable (<1 mg/kg) 2,7-dichloro- or 2,3,7,8-tetrachlorodibenzo-*para*-dioxin. No adverse effects were observed. Diets containing 1500 mg/kg 2,4-D, while

---

[1] lactation index: (pups weaned/pups alive on day 4) x 100

apparently affecting neither the fertility of either sex nor litter size, sharply reduced the percentage of pups surviving to weaning and the weights of the weanlings (Hansen et al., 1971).

Mutagenicity

2,4-D was not mutagenic in *Escherichia coli* WP2 hcr^+ or hcr^- or in *Salmonella typhimurium* strains TA1535, TA1536, TA1537 or TA1538 (Andersen et al., 1972; Nagy et al., 1975; Shirasu, 1975; Shirasu et al., 1976; Zetterberg et al., 1977).

In the rec assay, which is believed to give an indication of reparable DNA damage, 2,4-D was not more toxic to *Bacillus subtilis* M45 (rec^-) than to H17 (rec^+), suggesting that this compound does not damage DNA (Shirasu, 1975).

In *Saccharomyces cerevisiae* D4, gene conversion was increased by concentrations of 2,4-D above 400 µg/ml. Mitotic recombination in *S. cerevisiae* D5 was also increased by 2,4-D (300 µg/ml) (Siebert & Lemperle, 1974; Zetterberg et al., 1977). *S. cerevisiae* RAD 18 (a histidine-dependent haploid strain) was reverted to histidine independence by 250 µg/ml 2,4-D. Toxic and mutagenic effects in *S. cerevisiae* were dependent on low pH (4.3) (Zetterberg, 1977) [Metabolic activation systems were not included in any of these tests].

In host-mediated assays with *S. typhimurium* strains TA1530 or TA1531, or with *S. cerevisiae* D4, no mutagenic effects were observed when adult male mice were given 6 mg 2,4-D (200 mg/kg) by gavage (Zetterberg et al., 1977). Serum from orally dosed rats was not mutagenic to *S. typhimurium* (Styles, 1973).

The effect of 2,4-D on chromosome aberrations in cultured plant tissues is complex because 2,4-D is required as a plant growth regulator in tissue culture. Singh & Harvey (1975a,b) found an inverse correlation between 2,4-D concentration and chromosome aberrations in *Vicia hajastana* and *Haplopappus gracilis*. However, with a strain of *Nicotiana* that does not require 2,4-D it increased chromosome breakage (Ronchi et al., 1976).

2,4-D induced chromosome aberrations in a number of cultivated plants and weeds. The cytological abnormalities included chromosome bridges, fragments, lagging chromosomes, C-mitoses and chromatin bodies (Mohandas & Grant, 1972).

No increase in the number of recessive lethals was observed when 2-day-old adult male *Drosophila melanogaster* flies were fed 4.5 or 9.0 mM 2,4-D in sucrose (Vogel & Chandler, 1974).

In vitro exposure of embryonic bovine kidney cells and of bovine peripheral blood cells to concentrations of 1-1000 µg/ml 2,4-D for 6-96 hours resulted in stimulation of mitosis. Chromosomal aberrations were not detected in the peripheral blood cells, but nucleolar irregularities and polyploid mitotic stages were observed in the kidney cells (Bongso & Basrur, 1973).

Treatment of cultured human lymphocytes with 2.5×10^{-7}M (0.02 µg/ml) 2,4-D increased the number of chromatid aberrations (single acentric fragments) and, to a lesser extent, of chromosomal aberrations (paired acentric fragments). In mice, toxic concentrations (100-300 mg/kg bw) of 2,4-D administered as a single oral dose significantly increased the frequency of aberrant metaphases (2-4-fold); single fragments were the primary aberration (Pilinskaya, 1974). 2,4-D had no effect on cultured cells nor on bone marrow after its oral administration to rats (Styles, 1973).

There was no detectable increase of micronuclei in the erythrocytes of mouse bone marrow after i.p. administration of 100 mg/kg bw 2,4-D (Jenssen & Renberg, 1976).

2,4-D did not increase dominant lethal mutations in mice when given as a single i.p. injection of 125 mg/kg bw, or when given orally on 5 successive days for a total dose of 75 mg/kg bw (Epstein *et al.*, 1972).

(b) Man

In a case of suicide of a 23-year old farming student, the total amount of 2,4-D in the body was estimated to be no less than 6 g, corresponding to a dose of about 80 mg/kg bw. All organs showed marked acute congestion. Severe, degenerative changes of the ganglion cells were found in the central nervous system (Nielsen *et al.*, 1965).

A man who accidentally ingested about 30 ml of concentrated weedkiller containing 50% of a thiolcarbamate and 36% 2,4-D isooctyl ester in aqueous solution exhibited fibrillary twitching and paralysis of the intercostal muscles. There was evidence of generalized skeletal muscle damage, as indicated by marked elevation of the levels of several muscle enzymes, as well as haemoglobinuria and myoglobinuria. Recovery was complete after several months (Berwick, 1970).

No adverse effects were reported in a man who took 500 mg 2,4-D orally daily for 3 weeks (approximately 8 mg/kg bw/day) (E.J. Krauss, cited in Mitchell *et al.*, 1946).

When 2,4-D was used as a treatment for a patient in the terminal stages of disseminated coccidiodomycosis, no side-effects were observed following 18 i.v. doses over 33 days: in the 7th to the 17th injection the dose of 2,4-D was 800-960 mg (about 15 mg/kg bw), and the 18th dose was 2000 mg (about 37 mg/kg bw). A 19th and final dose of 3600 mg (67 mg/kg bw) produced symptoms of toxicity comprising a semi-stuporous status, fibrillar movements, hyporeflexia and urinary incontinence, which persisted for 24 hours. Seventeen days after the last administration, the patient died (Seabury, 1963).

Three cases of peripheral neuropathy have been reported following spraying of 2,4-D. Initial symptoms were nausea, vomiting, muscular weakness, diarrhoea and swelling or aching of the feet and legs, with malaise and headache, which persisted for 10-20 days. In one case, paresthesia in the extremities and pain in the legs appeared within 4-5 days, followed by twitching of the muscles in the calves and arms; fasciculations became generalized, without neurological or electromyographical changes. In the second case, one week after a second exposure to 2,4-D, numbness and aching of the fingers and toes occurred, followed 6 weeks later by a well-developed neuropathy. In the third case, after a second exposure, severe pains occurred in the legs, with swelling of the metacarpal joints of both hands; 5 months later flaccid paraparesis was seen (Goldstein *et al.*, 1959).

Similar case reports of poisoning in agricultural workers have been reported following spraying of 2,4-D (Monarca & Di Vito, 1961; Paggiaro et al., 1974; Todd, 1962). The main initial symptoms were muscular weakness, vomiting, diarrhoea, fever, hyperthermia and tachycardia. In two cases, neurological symptoms occurred, which continued for 40 days to 2 years after exposure and included loss of deep-tendon reflexes and paralysis of thigh and leg muscles.

Assouly (1951) reported that workers employed in the fabrication of 2,4-D developed symptoms of somnolence, anorexia and gastralgia, increased salivation, a sweet taste in the mouth, a sensation of drunkenness, heaviness of the legs and hyperacusia.

Subjective clinical symptoms reported among workers using various esters and salts of 2,4-D included rapid fatigue, headache, loss of appetite and pains in the region of the liver and stomach. Sensitivity to taste and smell was lowered (Fetisov, 1966).

Bashirov (1969) examined 292 persons (248 men and 44 women) engaged in the manufacture of the amine salt and butyl ester of 2,4-D, with exposure ranging from under 5 years to 6-10 years (for 194 and 98 persons, respectively); 63% of these workers complained frequently of weakness, rapid fatigue, headache or vertigo. About 20% had disturbances of the cardiovascular system (mainly hypotension and bradycardia) and of the digestive organs (dyspeptic symptoms and gastritis). The various liver dysfunctions that were found were more pronounced in workers with longer exposures to the herbicides.

Changes in metabolic processes were observed in workers engaged in the production of 2,4-D, in particular, increases in blood cholesterol content, with no change in the lecithin:cholesterol ratio. Decreases in serum albumins, increases in globulins, decreases in blood sugar levels and altered responses to sugar loads were also noted (Lukoshkina et al., 1970).

In a report on 220 workers exposed in a manufacturing plant to 30-40 mg/day 2,4-D for periods ranging from 0.5 to 22 years, Johnson (1971) stated [without providing any supporting evidence] that no 'meaningful' differences were observed in [unspecified] clinical assessment, in comparison to a control group of 4600 men, and that no chromosomal effects were observed in 10 workers whose chromosomes were karyotyped.

Feldmann & Maibach (1974) studied the absorption through the skin of 4 μg/cm² ^{14}C-labelled 2,4-D dissolved in a small amount of acetone. ^{14}C activity was measured in urine over a 5-day period and compared with that in urine after i.v. administration of the compound: urinary excretion of 2,4-D after i.v. administration was 100% of the dose in 120 hours, while excretion after topical administration was 5.8% of the dose.

Kohli et al. (1974) administered 5 mg/kg bw pure 2,4-D in a gelatin capsule with water to 6 healthy male volunteers, aged 22-30 years. None of the subjects complained of any ill-effects; no changes in blood pressure, pulse rate, haemoglobin content or total or differential white cell counts were observed. 2,4-D was absorbed fairly rapidly; the highest concentration in blood was reached in 7-24 hours. In urine, 2,4-D was present as early as 2 hours after ingestion, and more than 75% was excreted in 96 hours without undergoing transformation in the body.

In 5 male volunteers given a single oral dose of 5 mg/kg bw 2,4-D, the half-life in the plasma was 11.7 hours, and elimination in the urine occurred with a half-life of 17.7 hours. About 82% was excreted as such and 12.8% as a conjugate (Sauerhoff et al., 1976).

For details of adverse toxicological effects resulting from the spraying of 'Agent Orange' (a 50:50 mixture of the n-butyl esters of 2,4-D and 2,4,5-T, contaminated with up to 30 mg/kg or more TCDD) and other herbicides in Vietnam, see monograph on chlorinated dibenzodioxins, p. .

3.3 Case reports and epidemiological studies

Axelson & Sundell (1974) reported that in a cohort study of Swedish railway workers exposed to a variety of herbicides a significant, two-fold excess of all cancers was observed in exposed workers, as compared with the national average. The situation was difficult to evaluate because of the combined exposure of many workers to more than one herbicide. Most of the excess, however, seemed to be due to exposure to 3-amino-1,2,4-triazole (amitrole); within the subgroups that had been exposed to phenoxyacids (2,4-D and/or 2,4,5-T), only a small difference was detected: 5 cancers at all sites observed *versus* 2.8 expected. The authors stated, however, that use of 2,4-D and 2,4,5-T had probably been higher than that they could trace.

See also monograph on chlorinated dibenzodioxins, p. 41.

4. Comments on Data Reported and Evaluation

4.1 Animal data

2,4-D and several of its esters were tested in rats and mice by oral administration and in mice by subcutaneous administration. All of these studies had limitations, due either to inadequate reporting or to the small number of animals used. Therefore, although increased incidences of tumours were observed in one study in which rats received 2,4-D orally and in another in which mice received its isooctyl ester by subcutaneous injection, no evaluation of the carcinogenicity of this compound could be made.

4.2 Human data

The results of the single cohort study of a small number of workers exposed to various herbicides, including 2,4-D, 2,4,5-T and 3-amino-1,2,4-triazole (amitrole)[1], are not sufficient to evaluate the carcinogenicity of 2,4-D to man [Because 2,4-D may be used with 2,4,5-T, which is contaminated with 2,3,7,8-tetrachlorodibenzo-*para*-dioxin, see also monograph on chlorinated dibenzodioxins, p. 41].

---

[1] See also IARC, 1974.

5. References

Andersen, K.J., Leighty, E.G. & Takahashi, M.T. (1972) Evaluation of herbicides for possible mutagenic properties. J. agric. Fd Chem., 20, 649-656

Arkhipov, G.N. & Koslova, I.N. (1974) The study of the carcinogenic properties of the amine salt of 2,4-D. Vop. Pitan., 5, 83-84

Assouly, M. (1951) Désherbants sélectifs et substances de croissance. Aperçu technique. Effet pathologique sur l'homme au cours de la fabrication de l'ester du 2,4-D. Arch. Mal. prof., 12, 26-30

Axelson, O. & Sundell, L. (1974) Herbicide exposure, mortality and tumor incidence. An epidemiological investigation on Swedish railroad workers. Work-environm.-hlth, 11, 21-28

Bashirov, A.A. (1969) Health condition of workers producing herbicides of amine salt and butyl ether of 2,4-D acid. Vrach. Delo, 10, 92-95

Beroza, M., ed. (1976) Changes in official methods of analysis made at the eighty-ninth annual meeting, October 13-16, 1975. J. Ass. off. analyt. Chem., 59, 456-457

Berwick, P. (1970) 2,4-Dichlorophenoxyacetic acid poisoning in man. Some interesting clinical and laboratory findings. J. Amer. med. Ass., 214, 1114-1117

Björklund, N.-E. & Erne, K. (1966) Toxicological studies of phenoxyacetic herbicides in animals. Acta vet. scand., 7, 364-390

Bjorn, M.K. & Northen, H.T. (1948) Effects of 2,4-dichlorophenoxyacetic acid on chicks. Science, 108, 479-480

Bongso, T.A. & Basrur, P.K. (1973) *In vitro* response of bovine cells to 2,4-dichlorophenoxy acetic acid. In Vitro, 8, 416-417

Brody, T.M. (1952) Effect of certain plant growth substances on oxidative phosphorylation in rat liver mitochondria. Proc. Soc. exp. Biol. (N.Y.), 80, 533-536

Bucher, N.L.R. (1946) Effects of 2,4-dichlorophenoxyacetic acid on experimental animals. Proc. Soc. exp. Biol. (N.Y.), 63, 204-205

Chau, A.S.Y. & Terry, K. (1976) Analysis of pesticides by chemical derivatization. III. Gas chromatographic characteristics and conditions for the formation of pentafluorobenzyl derivatives of ten herbicidal acids. J. Ass. off. analyt. Chem., 59, 633-636

Collier, R.H. & Grimes, G.S. (1974) Determination of chlorophenoxy acids in formulations by gas-liquid chromatography of their trimethylsilyl derivatives. J. Ass. off. analyt. Chem., 57, 781-784

Collins, T.F.X. & Williams, C.H. (1971) Teratogenic studies with 2,4,5-T and 2,4-D in the hamster. Bull. environm. Contam. Toxicol., 6, 559-567

Committee on the Effects of Herbicides in Vietnam (1974) The Effects of Herbicides in South Vietnam, Part A, Summary and Conclusions, Washington DC, National Academy of Sciences

Dalgaard-Mikkelsen, S. & Poulsen, E. (1962) Toxicology of herbicides. Pharmacol. Rev., 14, 225-250

Davis, D.E. (1974) The 2,4,5-T story. Weeds Today, spring, pp. 12-13, 18

Drill, V.A. & Hiratzka, T. (1953) Toxicity of 2,4-dichlorophenoxyacetic acid and 2,4,5-trichlorophenoxyacetic acid: a report on their acute and chronic toxicity in dogs. Arch. industr. Hyg. occup. Med., 7, 61-67

Duffy, J.R. & Shelfoon, P. (1967) Determination of 2,4-D and its butoxyethanol ester in oysters by gas chromatography. J. Ass. off. analyt. Chem., 50, 1098-1102

Duggan, R.E., Barry, H.C. & Johnson, L.Y. (1966) Pesticide residues in total-diet samples. Science, 151, 101-104

Epstein, S.S., Arnold, E., Andrea, J., Bass, W. & Bishop, Y. (1972) Detection of chemical mutagens by the dominant lethal assay in the mouse. Toxicol. appl. Pharmacol., 23, 288-325

Erne, K. (1966a) Distribution and elimination of chlorinated phenoxyacetic acids in animals. Acta vet. scand., 7, 240-256

Erne, K. (1966b) Studies on the animal metabolism of phenoxyacetic herbicides. Acta vet. scand., 7, 264-271

Fedorova, L.M. & Belova, R.S. (1974) Incorporation of 2,4-dichlorophenoxyacetic acid into the organs of animals: paths and dynamics of its excretion. Gig. i Sanit., 2, 105-107

Feldmann, R.J. & Maibach, H.I. (1974) Percutaneous penetration of some pesticides and herbicides in man. Toxicol. appl. Pharmacol., 28, 126-132

Fetisov, M.I. (1966) Problems of occupational hygiene in work with herbicides of 2,4-D group. Gig. i Sanit., 31, 28-30

Fine, D.H., Ross, R., Rounbehler, D.P. & Fan, S. (1977) N-Nitroso compound impurities in herbicide formulations. J. agric. Fd Chem. (in press)

Finkelstein, H. (1969) *Preliminary Air Pollution Survey of Pesticides*, Raleigh, North Carolina, US Department of Health, Education and Welfare, pp. 52, 136

Florsheim, W.H. & Velcoff, S.M. (1962) Some effects of 2,4-dichlorophenoxyacetic acid on thyroid function in the rat: effects on iodine accumulation. *Endocrinology*, 71, 1-6

Goldstein, N.P., Jones, P.H. & Brown, J.R. (1959) Peripheral neuropathy after exposure to an ester of dichlorophenoxyacetic acid. *J. Amer. med. Ass.*, 171, 1306-1309

Gore, R.C., Hannah, R.W., Pattacini, S.C. & Porro, T.J. (1971) Infrared and ultraviolet spectra of seventy-six pesticides. *J. Ass. off. analyt. Chem.*, 54, 1040-1082

Grunow, W. & Böhme, C. (1974) Über den Stoffwechsel von 2.4.5-T und 2.4-D bei Ratten und Mäusen. *Arch. Toxicol.*, 32, 217-225

Hammond, H. (1973) Free acid in esters of 2,4-dichlorophenoxyacetic acid and 2,4,5-trichlorophenoxyacetic acid and their formulations. *J. Ass. off. analyt. Chem.*, 56, 596-597

Hansen, W.H., Quaife, M.L., Habermann, R.T. & Fitzhugh, O.G. (1971) Chronic toxicity of 2,4-dichlorophenoxyacetic acid in rats and dogs. *Toxicol. appl. Pharmacol.*, 20, 122-129

Hill, E.V. & Carlisle, H. (1947) Toxicity of 2,4-dichlorophenoxyacetic acid for experimental animals. *J. industr. Hyg. Toxicol.*, 29, 85-95

Horwitz, W., ed. (1975) *Official Methods of Analysis of the Association of Official Analytical Chemists*, 12th ed., Washington DC, Association of Official Analytical Chemists, pp. 110-111

Huston, B.L. (1972) Identification of three neutral contaminants in production grade 2,4-D. *J. agric. Fd Chem.*, 20, 724-727

IARC (1972) *IARC Monographs on the Evaluation of Carcinogenic Risk of Chemicals to Man*, 1, Lyon, pp. 95-106

IARC (1974) *IARC Monographs on the Evaluation of Carcinogenic Risk of Chemicals to Man, 7, Some Anti-thyroid and Related Substances, Nitrofurans and Industrial Chemicals*, pp. 31-43

Innes, J.R.M., Ulland, B.M., Valerio, M.G., Petrucelli, L., Fishbein, L., Hart, E.R., Pallotta, A.J., Bates, R.R., Falk, H.L., Gart, J.J., Klein, M., Mitchell, I. & Peters, J. (1969) Bioassay of pesticides and industrial chemicals for tumorigenicity in mice: a preliminary note. *J. nat. Cancer Inst.*, 42, 1101-1114

Jenssen, D. & Renberg, L. (1976) Distribution and cytogenetic test of 2,4-D and 2,4,5-T phenoxyacetic acids in mouse blood tissues. Chem.-biol. Interact., 14, 291-299

Johnson, J.E. (1971) The public health implications of widespread use of the phenoxy herbicides and picloram. Bioscience, 21, 899-905

Johnson, L.D., Waltz, R.H., Ussary, J.P. & Kaiser, F.E. (1976) Automated gel permeation chromatographic cleanup of animal and plant extracts for pesticide residue determination. J. Ass. off. analyt. Chem., 59, 174-187

Kay, J.H., Palazzolo, R.J. & Calandra, J.C. (1965) Subacute dermal toxicity of 2,4-D. Arch. environm. Hlth, 11, 648-651

Khan, S.U. (1975) Electron capture gas-liquid chromatographic method for the simultaneous analysis of 2,4-D, dicamba, and mecoprop residues in soil, wheat, and barley. J. Ass. off. analyt. Chem., 58, 1027-1031

Khanna, S. & Fang, S.C. (1966) Metabolism of C^{14}-labeled 2,4-dichlorophenoxyacetic acid in rats. J. agric. Fd Chem., 14, 500-503

Khera, K.S. & McKinley, W.P. (1972) Pre- and postnatal studies on 2,4,5-trichlorophenoxyacetic acid, 2,4-dichlorophenoxyacetic acid and their derivatives in rats. Toxicol. appl. Pharmacol., 22, 14-28

Kohli, J.D., Khanna, R.N., Gupta, B.N., Dhar, M.M., Tandon, J.S. & Sircar, K.P. (1974) Absorption and excretion of 2,4-dichlorophenoxyacetic acid in man. Xenobiotica, 4, 97-100

Konstantinova, T.K. (1970) Toxicology and some problems of the embryotropic action of the butyl ester of 2,4-D. In: Vygodchikov, G.V., ed., Proceedings of a Conference on Problems on Hygiene and Toxicology of Pesticides, USSR, 1967, Moscow, Meditsina, pp. 177-179

Lukoshkina, L.P., Guseinova, R.S. & Melik-Zade, T.M. (1970) Lipid-protein-carbohydrate metabolism in workers during 2,4-dichlorophenoxyacetic acid production. Proc. Res. Inst. Occup. Hlth, Azerbaijan, 5, 146-149

Lutz-Ostertag, Y. & Lutz, H. (1970) Action néfaste de l'herbicide 2,4-D sur le développement embryonnaire et la fécondité du gibier à plumes. C.R. Acad. Sci. (Paris), Ser. D, 271, 2418-2421

Malina, M. (1971) Collaborative study of infrared analysis of dicamba-2-methyl-4-chlorophenoxyacetic acid and dicamba-2,4-dichlorophenoxyacetic acid formulations. J. Ass. off. analyt. Chem., 54, 706-710

McLeod, H.A. & Wales, P.J. (1972) A low temperature cleanup procedure for pesticides and their metabolites in biological samples. J. agric. Fd Chem., 20, 624-627

Mitchell, J.W., Hodgson, R.E. & Gaetjens, C.F. (1946) Tolerance of farm animals to feed containing 2,4-dichlorophenoxyacetic acid. J. Animal Sci., 5, 226-232

Mohandas, T. & Grant, W.F. (1972) Cytogenetic effects of 2,4-D and amitrole in relation to nuclear volume and DNA content in some higher plants. Canad. J. Genet. Cytol., 14, 773-783

Monarca, G. & Di Vito, G. (1961) Sull'intossicazione acuta da diserbante (acido 2-4 dichlorofenossiacetico): contributo clinico. Folia med., 44, 480-485

Nagy, Z., Mile, I. & Antoni, F. (1975) The mutagenic effect of pesticides on *Escherichia coli* WP2 try. Acta microbiol. acad. sci. hung., 22, 309-314

Nielsen, K., Kaempe, B. & Jensen-Holm, J. (1965) Fatal poisoning in man by 2,4-dichlorophenoxyacetic acid (2,4-D): determination of the agent in forensic materials. Acta pharmacol. toxicol., 22, 224-234

NTIS (National Technical Information Service) (1968a) Evaluation of Carcinogenic, Teratogenic and Mutagenic Activities of Selected Pesticides and Industrial Chemicals, Vol. 1, Carcinogenic Study, Washington DC, US Department of Commerce

NTIS (National Technical Information Service)(1968b) Evaluation of Carcinogenic, Teratogenic and Mutagenic Activities of Selected Pesticides and Industrial Chemicals, Vol. 2, Teratogenic Study in Mice and Rats, Washington DC, US Department of Commerce

Paggiaro, P.L., Martino, E. & Mariotti, S. (1974) Su un caso di intossicazione da acido 2,4-diclorofenossiacetico. Med. Lavoro, 65, 128-135

Palmer, J.S. & Radeleff, R.D. (1964) The toxicologic effects of certain fungicides and herbicides on sheep and cattle. Ann. N.Y. Acad. Sci., 111, 729-736

Pilinskaya, M.A. (1974) Cytogenetic effect of the herbicide 2,4-D on human and animal chromosomes. Tsitol. Genet., 8, 202-206

Pokorny, R. (1941) Some chlorophenoxyacetic acids. J. Amer. chem. Soc., 63, 1768

Ronchi, V.N., Martini, G. & Buiatti, M. (1976) Genotype-hormone interaction in the induction of chromosome aberrations: effect of 2,4-dichlorophenoxyacetic acid (2,4-D) and kinetin on tissue cultures from *Nicotiana* spp. Mutation Res., 36, 67-72

Rowe, V.K. & Hymas, T.A. (1954) Summary of toxicological information on 2,4-D and 2,4,5-T type herbicides and an evaluation of the hazards to livestock associated with their use. Amer. J. vet. Res., 15, 622-629

Sauerhoff, M.W., Braun, W.H., Blau, G.E. & LeBeau, J.E. (1976) The fate of 2,4-dichlorophenoxyacetic acid (2,4-D) following oral administration to man. Toxicol. appl. Pharmacol., 37, 136-137

Schillinger, J.I. (1960) Hygienische Wertung von landwirtschaftlichen Erzeugnissen, angebaut unter Anwendung von Herbiziden. J. Hyg. Epidemiol. (Praha), 4, 243-252

Schultz, D.P. & Harman, P.D. (1974) Residues of 2,4-D in pond waters, mud, and fish, 1971. Pest. Monit. J., 8, 173-179

Schwetz, B.A., Sparschu, G.L. & Gehring, P.J. (1971) The effect of 2,4-dichlorophenoxyacetic acid (2,4-D) and esters of 2,4-D on rat embryonal, foetal and neonatal growth and development. Fd Cosmet. Toxicol., 9, 801-817

Seabury, J.H. (1963) Toxicity of 2,4-dichlorophenoxyacetic acid for man and dog. Arch. environm. Hlth, 7, 202-209

Shirasu, Y. (1975) Significance of mutagenicity testing on pesticides. Environm. Qual. Saf., 4, 226-231

Shirasu, Y., Moriya, M., Kato, K., Furuhashi, A. & Kada, T. (1976) Mutagenicity screening of pesticides in the microbial system. Mutation Res., 40, 19-30

Siebert, D. & Lemperle, E. (1974) Genetic effects of herbicides: induction of mitotic gene conversion in *Saccharomyces cerevisiae*. Mutation Res., 22, 111-120

Singh, B.D. & Harvey, B.L. (1975a) Does 2,4-D induce mitotic irregularities in plant tissue cultures? Experientia, 31, 785-787

Singh, B.D. & Harvey, B.L. (1975b) Effects of different 2,4-D concentrations on the cytogenetic behaviour of plant cells cultured *in vitro*. Biol. plant. (Praha), 17, 167-174

Skelly, N.E., Russell, R.J. & Porter, D.F. (1976) Collaborative study of the high-pressure liquid chromatographic analysis of picloram-2,4-D formulations. J. Ass. off. analyt. Chem., 59, 748-752

Styles, J.A. (1973) Cytotoxic effects of various pesticides *in vivo* and *in vitro*. Mutation Res., 21, 50-51

Szöcs, J., Molnar, V., Balogh, E., Ajtay, M. & Fülöp, I. (1970) Experimental data on the toxicity of the herbicide 2,4-D (dichloroden). Rev. Med. (Tirgu-Mures), 16, 94-97

Todd, R.L. (1962) A case of 2-4D intoxication. J. Iowa med. Soc., 52, 663-664

US Bureau of Foods (1975) Compliance Program Evaluation. Total Diet Studies: FY 1973 (7320.08) Washington DC, US Government Printing Office, p. 19

US Department of Agriculture (1973) The Pesticide Review, 1972, Agricultural Stabilization and Conservation Service, Washington DC, US Government Printing Office, p. 44

US Department of Commerce (1975) US Exports, Schedule B, Commodity by Country, Domestic Merchandise, FT 410/December 1975, Washington DC, US Government Printing Office, p. 2-74

US Food and Drug Administration (1975a) Pesticide Analytical Manual, Vol. I, Methods Which Detect Multiple Residues, Rockville, Md, US Department of Health, Education and Welfare, sections 221.12a, 221.12b, 221.14, 221.15, 221.18, 222.12a, 222.12b, 222.18

US Food and Drug Administration (1975b) Pesticide Analytical Manual, Vol. II, Methods for Individual Pesticide Residues, Rockville, Md, US Department of Health, Education and Welfare, section 120.142

US International Trade Commission (1976a) Synthetic Organic Chemicals, US Production and Sales, 1974, ITC Publication 776, Washington DC, US Government Printing Office, p. 189

US International Trade Commission (1976b) Imports of Benzenoid Chemicals and Products, 1974, ITC Publication 762, Washington DC, US Government Printing Office, p. 96

US Tariff Commission (1946) Synthetic Organic Chemicals, US Production and Sales, 1944, Report No. 155, Second Series, Washington DC, US Government Printing Office, p. 116

US Tariff Commission (1974) Imports of Benzenoid Chemicals and Products, 1973, TC Publication 688, Washington DC, US Government Printing Office, p. 92

Vogel, E. & Chandler, J.L.R. (1974) Mutagenicity testing of cyclamate and some pesticides in *Drosophila melanogaster*. Experientia, 30, 621-623

Weed Science Society of America (1974) Herbicide Handbook, 3rd ed., Champaign, Illinois, pp. 116-122

WHO (1975) 1974 Evaluations of some pesticide residues in food. Wld Hlth Org. Pest. Res. Ser., No. 4, pp. 159-183

WHO (1977) 1975 Evaluations of some pesticide residues in food. Wld Hlth Org. Pest. Res. Ser., No. 5 (in press)

Winell, M.A. (1975) An international comparison of hygienic standards for chemicals in the work environment. Ambio, 4, 34-36

Woolson, E.A., Thomas, R.F. & Ensol, P.D. (1972) Survey of polychlorodibenzo-*p*-dioxin content in selected pesticides. J. agric. Fd Chem., 20, 351-354

Zetterberg, G. (1977) Experimental results of phenoxy acids on microorganisms. In: Ramel, C., ed., Chlorinated Phenoxy Acids and their Dioxins: Mode of Action, Health Risks and Environmental Effects. Ecol. Bull. (Stockholm), 27 (in press)

Zetterberg, G., Busk, L., Elovson, R., Starec-Nordenhammar, I. & Ryttman, H. (1977) The influence of pH on the effects of 2,4-D (2,4-dichlorophenoxyacetic acid, Na salt) on *Saccharomyces cerevisiae* and *Salmonella typhimurium*. Mutation Res., 42, 3-18

Zielinski, W.L., Jr. & Fishbein, L. (1967) Gas chromatographic measurement of disappearance rates of 2,4-D and 2,4,5-T acids and 2,4-D esters in mice. J. agric. Fd Chem., 15, 841-844

Zweig, G., ed. (1972) Analytical Methods for Pesticides and Plant Growth Regulators, Vol. VI, Gas Chromatographic Analysis, New York, Academic Press, pp. 630-635

1,2-DIBROMO-3-CHLOROPROPANE

1. Chemical and Physical Data

1.1 Synonyms and trade names

Chem. Abstr. Services Reg. No.: 96-12-8

Chem. Abstr. Name: 1,2-Dibromo-3-chloropropane

3-Chloro-1,2-dibromopropane; dibromochloropropane

DBCP; Fumazone; Nemafume; Nemagon; Nemagon 20; Nemagon 20G; Nemagon 90; Nemagon Soil Fumigant; Nemapaz; Nemazon

1.2 Chemical formula and molecular weight

$$\begin{array}{c} \text{H} \quad \text{H} \quad \text{H} \\ | \quad | \quad | \\ \text{H}-\text{C}-\text{C}-\text{C}-\text{Cl} \\ | \quad | \quad | \\ \text{Br} \quad \text{Br} \quad \text{H} \end{array}$$

$C_3H_5Br_2Cl$ Mol. wt: 236.4

1.3 Chemical and physical properties of the pure substance

From Spencer (1973), unless otherwise specified

(a) Description: Dark-amber to dark-brown liquid with pungent odour

(b) Boiling-point: 196°C

(c) Density: d_{20}^{20} 2.08 (Martin, 1971)

(d) Refractive index: n_D^{25} 1.5518

(e) Solubility: Slightly soluble in water (0.1% w/w); miscible with liquid hydrocarbons, ethanol, methanol, isopropyl alcohol and halogenated hydrocarbons

(f) Volatility: Vapour pressure is 0.8 mm at 21°C.

(g) Stability: Stable in neutral and acidic media; hydrolysed by alkali to 2-bromoallyl alcohol

(h) Reactivity: Corrodes aluminium, magnesium and tin and alloys containing these metals

1.4 Technical products and impurities

1,2-Dibromo-3-chloropropane is available in the US as a technical grade containing not less than 95% of the pure chemical (Johnson & Lear, 1969), as emulsifiable concentrates containing 70.7-87.8%, as solutions containing 47.2%, as granules containing 5.25-34% and in fertilizer mixes containing 0.6-5% (US Environmental Protection Agency, 1974).

A technical grade available in the USSR contains 97-98% of the pure chemical and 1-3% of other halogenated hydrocarbons (Vengerskaya & Rakhmatullaev, 1970).

2. Production, Use, Occurrence and Analysis

For background information on this section, see preamble, p. 17.

2.1 Production and use

(a) Production

1,2-Dibromo-3-chloropropane was first prepared by Oppenheim in 1833 by the addition of bromine to allyl chloride (Prager & Jacobson, 1918), and this is the method used currently for its production.

1,2-Dibromo-3-chloropropane was first produced commercially in the US in 1955 (US Tariff Commission, 1956). In 1969, US production was 3.9 million kg (US Tariff Commission, 1971), and in 1975, three US companies were producing the chemical (see preamble, p. 17) (US International Trade Commission, 1976).

It is produced in the Benelux, France, Italy, Spain, Switzerland and the UK, and production in these countries has been estimated to be 3-30 million kg annually.

1,2-Dibromo-3-chloropropane was first produced commercially in Japan in 1960 (Sakurai, 1973). In 1974, the single Japanese producer manufactured 496 thousand kg; in 1975, production dropped to 159 thousand kg (Muto, 1976).

(b) Use

1,2-Dibromo-3-chloropropane is used as a soil fumigant and nematicide; its nematicidal activity was first reported in 1955 (McBeth & Bergeson, 1955). In the US, it is registered for use on a variety of fruit, vegetable, nut and ornamental crops as well as for garden use (US Environmental Protection Agency, 1974). In 1971, US farmers used 1.6 million kg on crops (US Department of Agriculture, 1974), and in 1975, 285 thousand kg were used in California alone (California Department of Food and Agriculture, 1976).

A decision on a rebuttable presumption against renewal of registration (see 'General Remarks on Substances Considered', p. 28) is scheduled for October 1977.

2.2 Occurrence

1,2-Dibromo-3-chloropropane is not known to occur in nature.

It has been applied to various soil types in California by injection, flooding and sprinkling. Its distribution in soil was proportional to the size of soil particles; the greatest concentration was found in sandy soils and the lowest in clay (Hodges, 1972).

US tolerances for residues of inorganic bromides in or on raw agricultural commodities grown in soil treated with 1,2-dibromo-3-chloropropane are as follows: endives and lettuce, 130 mg/kg; bananas and soya beans, 125 mg/kg; almond hulls, carrots, celery, figs, broad beans, okra, parsnips, radishes, French beans and turnips, 75 mg/kg (US Environmental Protection Agency, 1976).

1,2-Dibromo-3-chloropropane occurs at a level of 0.05% in the flame retardant, tris(2,3-dibromopropyl)phosphate (Blum & Ames, 1977).

2.3 Analysis

Gas chromatography with electron capture detection has been used to measure 1,2-dibromo-3-chloropropane extracted with acetone from soils containing as little as 1 mg/kg, with 84% recovery (Gutenmann & Lisk, 1968).

A method of recovering 1,2-dibromo-3-chloropropane from soils by extraction with hexane and subsequent gas chromatographic determination with electron capture detection gave excellent recovery. The method is applicable for determining 1-100 mg/kg in soil and water (Johnson & Lear, 1969).

Polarography has been used to determine 1,2-dibromo-3-chloropropane in water, with a ±10-15% error (Novik & Kozlova, 1971). Concentrations as low as 0.1-0.15 mg/kg of soil (Novik & Kozlova, 1973) and 0.07-0.10 mg/l of air (Novik & Plyngyu, 1973) have been determined polarographically.

With a simple instrumental method, 1,2-dibromo-3-chloropropane has been determined nephelometrically in water as a silver chloride suspension after extraction into ether, followed by evaporation and alkaline hydrolysis. The limit of detection is 5 μg in the final solution (Vengerskaya & Rakhmatullaev, 1970).

3. Biological Data Relevant to the Evaluation of Carcinogenic Risk to Man

3.1 Carcinogenicity and related studies in animals[1]

Oral administration

Mouse: According to a report of an experiment in progress, two groups of 50 male and 50 female (C57BlxC3H)F_1 mice had received 1,2-dibromo-3-chloropropane (purity at least 96%) in corn oil by gavage 5 times per week for 42 weeks. The initial dose levels were 80 and 160 mg/kg bw/day for males and 60 and 120 mg/kg bw/day for females. After 14 weeks, the doses were increased to 100 and 200 mg/kg bw for both sexes; after an additional 14 weeks they were increased to 130 mg/kg bw (described by the authors as half the maximal tolerated dose, ½ MTD) and 260 mg/kg bw (MTD). At the time of reporting (42 weeks), 14 male and 9 female mice treated with

---

[1]The Working Group was aware of a carcinogenicity study in progress involving i.p. injection in mice and of a planned inhalation study in mice and rats (IARC, 1976).

the higher dose and 3 male and 3 female mice treated with the lower dose had developed squamous-cell carcinomas of the forestomach. No tumours had developed in 20 male and 20 female controls (Olson et al., 1973). A later report stated that the incidence of squamous-cell carcinomas of the forestomach after 78 weeks was over 90% in the treated animals; the tumours were invasive and had metastasized (Powers et al., 1975).

Rat: According to a report of an experiment in progress, groups of 50 male and 50 female Osborne-Mendel rats had received 1,2-dibromo-3-chloropropane in corn oil by gavage 5 times per week for 54 weeks. The initial dose levels were 12 and 24 mg/kg bw; these were increased after 14 weeks to 15 and 30 mg/kg bw (½ MTD and MTD). After 54 weeks, of those receiving the higher dose 17 males and 33 females had developed squamous-cell carcinomas of the forestomach, and 12 females had developed mammary carcinomas; of those receiving the lower dose 4 males and 14 females had developed squamous-cell carcinomas of the forestomach, and 5 females had mammary carcinomas. One lipoma (site not specified) was observed in 20 male and 20 female controls receiving corn oil only (Olson et al., 1973). In a later report, it was stated that after 78 weeks more than 60% of treated rats had developed squamous-cell carcinomas of the forestomach, and 54% of the treated females had developed mammary carcinomas. The first tumour was noted after 10 weeks; the tumours were invasive and metastasized (Powers et al., 1975).

3.2 Other relevant biological data

(a) Experimental systems

The percutaneous LD_{50} of 1,2-dibromo-3-chloropropane in rabbits is 1.4 g/kg bw; it induces minimal skin irritation and moderate irritation of the eyes in this species (Kodama & Dunlap, 1956).

The LC_{50}'s in rats administered the compound by inhalation for 1, 2, 4 and 8 hours are 368 (3.5), 232 (2.4), 154 (1.6) and 103 ppm (0.9 mg/l) in air, respectively (Kodama & Dunlap, 1956). In rats exposed 50 times by inhalation over 10 weeks to 5 (0.05), 10 (0.1), 20 (0.2) or 50 ppm (0.5 mg/l) in air, no apparent visceral damage was observed, but growth was retarded with all but the 10 ppm (0.1 mg/l) level (Kodama & Dunlap, 1956).

Daily oral intake of 70 mg/kg bw (20% of the acute oral LD_{50}) was lethal to rats after 3 weeks (Faidysh et al., 1970). In a 90-day feeding study, rats were fed 5, 20, 150, 450 or 1350 mg/kg 1,2-dibromo-3-chloropropane in the diet. The lowest levels that retarded growth were 150 mg/kg of diet for females and 450 mg/kg of diet for males. In those receiving 1350 mg/kg, mortality exceeded 50% (Kodama & Dunlap, 1956).

No data on embryotoxicity or teratogenicity were available to the Working Group.

In the polymerase assay, which is believed to give an indication of reparable DNA damage, 1,2-dibromo-3-chloropropane was more toxic to *Escherichia coli* p3478 ($pol\ A_1^-$) than to W3110 ($pol\ A^+$), suggesting that this compound can damage DNA. 1,2-Dibromo-3-chloropropane increased base-pair substitution mutations in *Salmonella typhimurium* TA1530, but did not increase frameshift mutations in TA1538 (Rosenkranz, 1975). Prival et al. (1977) found that this compound increased the reversion of *S. typhimurium* TA1535 (but not TA1538) when 0.01 µl was incorporated into the agar. A hepatic microsomal fraction from Aroclor 1254-pretreated rats increased the number of revertants.

(b) Man

No data were available to the Working Group.

3.3 Case reports and epidemiological studies

No data were available to the Working Group.

4. Comments on Data Reported and Evaluation[1]

4.1 Animal data

1,2-Dibromo-3-chloropropane is carcinogenic in mice and rats after its oral administration, the only route tested; it produced squamous-cell carcinomas of the forestomach in both species and mammary carcinomas in rats.

---

[1]See also the section, 'Animal Data in Relation to the Evaluation of Risk to Man' in the introduction to this volume, p. 15.

4.2 Human data

No case reports or epidemiological studies were available to the Working Group.

5. References

Blum, A. & Ames, B.N. (1977) Flame-retardant additives as possible cancer hazards. *Science*, 195, 17-23

California Department of Food and Agriculture (1976) *Pesticide Use Report 1975*, Sacramento, pp. 51-53

Faidysh, E.V., Rakhmatullaev, N.N. & Varshaveskii, V.A. (1970) Cytotoxic action of Nemagon in a subacute experiment. *Med. Zh. Uzb.*, 1, 64-65

Gutenmann, W.H. & Lisk, D.J. (1968) Gas chromatographic analysis of Nemagon fumigant in extracts of soil on porous polymer beads. *J. Gas Chromat.*, 6, 124-125

Hodges, L.R. (1972) Distribution and persistence of 1,2-dibromo-3-chloropropane in soil. *Diss. Abstr. Int.*, 32, 4968B

IARC (1976) *IARC Information Bulletin on the Survey of Chemicals Being Tested for Carcinogenicity*, No. 6, Lyon, pp. 198, 268

Johnson, D.E. & Lear, B. (1969) 1,2-Dibromo-3-chloropropane: recovery from soil and analysis by GLC. *J. chromat. Sci.*, 7, 384-385

Kodama, J.K. & Dunlap, M.K. (1956) Toxicity of 1,2-dibromo-3-chloropropane. *Fed. Proc.*, 15, 448

Martin, H., ed. (1971) *Pesticide Manual. Basic Information on the Chemicals used as Active Components of Pesticides*, 2nd ed., Ombersley, British Crop Protection Council, p. 148

McBeth, C.W. & Bergeson, G.B. (1955) 1,2-Dibromo-3-chloropropane - a new nematocide. *Plant Disease Reporter*, 39, 223-225

Muto, T. (1976) *Nayaku Yoran*, Tokyo, Nippon Plant Boeki Association

Novik, R.M. & Kozlova, I.V. (1971) Polarographic method of determining the insecticide Nemagon in water. *Fiz.-Khim. Metody Anal.*, 84-91

Novik, R.M. & Kozlova, I.V. (1973) *Possibility of determining Nemagon in soil*. In: Lyalikov, Y.S. & Novik, R., eds, *Theory and Practice of Polarographic Analyses*, Kishinev, Shtiintsa, pp. 71-76

Novik, R.M. & Plyngyu, N.I. (1973) *Use of ac polarography to determine the insecticide Nemagon in air*. In: Lyalikov, Y.S. & Novik, R., eds, *Theory and Practice of Methods of Polarographic Analyses*, Kishinev, Shtiintsa, pp. 19-24

Olson, W.A., Habermann, R.T., Weisburger, E.K., Ward, J.M. & Weisburger, J.H. (1973) Induction of stomach cancer in rats and mice by halogenated aliphatic fumigants. J. nat. Cancer Inst., 51, 1993-1995

Powers, M.B., Voelker, R.W., Page, N.P., Weisburger, E.K. & Kraybill, H.F. (1975) Carcinogenicity of ethylene dibromide (EDB) and 1,2-dibromo-3-chloropropane (DBCP) after oral administration in rats and mice. Toxicol. appl. Pharmacol., 33, 171-172

Prager, B. & Jacobson, P., eds (1918) Beilsteins Handbuch der Organischen Chemie, 4th ed., Vol. 1, Syst. 10, Berlin, Springer-Verlag, p. 111

Prival, M.J., McCoy, E.C., Gutter, B. & Rosenkranz, H.S. (1977) Tris(2,3-dibromopropyl)phosphate: mutagenicity of a widely used flame retardant. Science, 195, 76-78

Rosenkranz, H.S. (1975) Genetic activity of 1,2-dibromo-3-chloropropane, a widely-used fumigant. Bull. environm. Contam. Toxicol., 14, 8-12

Sakurai, T. (1973) Sengo Nippon Kagaku Kogyo Shi, Tokyo, Kagaku Daily Co., Ltd, p. 185

Spencer, E.Y. (1973) Guide to the Chemicals Used in Crop Protection, Publication 1093, 6th ed., London, Ontario, University of Western Ontario, Research Branch, Agriculture Canada, p. 172

US Department of Agriculture (1974) Farmers' Use of Pesticides in 1971... Quantities, Agriculture Economic Report No. 252, Washington DC, p. 54

US Environmental Protection Agency (1974) EPA Compendium of Registered Pesticides, Vol. II, Fungicides and Nematicides, Part II, Washington DC, US Government Printing Office, pp. D-25-00.01-D-25-00.13

US Environmental Protection Agency (1976) Inorganic bromides resulting from soil treatment with 1,2-dibromo-3-chloropropane; tolerances for residues. US Code of Federal Regulations, Title 40, part 180.197, pp. 180-181

US International Trade Commission (1976) Synthetic Organic Chemicals, US Production and Sales of Pesticides and Related Products, 1975 Preliminary, Washington DC, US Government Printing Office, p. 10

US Tariff Commission (1956) Synthetic Organic Chemicals, US Production and Sales, 1955, Report No. 198, Second Series, Washington DC, US Government Printing Office, p. 138

US Tariff Commission (1971) Synthetic Organic Chemicals, US Production and Sales, 1969, TC Publication 412, Washington DC, US Government Printing Office, p. 191

Vengerskaya, K.Y. & Rakhmatullaev, N.N. (1970) Determination of small amounts of Nemagon in water. Gig. i Sanit., 35, 59-60

trans-1,4-DICHLOROBUTENE

1. Chemical and Physical Data

1.1 Synonyms and trade names

Chem. Abstr. Services Reg. No.: 764-41-0

Chem. Abstr. Name: 1,4-Dichloro-2-butene

2-Butylene dichloride; 1,4-dichlorobutene

1.2 Chemical formula and molecular weight

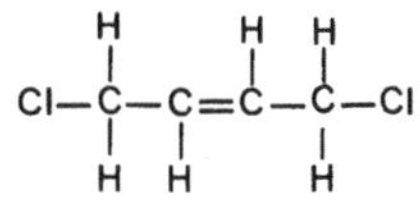

$$Cl-\underset{H}{\overset{H}{C}}-C=C-\underset{H}{\overset{H}{C}}-Cl$$

$C_4H_6Cl_2$ Mol. wt: 125

1.3 Chemical and physical properties of the pure substance

From Weast (1976), unless otherwise specified

(a) Description: Colourless liquid with a distinct odour (Hawley, 1971)

(b) Boiling-point: 155.5°C at 758 mm; 55.5°C at 20 mm

(c) Melting-point: 1-3°C

(d) Density: d_4^{25} 1.183

(e) Refractive index: n_D^{25} 1.4871

(f) Spectroscopy data: Nuclear magnetic resonance spectra are given by Van Duuren *et al.* (1975).

(g) Solubility: Insoluble in water; soluble in ethanol, diethyl ether, acetone, benzene and chloroform

1.4 Technical products and impurities

1,4-Dichlorobutene available in the US contains 95-98% *trans*-1,4-dichlorobutene and 2-5% of the *cis* isomer (Hawley, 1971).

2. Production, Use, Occurrence and Analysis

For background information on this section, see preamble, p. 17.

2.1 Production and use

(a) Production

The preparation of *trans*-1,4-dichlorobutene by the chlorination of butadiene was first reported in 1930 (Muskat & Northrup, 1930), and this method is used for its commercial production. The isomers 3,4-dichlorobutene, *cis*-1,4-dichlorobutene and *trans*-1,4-dichlorobutene are produced, and when the mixture is heated, an equilibrium results. The residue resulting from removal of the 3,4-isomer, which has a lower boiling-point, is normally used without further separation.

Although *trans*-1,4-dichlorobutene is reported to have been in use in the US as an intermediate since 1951, commercial production was not begun until 1963 (US Tariff Commission, 1964). Two US companies currently manufacture it (see preamble, p. 17).

Since *trans*-1,4-dichlorobutene is an intermediate, *via* 3,4-dichlorobutene, in one process for manufacturing chloroprene, and since chloroprene is produced in the Federal Republic of Germany, France, Italy, the UK and the USSR, *trans*-1,4-dichlorobutene may be produced in one or more of these countries.

Commercial production of this chemical was started in Japan in 1971, where it is currently manufactured by one company by the same process as used in the US. It is also reported to be produced on a small scale in the People's Republic of China.

(b) Use

In the US, virtually all of the *trans*-1,4-dichlorobutene is used as an intermediate in the manufacture of hexamethylenediamine and chloroprene. Total US production of hexamethylenediamine in 1975 was 340 million kg (US International Trade Commission, 1976a), but data on the amount derived from the dichlorobutenes are not available. Hexamethylenediamine is used as a chemical intermediate in the manufacture of nylon 66 and 612 polyamide resins.

Chloroprene is used in the production of polychloroprene rubber. US production of this product in 1975 was 143.9 million kg (US International Trade Commission, 1976b) and is estimated to have consumed an equal quantity of chloroprene. In Japan, the method primarily used to produce polychloroprene rubber involves acetylene rather than butadiene, although some is manufactured from butadiene *via* the dichlorobutenes. *trans*-1,4-Dichlorobutene is also consumed captively in that country to produce 1,4-butanediol by hydrolysis followed by hydrogenation. Japanese production of 1,4-butanediol in 1975 amounted to 1-1.5 million kg.

Although there is at least one process for producing adipic acid from dichlorobutenes, it is not being used commercially at present.

2.2 Occurrence

trans-1,4-Dichlorobutene is not known to occur as a natural product.

2.3 Analysis

Gas chromatography has been used to determine the products, including *trans*-1,4-dichlorobutene, resulting from the addition of chlorine to butadiene in acetic acid (Heasley *et al.*, 1972).

3. Biological Data Relevant to the Evaluation of Carcinogenic Risk to Man

3.1 Carcinogenicity and related studies in animals

(a) Skin application

Mouse: A group of 30 female ICR/Ha Swiss mice were given skin applications of 1 mg *trans*-1,4-dichlorobutene dissolved in 0.1 ml acetone thrice weekly for 77 weeks. No skin tumours were observed (Van Duuren *et al.*, 1975).

trans-1,4-Dichlorobutene was tested in a two-stage carcinogenesis experiment with phorbol myristyl acetate as a promoting agent in female ICR/Ha Swiss mice. Of 30 mice treated with 1 mg *trans*-1,4-dichlorobutene in 0.1 ml acetone plus 2.5 µg phorbol myristyl acetate in 0.1 ml acetone, 1 developed a skin papilloma, compared with 28 positive controls with 209 papillomas and 17 with squamous-cell carcinomas of the skin after treatment with 7,12-dimethylbenz[a]anthracene and phorbol myristyl acetate. Of 30 mice treated with phorbol myristyl acetate alone, 3 had skin papillomas and 1 a skin carcinoma (Van Duuren et al., 1975).

(b) Subcutaneous and/or intramuscular administration

Mouse: A group of 30 female ICR/Ha Swiss mice were given weekly s.c. injections of 0.05 mg trans-1,4-dichlorobutene dissolved in 0.05 ml tricaprylin for 77 weeks; the median survival time was 477 days. Three mice developed local sarcomas ($P<0.05$). No local tumours were observed in 50 control mice injected with tricaprylin alone, whose mean survival time was 436 days (Van Duuren et al., 1975) [The Working Group noted the low dose used].

(c) Intraperitoneal administration

Mouse: A group of 30 female ICR/Ha Swiss mice were given weekly i.p. injections of 0.05 mg trans-1,4-dichlorobutene dissolved in 0.05 ml tricaprylin for 77 weeks; the median survival time was 478 days. Two mice developed local sarcomas ($P>0.1$). No local tumours were observed in 30 control mice injected with tricaprylin alone, whose mean survival time was 513 days (Van Duuren et al., 1975) [The Working Group noted the low dose used].

3.2 Other relevant biological data

(a) Experimental systems

The oral LD_{50} of trans-1,4-dichlorobutene in rats is 89 mg/kg bw; 62 ppm (0.34 mg/l) given to rats by inhalation for 4 hours caused mortality in 2/6 animals in 14 days (Smith et al., 1951).

No data on the chronic toxicity, embryotoxicity or teratogenicity of this compound were available to the Working Group.

trans-1,4-Dichlorobutene caused reverse mutations in Salmonella typhimurium TA100; liver microsomal fractions from mice or humans enhanced the mutagenic effect (Bartsch et al., 1976). It was also reported to be mutagenic in Escherichia coli (Mukai & Hawryluk, 1973).

(b) Man

No data were available to the Working Group.

3.3 Case reports and epidemiological studies

No data were available to the Working Group.

4. Comments on Data Reported and Evaluation

4.1 Animal data

trans-1,4-Dichlorobutene has been tested in female mice by skin application and by subcutaneous and intraperitoneal injection. When injected subcutaneously or intraperitoneally, it produced low incidences of local sarcomas. The available data do not allow an evaluation of the carcinogenicity of this compound to be made.

4.2 Human data

No case reports or epidemiological studies were available to the Working Group.

5. References

Bartsch, H., Malaveille, C., Barbin, A., Planche, G. & Montesano, R. (1976) Alkylating and mutagenic metabolites of halogenated olefins produced by human and animal tissues. *Proc. Amer. Ass. Cancer Res.*, 17, 17

Hawley, G.G., ed. (1971) *The Condensed Chemical Dictionary*, 8th ed., New York, Van Nostrand Reinhold, p. 284

Heasley, V.L., Heasley, G.E., Loghry, R.A. & McConnell, M.R. (1972) Comparisons of the reactions of butadiene with chlorine, bromine, acetyl hypochlorite, and acetyl hypobromite. *J. org. Chem.*, 37, 2228-2231

Mukai, F.H. & Hawryluk, I. (1973) The mutagenicity of some halo-ethers and halo-ketones. *Mutation Res.*, 21, 228

Muskat, I.E. & Northrup, H.E. (1930) Studies of conjugated systems. V. The preparation and chlorination of butadiene. *J. Amer. chem. Soc.*, 52, 4043-4055

Smith, H.F., Carpenter, C.P. & Weil, C.S. (1951) Range-finding toxicity data: list IV. *Arch. industr. Hyg. occup. Med.*, 4, 119-122

US International Trade Commission (1976a) *Synthetic Organic Chemicals, US Production and Sales of Miscellaneous Chemicals, 1975 Preliminary*, Washington DC, US Government Printing Office, p. 6

US International Trade Commission (1976b) *Synthetic Organic Chemicals, US Production and Sales of Elastomers, 1975 Preliminary*, Washington DC, US Government Printing Office, p. 2

US Tariff Commission (1964) *Synthetic Organic Chemicals, US Production and Sales, 1963*, TC Publication 143, Washington DC, US Government Printing Office, p. 194

Van Duuren, B.L., Goldschmidt, B.M. & Seidman, I. (1975) Carcinogenic activity of di- and trifunctional α-chloro ethers and of 1,4-dichlorobutene-2 in ICR/HA Swiss mice. *Cancer Res.*, 35, 2553-2557

Weast, R.C., ed. (1976) *CRC Handbook of Chemistry and Physics*, 57th ed., Cleveland, Ohio, Chemical Rubber Co., p. C-230

DIHYDROXYBENZENES

1. Chemical and Physical Data

1.1 Synonyms and trade names

Catechol

Chem. Abstr. Services Reg. No.: 120-80-9

Chem. Abstr. Name: 1,2-Benzenediol

ortho-Benzenediol; 1,2-benzene diol; catechin; C.I. 76500; C.I. oxidation base 26; 1,2-dihydroxybenzene; *ortho*-dihydroxybenzene; *ortho*-dioxybenzene; *ortho*-hydroquinone; 2-hydroxyphenol; *ortho*-hydroxyphenol; oxyphenic acid; *ortho*-phenylenediol; pyrocatechin; pyrocatechine; pyrocatechol

Durafur Developer C; Fouramine PCH; Fourrine 68; Pelagol Grey C

Resorcinol

Chem. Abstr. Services Reg. No.: 108-46-3

Chem. Abstr. Name: 1,3-Benzenediol

meta-Benzenediol; C.I. 76505; C.I. Developer 4; C.I. oxidation base 31; 1,3-dihydroxybenzene; *meta*-dihydroxybenzene; *meta*-dioxybenzene; *meta*-hydroquinone; 3-hydroxycyclohexadien-1-one; 3-hydroxyphenol; *meta*-hydroxyphenol

Developer O; Developer R; Developer RS; Durafur Developer G; Fouramine RS; Fourrine 79; Fourrine EW; Nako TGG; Pelagol Grey RS; Pelagol RS; Resorcin; Resorcine

Hydroquinone

Chem. Abstr. Services Reg. No.: 123-31-9

Chem. Abstr. Name: 1,4-Benzenediol

para-Benzenediol; benzohydroquinone; benzoquinol; 1,4-dihydroxybenzene; *para*-dihydroxybenzene; *para*-dioxobenzene; *para*-dioxybenzene; hydroquinol; hydroquinole; α-hydroquinone; *para*-hydroquinone;

para-hydroxyphenol; quinol; β-quinol

Arctuvin; Eldopaque; Eldoquin; HE5; Tecquinol; Tenox HQ; Tequinol

1.2 <u>Chemical formulae and molecular weights</u>

Catechol

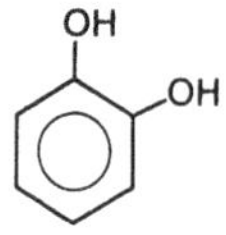

$C_6H_6O_2$ Mol. wt: 110.1

Resorcinol

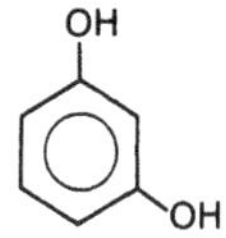

$C_6H_6O_2$ Mol. wt: 110.1

Hydroquinone

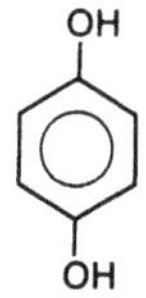

$C_6H_6O_2$ Mol. wt: 110.1

1.3 <u>Chemical and physical properties of the pure substance</u>

Catechol

(a) <u>Description</u>: Colourless crystals (Raff & Ettling, 1966)

(b) <u>Boiling-point</u>: 245°C at 750 mm (Weast, 1976)

(c) <u>Melting-point</u>: 105°C (Weast, 1976)

(d) <u>Density</u>: d_4^{15} 1.371 (Raff & Ettling, 1966)

(e) <u>Refractive index</u>: n_D^{20} 1.604 (Raff & Ettling, 1966)

(f) <u>Spectroscopy data</u>: λ_{max} 214 nm (E_1^1 = 614.6) in cyclohexane (Weast, 1976)

(g) <u>Solubility</u>: Very soluble in acetone, water and ethanol; soluble in ether, hot benzene, alkali, chloroform and carbon tetrachloride (Raff & Ettling, 1966)

(h) *Volatility*: Sublimes; volatile with steam (Raff & Ettling, 1966)

(i) *Stability*: Discolours in air and light (Windholz, 1976)

(j) *Reactivity*: Acts as a reducing agent (Windholz, 1976)

Resorcinol

(a) *Description*: Colourless crystals (Weast, 1976)

(b) *Boiling-point*: 178°C at 16 mm (Weast, 1976)

(c) *Melting-point*: 111°C (Weast, 1976)

(d) *Density*: d_4^{15} 1.272 (Raff & Ettling, 1966)

(e) *Spectroscopy data*: λ_{max} 220 nm (E_1^1 = 560.5) and 276 nm (E_1^1 = 194) in ethanol; infra-red, ultra-violet, nuclear magnetic resonance and mass spectra have been tabulated by Grasselli (1973).

(f) *Solubility*: Slightly soluble in benzene, chloroform and carbon tetrachloride; soluble in water, ethanol and acetone (Raff & Ettling, 1966)

(g) *Volatility*: Vapour pressure is 53 mm at 190°C (Raff & Ettling, 1966).

(h) *Stability*: Hygroscopic; acquires a pink tint when exposed to light and air (Raff & Ettling, 1966)

Hydroquinone

(a) *Description*: White crystals (Weast, 1976)

(b) *Boiling-point*: 285°C at 730 mm (Weast, 1976)

(c) *Melting-point*: 173-174°C (Weast, 1976)

(d) *Density*: d^{15} 1.328 (Weast, 1976)

(e) *Spectroscopy data*: λ_{max} 228 nm (E_1^1 = 208.2) in water; infra-red, ultra-violet, nuclear magnetic resonance and mass spectra have been tabulated by Grasselli (1973).

(f) Solubility: Slightly soluble in benzene; soluble in ether and in water (9.4 g/100 ml at 28.5°C) (Raff & Ettling, 1966); very soluble in ethanol, acetone and carbon tetrachloride (Weast, 1976)

(g) Stability: Solutions are oxidized in air (Windholz, 1976).

1.4 Technical products and impurities

Catechol

Catechol is available in the US in technical, chemically pure and extra pure grades. One manufacturer's specifications for the chemically pure grade are: white crystals or flakes with 99.3% min. purity, 0.35% max. water and a freezing-point of 103°C min.; for the extra pure grade: white crystals with 99.5% min. purity, 0.3% max. water and a freezing-point of 103.2°C min.

In Japan, commercially available catechol has a 99% min. purity and a melting-point of 103°C min. It contains the other hydroquinone isomers as impurities.

Resorcinol

Resorcinol is available in the US in USP and technical grades. Specifications for the USP grade are: 99-100.5% active ingredient; melting range, 109-111°C; 1% max. weight loss on drying over silica gel for 4 hours; 0.05% max. ignition residue; and containing no phenol or catechol (US Pharmacopeial Convention, Inc., 1975). Technical grade resorcinol has a 99% min. resorcinol content and contains small amounts of phenol and catechol as impurities.

In Japan, technical resorcinol has the following specifications: a freezing-point of 108.5°C min.; 0.5% max. water; and 0.1% max. residue on ignition. The chief impurities are the other hydroquinone isomers.

Hydroquinone

Hydroquinone is available in the US in photographic and technical grades; specifications for the technical grade are: appearance, light-tan to light-grey crystals; 98.5% min. active ingredient; 1% max. water;

0.07% max. ash; a melting-point of 169°C min.; and miscible with water (Raff & Ettling, 1966).

In Japan, commercially available hydroquinone has 99% min. active ingredient; 0.05% max. ignition residue; 30 mg/kg max. lead; 30 mg/kg max. iron; and a melting-point of 169-174°C.

2. Production, Use, Occurrence and Analysis

For background information on this section, see preamble, p. 17. A review on catechol, resorcinol and hydroquinone has been published (Raff & Ettling, 1966).

2.1 Production and Use

Catechol

(a) *Production*

Catechol was prepared by Reinsch in 1839 by distilling catechin (Raff & Ettling, 1966). Although catechol can be prepared by the alkaline fusion or dry distillation of a variety of naturally occurring materials, commercial production in the US is reported to be based on either the alkaline fusion of *ortho*-chlorophenol or recovery from lignin-containing wastes from wood pulping operations. Since 1973, production of catechol in Japan has been carried out solely by oxidation of benzene with hydrogen peroxide to produce a mixture of products from which both hydroquinone and catechol are isolated. A factory using an oxidation process started production in France in 1973.

In the US, catechol has been produced in commercial quantities since 1920 (US Tariff Commission, 1921). In 1974, only one US company reported commercial production (see preamble, p. 17) (US International Trade Commission, 1976a); at present, one other company is reported to produce the chemical for captive use, and another produces it on command. Imports of catechol through the principal US customs districts in 1974 amounted to 502 thousand kg (US International Trade Commission, 1976b).

Catechol is produced in the Federal Republic of Germany, France, Switzerland and the UK. It was formerly produced in Czechoslovakia

(Anon., 1973a,b). Production in western Europe is estimated to be in the range of 4-40 million kg annually.

Catechol was first produced in Japan in 1955. In 1975, the sole Japanese manufacturer produced an estimated 600 thousand kg, of which about 200 thousand kg were exported. Japanese imports of catechol in 1975 were about 10-20 thousand kg, primarily from France.

(b) Use

World-wide use of catechol in 1973 has been estimated to have been 1.4-2.3 million kg (Anon., 1973b); that in the US in 1970 was more than 545 thousand kg (Anon., 1973a).

Some of the more important present and potential applications of catechol are in polymerization inhibitors and antioxidants, in electro-sensitive copying papers, in the synthesis of pharmaceuticals and pesticides, in photography and in rubber compounding aids.

The major use is in the synthesis of 4-tertiary-butyl-catechol (4-tertiary-butylpyrocatechol), and about 270 thousand kg were used for this purpose in the US in 1970. 4-Tertiary-butyl-catechol is used primarily as a polymerization inhibitor in styrene (Anon., 1973a).

Other important uses are as a photographic developing agent, as an oxidation base in fur and hair dye preparations, and as a chemical intermediate for a rubber accelerator, the di-*ortho*-tolylguanidine salt of dicatechol borate. Small amounts may also be used as an analytical reagent.

Catechol has been used to synthesize certain chlorinated dibenzo-*para*-dioxins (Pohland & Yang, 1972).

In Japan, use of catechol in 1975 is estimated to have been as follows: 75% for synthesis of 4-tertiary-butyl-catechol, 5% for medicinal uses and 20% for other uses (including synthesis of perfumes and as an additive in metal plating baths).

Resorcinol

(a) Production

Resorcinol was prepared by Hlasiwetz & Barth in 1864 by fusing galbanum and asafetida resins with alkali (Raff & Ettling, 1966). It is produced commercially in the US and Japan by fusion of the sodium salt of *meta*-benzenedisulphonic acid with sodium hydroxide, followed by acidification (Raff & Ettling, 1966).

In the US, resorcinol has been produced in commercial quantities since 1918 (US Tariff Commission, 1919). In 1974, only one US company reported commercial production (see preamble, p. 17) (US International Trade Commission, 1976a) of about 16 million kg. Imports of pharmaceutical grade resorcinol through the principal US customs districts in 1974 were 4.5 thousand kg (US International Trade Commission, 1976b); exports in 1975 totalled 3.56 million kg, primarily to the following countries (in order of decreasing imports): The Netherlands, Japan and the UK (US Department of Commerce, 1976).

Resorcinol is produced by two companies in each of the following countries: the Federal Republic of Germany, France and the UK, and by one company in Italy. It is also produced in Switzerland and in India. Annual production in western Europe is estimated to be 4-40 million kg.

Resorcinol has been produced commercially in Japan since 1945. The sole Japanese manufacturer produced an estimated 1 million kg in 1975, of which about 100 thousand kg were exported; imports in that year were 1.2-1.8 million kg, primarily from the Federal Republic of Germany and the US.

(b) Use

Use of resorcinol in the US in 1974 was as follows: 67% in the manufacture of rubber products, 20% in the manufacture of wood adhesives and 13% for miscellaneous uses.

Resorcinol (alone or in combination with phenol) is used to make resins or resin intermediates by reaction with formaldehyde. In the manufacture of rubber products, these are primarily used in tire-cord adhesive dips and as additives to the tire carcass rubber to improve adhesion and physical properties. In the manufacture of wood adhesives, these resins are formulated with other ingredients to produce adhesives that find a variety of uses because they can be cured at low or intermediate temperatures to give durable, waterproof bonding (e.g., in laminated beams and marine plywood).

Miscellaneous uses of resorcinol are as a chemical intermediate and as a pharmaceutical. It is used to produce (i) the 2-hydroxy-4-alkyl (C_8-C_{12})oxybenzophenones (ultra-violet absorbers in plastics to retard light-induced degradation); (ii) β-methylumbelliferone (an optical brightener); (iii) modified fur and hair dyes (it is used as a developer in combination with other oxidation bases), xanthene dyes (e.g., fluorescein and eosin) and azo dyes (e.g., Fast brown BRL and Resorcin Brown); (iv) 4-n-hexylresorcinol (an antiseptic and anthelmintic); (v) dibromohydroxy-mercurifluorescein, disodium salt (an antiseptic); (vi) *para*-aminosalicylic acid (an analgesic agent); (vii) condensation products with aldehydes (used as tanning agents and as resins in adhesives other than for rubber and wood products); (viii) its diglycidyl ether by reaction with epichlorohydrin[1] (resin intermediate); and (ix) the lead salt of 2,4,6-trinitroresorcinol (a primer for explosives).

Resorcinol and its acetic acid ester are used for external treatment of a variety of skin conditions.

In Japan, use of resorcinol in 1975 is estimated to have been as follows: 55% for rubber products, 20% for wood adhesives, 10% for ultra-violet absorbers, and 15% for dyes and pharmaceuticals.

In 1976, the American Conference of Governmental Industrial Hygienists adopted a time-weighted average value of 45 mg/m^3 (10 ppm) as a threshold limit value for resorcinol in the working atmosphere over any eight-hour workshift of a forty-hour working week (ACGIH, 1976).

---

[1]See also IARC, 1976.

Hydroquinone

(a) Production

Hydroquinone was prepared by Pelletier & Caventon in 1820 by the dry distillation of quinic acid (Raff & Ettling, 1966). Although it can be produced by the oxidation of benzene or of numerous benzene derivatives, followed by reduction of the resulting quinone, the method used for its commercial production in the US and Japan until recently has been the oxidation of aniline (with manganese dioxide and sulphuric acid), followed by reduction with iron dust and water (Raff & Ettling, 1966). A Japanese factory that used this method was closed in 1974, but it is still used for most production in the US.

Of current Japanese production, over 80% is by the alkylation of benzene with propylene to produce a mixture of di-isopropylbenzene isomers from which the *para*-isomer is isolated. This is oxidized with oxygen to produce the corresponding dihydroperoxide, which is treated with acid to produce acetone and hydroquinone (Anon., 1974). Only a small proportion of US production is based on this process.

Another process, which is estimated to represent 15-20% of current Japanese production, is based on the oxidation of phenol with hydrogen peroxide to produce a mixture of products from which both hydroquinone and catechol are isolated.

Commercial production of hydroquinone was first reported in the US in 1918, when combined US production of hydroquinone and chlorhydroquinone was 139 thousand kg (US Tariff Commission, 1919). Three US companies now produce the technical grade, and total production in 1975 amounted to 7.5 million kg (US International Trade Commission, 1976c). US imports of technical hydroquinone through the principal customs districts in 1974 were 500 kg (US International Trade Commission, 1976b).

Hydroquinone is produced in the Federal Republic of Germany, France, Switzerland and the UK, and annual production in these countries is estimated to be 4-40 million kg.

Hydroquinone was first produced in Japan in 1938 or 1939. In 1975, two Japanese producers manufactured an estimated 2.9 million kg, and another 200 thousand kg were imported, primarily from France.

About 50,000 kg were imported into Australia in 1975-1976.

(b) Use

The major use of hydroquinone is as a developer in black-and-white photography. It has also been used as an antioxidant and polymerization inhibitor, as a chemical intermediate and as a laboratory reagent.

Its use in photography is based on its ability to reduce exposed grains of silver halide in the photographic emulsion rapidly and selectively, frequently in combination with *para*-methylaminophenol sulphate. It has also been used as an antioxidant and polymerization inhibitor in fats, oils, turpentine, paints, vitamins, unsaturated monomers and petrol (Raff & Ettling, 1966).

It is used as a component of dermatological preparations designed to bleach hyperpigmented skin blemishes (Blacow, 1972). It is reportedly used for the production of its mono- and dialkyl ethers, e.g., *para*-methoxyphenol, which is used as an intermediate for butylated hydroxyanisole; in several rubber-processing chemicals, e.g., *para*-aminophenol and N,N-diphenyl-*para*-phenylenediamine, both of which are used as antioxidants; and in ring-substituted alkyl derivatives, e.g., di-tert-butyl hydroquinone, which is used as an intermediate in another synthesis route for butylated hydroxyanisole.

Use of hydroquinone in Japan is estimated to be as follows: polymerization inhibitor, 35%; intermediate for rubber-processing chemicals, 27%; photographic developer, 19%; dye intermediate, 13%; and other uses, 6%.

The US Occupational Safety and Health Administration's health standards for exposure to air contaminants require that an employee's exposure to hydroquinone does not exceed an eight-hour time-weighted average of 2 mg/m^3 (0.45 ppm) in the working atmosphere during any eight-hour workshift of a forty-hour working week (US Occupational Safety & Health Administration, 1976). This level is also recommended in Australia.

2.2 Occurrence

Catechol

Catechol has been found in onions, in crude beet sugar, in crude wood tar, in drainage water from bituminous shale, in coal and in cigarette smoke (Raff & Ettling, 1966). It has also been found in the effluents resulting from the production of coal-tar chemicals (Umpelev *et al.*, 1974).

It occurs as its sulphuric acid ester in the urine of some mammals (e.g., horse and man) (Raff & Ettling, 1966).

Resorcinol

Resorcinol has been found in wood smoke and cigarette smoke (Commins & Lindsey, 1956a,b). It was found as a pollutant in filtered surface and ground water at a water-treatment plant (Thielemann, 1969) and has also been found in the effluents resulting from the production of coal-tar chemicals (Umpelev *et al.*, 1974).

Hydroquinone

Hydroquinone has been found in cigarette smoke (Raff & Ettling, 1966) and in the effluents resulting from the production of coal-tar chemicals (Umpelev *et al.*, 1974).

A glucoside of hydroquinone, arbutin, occurs widely in the leaves of many plants (e.g., bearberry, mountain cranberry, bilberry), in fruit (Chinese anise) and in the bark and buds of pear trees (Raff & Ettling, 1966).

2.3 Analysis

A brief review of analytical methods for catechol, resorcinol and hydroquinone is given by Raff & Ettling (1966).

A non-aqueous oxidation-reduction titrimetric method for their determination has a relative error of 2% or less (Kreshkov *et al.*, 1973).

Phenols, including catechol, resorcinol and hydroquinone, can be determined at concentrations of 0.1 mg/l in biologically treated aqueous effluents, resin effluents, tar-works effluents and in river waters. The phenols are extracted from the sample with methyl isobutyl ketone, converted to the trimethylsilyl ether derivative, separated by gas chromatography and detected by flame ionization (Cooper & Wheatstone, 1973). A similar method was used on an ether or chloroform extract to give a preliminary identification of drugs, including resorcinol, extracted from tissue samples (Koempe, 1974).

Potassium metaperiodate has been tried as a reagent in detecting microgram quantities of catechol or hydroquinone by paper chromatography (Clifford & Wight, 1973). Thin-layer chromatography has been used to detect polyhydric phenols, including catechol, resorcinol and hydroquinone, in effluents resulting from the production of coal-tar chemicals (Umpelev et al., 1974). An investigation of ten different spray reagents for thin-layer chromatography of seven phenols, including catechol, resorcinol and hydroquinone, gave detection limits ranging from 0.008-4 µg (Thielemann, 1975).

In a method for determining catechol in $1 \times 10^{-5} - 1 \times 10^{-4}$ M concentrations, its iron complex is formed, extracted by ion-exchange and determined spectrophotometrically (Berenguer, 1975).

A method for assaying resorcinol-phenol-boric solution, used as an antifungal preparation, has been described by Gupta & Cates (1974); thin-layer chromatography has been used to detect polyhydric phenols, including resorcinol, in cosmetic products at levels below 0.01% (Wilson, 1975).

The US Pharmacopeia has published methods for the identification and assay of hydroquinone (US Pharmacopeial Convention, Inc., 1975), and an aqueous iodometrical titration method has been investigated (Sharma et al., 1976). Concentrations of 5-25 mg/kg hydroquinone have been determined in vinyl acetate monomer, with a relative error of 2% or less, by measuring the ultra-violet absorption at 293 nm spectrophotometrically (Barer et al., 1975).

3. Biological Data Relevant to the Evaluation of Carcinogenic Risk to Man

3.1 Carcinogenicity and related studies in animals

(a) Skin application

Mouse: A group of 50 7-week old female ICR/Ha Swiss mice received 2 mg catechol in 0.1 ml acetone by skin painting together with 5 µg benzo[a]pyrene in 0.1 ml acetone thrice weekly for 52 weeks, at which time 26 mice were still alive. A total of 86 skin papillomas occurred in 35 mice, and squamous-cell carcinomas of the skin were observed in 31 A further group of 50 mice were treated with 5 µg benzo[a]pyrene alone thrice weekly for 52 weeks, at which time 41 mice were still alive. A total of 14 papillomas were observed in 13 mice, and 10 had squamous-cell carcinomas of the skin. No skin tumours occurred in similar groups of controls that were either untreated or painted with acetone only (Van Duuren et al., 1973).

Three groups of 50 7-week old female Swiss mice were painted with 0.02 ml of a 5, 25 or 50% solution of resorcinol in acetone twice weekly for 100 weeks; a group of 150 mice were untreated, and a further group of 100 mice were painted with acetone alone. About half of the mice treated with resorcinol were still alive after 75 weeks. The percentages of tumour-bearing animals were similar in all groups; the tumours that occurred were mainly lymphomas, lung adenomas and liver haemangiomas. Skin tumours occurred in 2 mice painted with resorcinol in acetone, in 2 painted with acetone alone and in 3 untreated animals (Stenbäck & Shubik, 1974).

A group of 24 stock albino male mice of the 'S' strain, 7-9 weeks old, received a single skin application of 0.3 ml of a 6.7% solution of hydroquinone in acetone (20 mg dose). Three weeks later, croton oil was painted in 18 weekly applications of 0.3 ml of a 0.5% solution in acetone on the same area of the skin. One week after the end of the croton oil treatment all 22 survivors were killed and autopsied. One mouse had developed a skin papilloma (Roe & Salaman, 1955).

(b) *Other experimental systems*

Bladder implantation: In two groups of mice, 10 mg cholesterol pellets containing 20% catechol or hydroquinone were implanted into the bladder. Nineteen mice in each group survived 25 weeks. Of those given catechol, 1 mouse developed a papilloma and 3 developed carcinomas (P=0.03); of those mice treated with hydroquinone, 6 mice developed bladder carcinomas [P<0.01]. Of 77 mice given implants of cholesterol alone and surviving 25 weeks, 4 developed adenomas or papillomas and 5 developed carcinomas of the bladder (Boyland *et al.*, 1964).

3.2 Other relevant biological data

The toxicity of catechol, resorcinol and hydroquinone in animals and man has been reviewed by Deichmann & Keplinger (1963).

(a) *Experimental systems*

The oral LD_{50} of catechol in rats was reported to be 3900 mg/kg bw (Windholz, 1976). The s.c. LD_{50} in mice was 179 mg/kg bw (Lipkan, 1971).

The oral LD_{50} of resorcinol in rats and guinea-pigs was 370 mg/kg bw and that in rabbits, 750 mg/kg bw (Deichmann & Keplinger, 1963). The LD_{50} by s.c. injection in rats was 450 mg/kg bw (Stecher, 1968).

The LD_{50} of hydroquinone given by stomach tube to rats of various strains was approximately 1000 mg/kg bw. Fasting the animals for 18 hours prior to administration of the compound produced a 2-3-fold increase in its toxicity (Carlson & Brewer, 1953). A s.c. dose of 160 mg/kg bw was lethal to mice (Deichmann & Keplinger, 1963).

Exposure of experimental animals (unspecified) to lethal doses of hydroquinone induced signs of increased motor activity, followed by convulsions and methaemoglobinaemia. Subacute poisoning is characterized by haemolytic icterus, anaemia, leucocytosis, hypoglycaemia and, later, cachexia (Deichmann & Keplinger, 1963).

In a 2-year feeding study in rats, no effects on final body weight were observed in animals receiving a diet containing up to 1% hydroquinone, nor were any haematological or pathological changes reported. When 5% of the compound was administered, a 46% loss of body weight was observed within 9 weeks; the animals also developed aplastic anaemia, depletion of the bone marrow, liver cord-cell atrophy, superficial ulceration and haemorrhage of the gastric mucosa. Dogs treated with 40 mg/kg bw/day hydroquinone for 80 weeks (pups) or with 100 mg/kg bw/day for 26 weeks (adults) grew normally and showed no pathological signs at autopsy (Carlson & Brewer, 1953). Calder *et al.* (1973) reported that hydroquinone causes renal tubular necrosis in rats when administered intravenously at a dose of 198 mg/kg bw.

All three compounds are absorbed from the gastrointestinal tract and possibly through the skin. Oxidation to the more toxic quinones occurs. Hydroquinones, like other phenols, are partially excreted in the urine as such and in conjugation with hexuronic, sulphuric and other acids (Deichmann & Keplinger, 1963).

Free catechol and its glucuronide and sulphate conjugates were detected in the urine of chickens and dogs given injections of ^{3}H-catechol into the renal artery (Rennick & Quebbemann, 1970).

No data on embryotoxicity or teratogenicity were available to the Working Group.

In the polymerase assay, which is believed to give an indication of reparable DNA damage, hydroquinone was less toxic to *Escherichia coli* W3100 (*pol* A^+) than to p3478 (*pol* A^-), suggesting that this compound can damage DNA (Bilimoria, 1975). Resorcinol was not mutagenic to *Salmonella typhimurium* strains TA1535, TA1537, TA98 or TA100 in the presence or absence of a rat liver postmitochondrial supernatant fraction at a dose of up to 1000 µg/plate (McCann *et al.*, 1975).

The hydroquinones induced chromosome aberrations or karyotypic effects in *Allium cepa* (catechol, hydroquinone and resorcinol) (Levan & Tjio, 1948a,b), *Chara zeylanica* (resorcinol and hydroquinone) (Chatterjee & Sharma, 1972), *Vicia faba* (hydroquinone) (Sharma & Chatterjee, 1964; Valadaud-Barrieu & Izard, 1973), *Callisia fragrans* (hydroquinone) (Roy, 1973), *Trigonella foenum-graecum* (hydroquinone) (Sharma & Chatterjee, 1964), *Allium sativum* (hydroquinone) (Sharma & Chatterjee, 1964) and *Tulbaghia violacea* (resorcinol) (Riley & Hoff, 1960).

(b) Man

Skin contact with catechol causes dermatitis, and absorption through the skin may give rise to symptoms similar to those seen in phenol poisoning (Deichmann & Keplinger, 1963).

Application of a 3-25% solution of resorcinol to the skin may cause redness, itching, dermatitis, oedema or corrosion of the affected area. Ingestion of 8 g resorcinol by a child resulted in hypothermia, hypotension, decreased respiration, tremors, icterus and haemoglobinuria (Deichmann & Keplinger, 1963).

Ingestion of 1 g hydroquinone by an adult caused tinnitus, nausea, dizziness, a sense of suffocation, an increased rate of respiration, vomiting, pallor, muscular twitching, headache, dyspnoea, cyanosis, delirium and collapse. Ingestion of 5-12 g hydroquinone has been reported to be fatal. Exposure to 30 mg/m^3 hydroquinone in air has been shown to result in dermatitis, keratitis and depigmentation, as well as certain corneal changes, including disappearance of pigment (Deichmann & Keplinger, 1963).

Ingestion of 100-150 mg hydroquinone by 17 male volunteers thrice daily for 3-5 months produced no significant pathological changes in the blood or urine (Carlson & Brewer, 1953).

3.3 Case reports and epidemiological studies

No data were available to the Working Group.

4. Comments on Data Reported and Evaluation[1]

4.1 Animal data

In skin painting studies in mice, catechol increased the carcinogenic effects of benzo[*a*]pyrene on the skin; hydroquinone was inactive as an

---

[1]See also the section, 'Animal Data in Relation to the Evaluation of Risk to Man' in the introduction to this volume, p. 15.

initiator of skin carcinogenesis. When tested by repeated skin application, resorcinol showed no carcinogenic effect in mice. In bladder implantation studies, hydroquinone in cholesterol pellets increased the incidence of bladder carcinomas in mice (see also preamble, p. 21). The available data do not allow an evaluation of the carcinogenicity of these compounds.

4.2 Human data

No case reports or epidemiological studies were available to the Working Group.

5. References

ACGIH (American Conference of Governmental Industrial Hygienists) (1976) Actions on threshold limit values of air contaminants and physical agents. Occupational Safety & Health Reporter, 27 May, p. 1852

Anon. (1973a) Aromatic organics. Chemical Marketing Reporter, 16 April, p. 11

Anon. (1973b) Aromatic organics. Chemical Marketing Reporter, 13 August, pp. 11-12

Anon. (1974) Cheaper route to hydroquinone. Chemical Week, 11 December, p. 51

Barer, V.E., Buzina, I.N. & Faidel, G.I. (1975) Determination of small amounts of inhibitor in industrial samples of vinyl acetate. Plast. Massy, 8, 73

Berenguer, N.V. (1975) Spectrophotometric determination of catechol via the extraction of iron complexes with liquid ion exchangers. Fresenius' Z. analyt. Chem., 275, 128

Bilimoria, M.H. (1975) The detection of mutagenic activity of chemicals and tobacco smoke in a bacterial system. Mutation Res., 31, 328

Blacow, N.W., ed. (1972) Martindale, The Extra Pharmacopoeia, 26th ed., London, The Pharmaceutical Press, p. 564

Boyland, E., Busby, E.R., Dukes, C.E., Grover, P.L. & Manson, D. (1964) Further experiments on implantation of materials into the urinary bladder of mice. Brit. J. Cancer, 18, 575-581

Calder, I.C., Creek, M.J., Williams, P.J., Funder, C.C., Green, C.R., Ham, K.N. & Tange, J.D. (1973) N-Hydroxylation of p-acetophenetidide as a factor in nephrotoxicity. J. med. Chem., 16, 499-502

Carlson, A.J. & Brewer, N.R. (1953) Toxicity studies on hydroquinone. Proc. Soc. exp. Biol. (N.Y.), 84, 684-688

Chatterjee, P. & Sharma, A.K. (1972) Effect of phenols on nuclear division in *Chara zeylanica*. Nucleus, 15, 214-218

Clifford, M.N. & Wight, J. (1973) Metaperiodate - a new structure-specific locating reagent for phenolic compounds. J. Chromat., 86, 222-224

Commins, B.T. & Lindsey, A.J. (1956a) Determination of phenols by chromatography and spectrophotometry of their methyl ethers. III. The determination of phenols in wood smoke. Analyt. chim. acta, 15, 554-556

Commins, B.T. & Lindsey, A.J. (1956b) Determination of phenols by chromatography and spectrophotometry of their methyl ethers. IV. Determination of phenols in cigaret smoke. Analyt. chim. acta, 15, 557-558

Cooper, R.L. & Wheatstone, K.C. (1973) The determination of phenols in aqueous effluents. Water Res., 7, 1375-1384

Deichmann, W.B. & Keplinger, M.L. (1963) Phenols and phenolic compounds. In: Patty, F.A., ed., Industrial Hygiene and Toxicology, Vol. II, Toxicology, New York, Interscience, pp. 1363-1383

Grasselli, J.G., ed. (1973) CRC Atlas of Spectral Data and Physical Constants for Organic Compounds, Cleveland, Ohio, Chemical Rubber Co., p. B-229

Gupta, V.D. & Cates, L.A. (1974) Quantitative determination of resorcinol and phenol in resorcinol-phenol-boric acid solution. J. pharm. Sci., 63, 93-95

IARC (1976) IARC Monographs on the Evaluation of Carcinogenic Risk of Chemicals to Man, 11, Cadmium, Nickel, Some Epoxides, Miscellaneous Industrial Chemicals and General Considerations on Volatile Anaesthetics, Lyon, pp. 131-139

Koempe, B. (1974) A GLC-system for the identification of an unknown drug in forensic chemistry. Arch. pharm. chem. Sci., 2, 145-152

Kreshkov, A.P., Balyatinskaya, L.N., Kurchenko, T.V. & Dorofeev, A.A. (1973) Oxidation-reduction mercurimetric determination of pyrocatechol, resorcinol and hydroquinone in nonaqueous media. Zh. analit. Khim., 28, 2446-2449

Levan, A. & Tjio, J.H. (1948a) Chromosome fragmentation induced by phenols. Hereditas, 34, 250-252

Levan, A. & Tjio, J.H. (1948b) Induction of chromosome fragmentation by phenols. Hereditas, 34, 453-484

Lipkan, G.N. (1971) Determination of the acute toxicity of some preparations possessing vitamin activity. Farmakol. Toksikol. (Kiev), 6, 127-131

McCann, J., Choi, E., Yamasaki, E. & Ames, B.N. (1975) Detection of carcinogens as mutagens in the *Salmonella*/microsome test: assay of 300 chemicals. Proc. nat. Acad. Sci. (Wash.), 72, 5135-5139

Pohland, A.E. & Yang, G.C. (1972) Preparation and characterization of chlorinated dibenzo-*p*-dioxins. J. agric. Fd Chem., 20, 1093-1099

Raff, R. & Ettling, B.V. (1966) Hydroquinone, resorcinol and pyrocatechol. In: Kirk, R.E. & Othmer, D.F., eds, Encyclopedia of Chemical Technology, 2nd ed., Vol. 11, New York, John Wiley and Sons, pp. 462-492

Rennick, B. & Quebbemann, A. (1970) Site of excretion of catechol and catecholamines: renal metabolism of catechol. Amer. J. Physiol., 218, 1307-1312

Riley, H.P. & Hoff, V.J. (1960) Chromosome breakage in *Tulbaghia violacea* by radiation and chemicals. Nucleus, 3, 1-18

Roe, F.J.C. & Salaman, M.H. (1955) Further studies on incomplete carcinogenesis: triethylene melamine (T.E.M.), 1,2-benzanthracene and β-propiolactone as initiators of skin tumour formation in the mouse. Brit. J. Cancer, 9, 177-203

Roy, S.C. (1973) Comparative effects of colchicine, caffeine and hydroquinone on nodal roots of *Callisia fragrans*. Biol. plant. (Praha), 15, 383-390

Sharma, A.K. & Chatterjee, T. (1964) Effect of oxygen on chromosomal aberrations induced by hydroquinone. Nucleus, 7, 113-124

Sharma, D.N., Sharma, P.D. & Gupta, Y.K. (1976) Iodimetric determination of hydrazine and hydroquinone with thallium(III) solutions. Analyt. chim. acta, 81, 437-438

Stecher, P.G., ed. (1968) The Merck Index, 8th ed., Rahway, NJ, Merck & Co., p. 913

Stenbäck, F. & Shubik, P. (1974) Lack of toxicity and carcinogenicity of some commonly used cutaneous agents. Toxicol. appl. Pharmacol., 30, 7-13

Thielemann, H. (1969) Thin-layer chromatographic results for identification of organic pollution components of shore-filtered surface and ground water (Halle-Beesen waterworks). Z. Chem., 9, 189-190

Thielemann, H. (1975) Thin-layer chromatographic detection limits (semi-quantitative determination) of polyphenols on ready-made strips and silica gel G layers using various reagent sprays. Z. Chem., 15, 231-232

Umpelev, V.L., Kogan, L.A. & Gagarinova, L.M. (1974) Thin-layer-chromatographic separation of polyhydric phenols in effluents. Zh. analit. Khim., 29, 179-180

US Department of Commerce (1976) US Exports, Schedule B Commodity Groupings, Schedule B Commodity by Country, FT410/December 1975, Washington DC, Bureau of the Census, US Government Printing Office, p. 2-71

US International Trade Commission (1976a) Synthetic Organic Chemicals, US Production and Sales, 1974, ITC Publication 776, Washington DC, US Government Printing Office, pp. 44, 103, 208

US International Trade Commission (1976b) *Imports of Benzenoid Chemicals and Products, 1974*, ITC Publication 762, Washington DC, US Government Printing Office, pp. 20, 26, 85

US International Trade Commission (1976c) *Synthetic Organic Chemicals, US Production and Sales of Cyclic Intermediates, 1975 Preliminary*, Washington DC, US Government Printing Office, p. 4

US Occupational Safety & Health Administration (1976) Toxic and hazardous substances. *US Code of Federal Regulations*, Title 29, part 1910.1000, p. 29

US Pharmacopeial Convention, Inc. (1975) *The US Pharmacopeia*, 19th rev., Rockville, Md, pp. 440-441

US Tariff Commission (1919) *Report on Dyes and Related Coal-Tar Chemicals, 1918*, revised ed., Washington DC, US Government Printing Office, pp. 29, 43

US Tariff Commission (1921) *Census of Dyes and Coal-Tar Chemicals, 1920*, Tariff Information Series No. 23, Washington DC, US Government Printing Office, p. 30

Valadaud-Barrieu, D. & Izard, C. (1973) Modifications du cycle cellulaire sous l'influence de l'hydroquinone dans les méristèmes radiculaires de *Vicia faba*. *C.R. Acad. Sci. (Paris)*, *276*, 33-35

Van Duuren, B.L., Katz, C. & Goldschmidt, B.M. (1973) Cocarcinogenic agents in tobacco carcinogenesis. *J. nat. Cancer Inst.*, *51*, 703-705

Weast, R.C., ed. (1976) *CRC Handbook of Chemistry and Physics*, 57th ed., Cleveland, Ohio, Chemical Rubber Co., pp. C-158-C-159

Wilson, C.H. (1975) Identification of preservatives in cosmetic products by thin-layer chromatography. *J. Soc. Cosmet. Chem.*, *26*, 75-81

Windholz, M., ed. (1976) *The Merck Index*, 9th ed., Rahway, NJ, Merck & Co., pp. 635, 1037-1038

DIMETHOXANE

1. Chemical and Physical Data

1.1 Synonyms and trade names

Chem. Abstr. Services Reg. No.: 828-00-2

Chem. Abstr. Name: 2,6-Dimethyl-1,3-dioxan-4-ol acetate

Acetomethoxan; acetomethoxane; 6-acetoxy-2,4-dimethyl-*meta*-dioxane; 2,6-dimethyl-*meta*-dioxan-4-ol acetate; 2,6-dimethyl-*meta*-dioxan-4-yl acetate

Giv Gard DXN

1.2 Chemical formula and molecular weight

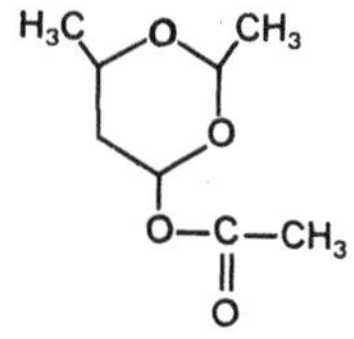

$C_8H_{14}O_4$ Mol. wt: 174.2

1.3 Chemical and physical properties of the pure substance

From Anon. (1962), unless otherwise specified

(a) Description: Light-amber liquid

(b) Freezing-point: <-25°C

(c) Boiling-point: 66°-68°C at 3 mm; 86°C at 10 mm (Windholz, 1976)

(d) Density: d_{25}^{25} 1.055-1.070

(e) Refractive index: n_D^{20} 1.4270-1.4320

(f) Solubility: Miscible with water and organic solvents

(g) Stability: Hydrolyses in aqueous solution to produce acetic acid and the corresponding free alcohol

1.4 Technical products and impurities

Dimethoxane is available in the US as a technical grade containing 93% of the pure chemical (US Environmental Protection Agency, 1973).

2. Production, Use, Occurrence and Analysis

For background information on this section, see preamble, p. 17.

2.1 Production and use

(a) Production

Dimethoxane was prepared in 1943 by the reaction of 2,4-dimethyl-6-hydroxy-*meta*-dioxane with acetic anhydride in pyridine (Späth et al., 1943). Commercial production was first reported in the US in 1962 (US Tariff Commission, 1963). Only one US company reported production of dimethoxane in 1974 (see preamble, p. 17) (US International Trade Commission, 1976).

(b) Use

Dimethoxane is an antimicrobial agent which can be used to protect against microbial spoilage due to bacteria, fungi and yeasts in a number of water-based paints and other industrial products. It can be used in water-based cutting oils, specialty textile chemical emulsions, dyestuffs, fabric softeners, latex emulsions, sizings, adhesives, antistatic lubricants and spinning emulsions at concentrations of 500-1500 mg/kg. Such concentrations are also used to prevent contamination of water-based printing inks and paints. It is also reported to be used as a petrol additive (Windholz, 1976). Dimethoxane was recommended for use in cosmetics in the past.

In the US, dimethoxane is registered as an antimicrobial agent 'for manufacturing use only' (US Environmental Protection Agency, 1973).

2.2 Occurrence

Dimethoxane is not known to occur in nature.

2.3 Analysis

No data were available to the Working Group.

3. Biological Data Relevant to the Evaluation of Carcinogenic Risk to Man

3.1 Carcinogenicity and related studies in animals

Oral administration

Rat: A group of 25 male Wistar rats (120-180 g bw) were given a 1% solution of dimethoxane in the drinking-water daily for 613 days, to give an average total dose of 237 g/animal. The solution was prepared daily by redistilling commercial dimethoxane and using the main fraction, which boiled at 86-87°C at 10 mm. The animals were given Terramycin® in the drinking-water for 1 week before the start of the experiment. All survivors were killed and autopsied 90 days after the end of treatment (703 days). Malignant tumours developed in 14/25 rats: 8 hepatomas, resembling in structure those produced by nitrosamine derivatives, 2 lymphosarcomas, 1 transitional-cell carcinoma of the kidney, 1 leukaemia, 1 epidermoid carcinoma of the neck and 1 subcutaneous fibrosarcoma. One lymphosarcoma was detected among the 14 controls, which had received Terramycin® only (Hoch-Ligeti et al., 1974).

3.2 Other relevant biological data

No data were available to the Working Group.

3.3 Case reports and epidemiological studies

No data were available to the Working Group.

4. Comments on Data Reported and Evaluation[1]

4.1 Animal data

Dimethoxane is carcinogenic in male rats after its oral administration, the only species, sex and route tested; it produced malignant tumours, predominantly in the liver.

---

[1] See also the section, 'Animal Data in Relation to the Evaluation of Risk to Man' in the introduction to this volume, p. 15.

4.2 **Human data**

No case reports or epidemiological studies were available to the Working Group.

5. References

Anon. (1962) Dimethoxane, a new preservative effective with nonionic agents. Amer. Perfum. Cosmet., 77, 32-34

Hoch-Ligeti, C., Argus, M.F. & Arcos, J.C. (1974) Oncogenic activity of an m-dioxane derivative: 2,6-dimethyl-m-dioxan-4-ol acetate (dimethoxane). J. nat. Cancer Inst., 53, 791-794

Späth, E., Lorenz, R. & Freund, E. (1943) Derivatives of aldol and of crotonaldehyde. V. An addition product of acetaldehyde with acetaldol. Ber. dtsch. chem. Ges., 76B, 57-68

US Environmental Protection Agency (1973) EPA Compendium of Registered Pesticides, Vol. II, Fungicides and Nematicides, Part I, Washington DC, US Government Printing Office, p. D-15-00.01

US International Trade Commission (1976) Synthetic Organic Chemicals, US Production and Sales, 1974, ITC Publication 776, Washington DC, US Government Printing Office, p. 205

US Tariff Commission (1963) Synthetic Organic Chemicals, US Production and Sales, 1962, TC Publication 114, Washington DC, US Government Printing Office, p. 173

Windholz, M., ed. (1976) The Merck Index, 9th ed., Rahway, NJ, Merck & Co., p. 428

EOSIN AND EOSIN DISODIUM SALT

1. Chemical and Physical Data

Eosin

1.1 Synonyms and trade names

Chem. Abstr. Services Reg. No.: 15086-94-9

Chem Abstr. Name: 2',4',5',7'-Tetrabromo-3',6'-dihydroxy-spiro[isobenzofuran-1(3H),9'-(9H)-xanthen]-3-one

Bromeosin; bromoeosin; bromofluoresceic acid; C.I. 45380:2; C.I. Solvent Red 43; D and C Red No. 21; eosine; 2,4,5,7-tetrabromo-3,6-fluorandiol; tetrabromofluorescein; 2',4',5',7'-tetrabromofluorescein

Eosine Acid; Red 11731

1.2 Chemical formula and molecular weight

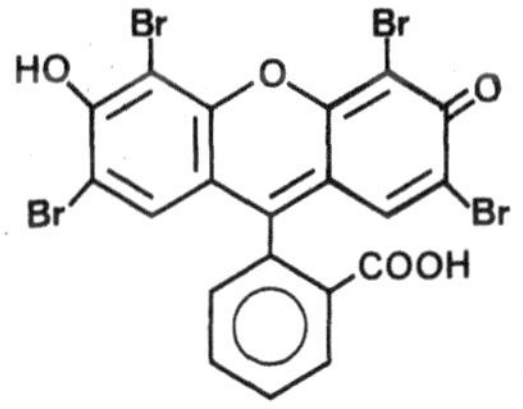

Quinonoid form $C_{20}H_8Br_4O_5$ Mol. wt: 647.9

1.3 Chemical and physical properties of the pure substance

From Weast (1976)

(a) Description: Yellow-red crystals

(b) Melting-point: 295-296°C

(c) Spectroscopy data: λ_{max} 520 (E_1^1 = 1942.8)

(d) Solubility: Insoluble in water and ether; soluble in ethanol

1.4 Technical products and impurities

The drug and cosmetic grade of eosin used in the US contains maximums of 2 mg/kg lead, 0.2 mg/kg arsenic, 3 mg/kg other heavy metals, 6.0% volatile matter (at 135°C), 1.0% insoluble matter (alkaline solution), 0.5% ether extracts (from alkaline solutions), 2.0% sodium chlorides and sulphates, 1.0% mixed oxides and 0.02% free bromine. It must contain a minimum of 93.0% of the pure dye (determined gravimetrically) (US Food and Drug Administration, 1976).

Eosin disodium salt

1.1 Synonyms and trade names

Chem. Abstr. Services Reg. No.: 17372-87-1

Chem. Abstr. Name: 2',4',5',7'-Tetrabromo-3',6'-dihydroxy-spiro[isobenzofuran-1(3H),9'-(9H)xanthen]-3-one, disodium salt

Bromo acid; bromoeosine; bromofluoresceic acid; bromo fluorescein; bromofluorescein; C.I. 45380; C.I. Acid Red 87; D and C Red No. 22; disodium eosin; disodium salt of 2,4,5,7-tetrabromo-9-*ortho*-carboxyphenyl-6-hydroxy-3-isoxanthone; eosin; eosine; eosine sodium salt; sodium eosinate; sodium eosine; 2,4,5,7-tetrabromo-3,6-fluorandiol; tetrabromofluorescein; 2',4',5',7'-tetrabromofluorescein, sodium salt; 2-(2,4,5,7-tetrabromo-6-hydroxy-3-oxo-3H-xanthene-9-yl)benzoic acid, disodium salt

Aizen Eosine GH; Bromo Acid J; Bromo Acid XL; Bromo B; Bromo 4D; Bromo 4DC; Bromo 4DL; Bromo FL; Bromo JPS; Bromo TS; Bromo X-100; Bromo XX; Bronze Bromo; Bronze Bromo ES; Certiqual Eosine; Cogilor Orange 212.00, 212.10, 212.42; D and C Red No. 23; Eosin Y; Eosin YS; Eosine; Eosine A; Eosine B; Eosine BPC; Eosine BS; Eosine BS-SF; Eosine DA; Eosine DH; Eosine DWC 73; Eosine Extra Conc. A Export; Eosine FA; Eosine G; Eosine 3G; Eosine GF; Eosine GGF; Eosine J; Eosine JSF; Eosine K Salt Free; Eosine L; Eosine Lake Red Y; Eosine OJ; Eosine S13; Eosine S extra; Eosine Salt Free; Eosine w/s; Eosine Y; Eosine 3Y; Eosine YB; Eosine Yellowish; Eosine YS; Eosine YY; Fenazo Eosine XG; Food Red No. 103;

Hidacid Boiling Bromo; Hidacid Bromo Acid Regular; Hidacid Dibromo Fluorescein; Hidacid Eosine Soda Salt; Hidacid White Bromo; Irgalite Bronze Red CL; Phloxine Red 20-7600; Phloxine Toner B; Phlox Red Toner X-1354; Pure Eosine YY; 11445 Red; 11731 Red; Symuler Eosin Toner; Tetrabromofluorescein D; Tetrabromofluorescein S; Tetrabromofluorescein soluble; Toyo Eosine G; 1903 Yellow Pink

1.2 Chemical formula and molecular weight

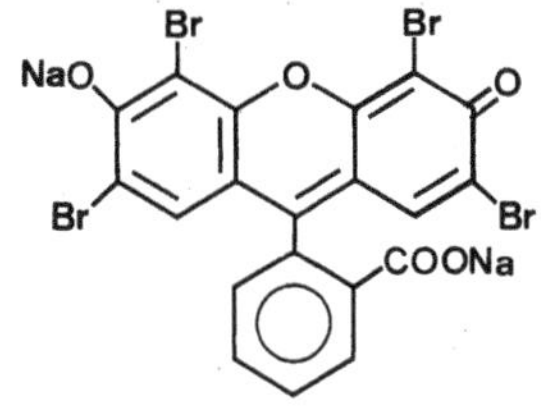

$C_{20}H_6Br_4Na_2O_5$ Mol. wt: 691.9

1.3 Chemical and physical properties of the decahydrate

From Weast (1976)

(a) Description: Red needles

(b) Spectroscopy data: λ_{max} 519 (E_1^1 = 1174.6); infra-red spectral data have been tabulated by Grasselli (1973).

(c) Solubility: Soluble in water and ethanol; insoluble in ether

1.4 Technical products and impurities

Eosin disodium salt is available in the US in reagent and indicator grades. The drug and cosmetic grade of eosin disodium salt used in the US contains maximums of 2 mg/kg lead, 0.2 mg/kg arsenic, 3 mg/kg other heavy metals, 10.0% volatile matter (at 135°C), 1.0% water-insoluble matter, 0.5% ether extracts, 5.0% sodium chlorides and sulphates, 1.0% mixed oxides and 0.02% free bromine. It must contain a minimum of 85.0% of the pure dye (determined gravimetrically) (US Food and Drug Administration, 1976).

2. Production, Use, Occurrence and Analysis

For background information on this section, see preamble, p. 17.

2.1 Production and use

(a) Production

Eosin was prepared in 1871 by Caro (Society of Dyers and Colourists, 1971a). One of the first reported methods for its preparation, carried out by Baeyer in 1876, involved the reaction of bromine with fluorescein in acetic acid or ethanol (Prager & Jacobson, 1934). It is still produced today by the bromination of fluorescein in aqueous or ethanolic solution and may be converted to the disodium salt with sodium hydroxide (Society of Dyers and Colourists, 1971a).

Eosin and eosin disodium salt have been produced commercially in the US for over 50 years (US Tariff Commission, 1919). In 1974, only two US companies reported production of eosin, and two other companies reported production of eosin disodium salt (see preamble, p. 17) (US International Trade Commission, 1976). In 1973, the latest year for which data are available, US imports of eosin disodium salt through the principal customs districts were reported to be about 160 kg (US Tariff Commission, 1974).

About 100 thousand to 1 million kg eosin are produced annually in Switzerland. Eosin disodium salt is reported to be produced in the Federal Republic of Germany, France, Italy, Switzerland and the UK.

In Japan, eosin is produced in negligible quantities by the acid treatment of eosin disodium salt. Eosin disodium salt has been produced commercially in Japan since 1944, and in 1975, four companies produced a combined total of 8.4 million kg.

(b) Use

Eosin is used as an intermediate in the production of eosin disodium salt and as a dye in cosmetics (Society of Dyers and Colourists, 1971b), such as lipsticks, rouges and face powders and talcums (Zuckerman, 1964); it is also used as an adsorption indicator in the titration of bromide or iodide ions with silver nitrate (Matsuyama, 1966).

Eosin disodium salt is used as a dye or as an intermediate in the production of red lakes and toners (Cesark, 1970) used in printing (Dunn et al., 1966).

It is used as a dye for fibres such as wool, nylon and silk, to dye paper, in inks, coloured pencils and in wood stains (Society of Dyers and Colourists, 1971c), in aqueous drug solutions and capsules, in soaps (Zuckerman, 1964), in lipsticks and nail polishes (Windholz, 1976), and also as a biological stain (Stenger & Atchison, 1964).

Eosin and eosin disodium salt are both certified as drug and cosmetic colours in the US and must meet the specifications (see sections 1.4) promulgated by law (US Food and Drug Administration, 1976).

2.2 Occurrence

Neither eosin nor eosin disodium salt is known to occur in nature.

2.3 Analysis

The Association of Official Analytical Chemists has published gravimetric and spectrophotometric methods of analysis for eosin and its disodium salt to be used in batch certification to meet specifications as defined by the US Food and Drug Administration (Horwitz, 1975).

Thin-layer chromatography has been used to determine variations in purity of batches of commercial dyes, including eosin and its disodium salt, employed for Romanowsky-type staining (Marshall & Lewis, 1974).

Polarography has been studied for use in determination of eosin in concentrations of 10^{-4}-10^{-3} M (Mizunoya & Omori, 1971).

In a method for determining various substances, including eosin disodium salt, the chemiluminescence produced by contact of the sample with a stream of ozone is measured; it has a sensitivity of 0.4 ng (Bowman & Alexander, 1966).

Separation on a liquid anion exchanger, followed by a colorimetric determination, has been used to analyse foods for various dyes, including eosin disodium salt (Tonogai, 1973).

A method has been described in which 20 water-soluble dyes, including eosin, were isolated from food products by means of DEAE-Sephadex adsorbent gel and detected by thin-layer chromatography on polyamide plates (Takeshita *et al.*, 1972). Thin-layer chromatography has also been used to identify eosin disodium salt in sweets after preliminary adsorption on bakers' yeast and extraction with ammonium hydroxide (Onozaki & Minami, 1971). Thin-layer and paper chromatography have been used to identify lipstick dyes, including eosin (Camacho & Duarte, 1971).

3. Biological Data Relevant to the Evaluation of Carcinogenic Risk to Man

3.1 Carcinogenicity and related studies in animals

(a) Oral administration

Rat: Ten male and 10 female Wistar rats, 45 days old, received 0.5 g eosin in the diet daily for 654 days. The maximum total dose was 304.5 g/animal, and the median survival times were 469 days for males and 778 days for females. The observation period was up to 829 days. One female rat developed a mammary fibrosarcoma. Among 10 female controls, one animal had a fibrosarcoma of the stomach (Hiller, 1962).

(b) Subcutaneous and/or intramuscular administration

Rat: Twenty male and female albino rats of a mixed strain (Saitama), weighing 200 g, were given weekly s.c. injections of 2 ml of a 5% solution of eosin disodium salt in water; from week 14, weekly s.c. injections of 1 ml of the same solution were given. The duration of the experiment was 671 days. One rat developed a cysticercus sarcoma of the liver, and two others developed mammary fibroadenomas. Two rats that received total doses of 2.8 and 3.65 g, that died on the 543rd and 671st days, respectively, developed sarcomas at the injection site. One of these animals also had a mammary fibroadenoma (Umeda, 1955, 1956) [The Working Group noted the small number of surviving animals and the absence of controls].

Ten male and 10 female Wistar rats, 45 days of age at the start of treatment, were given twice weekly s.c. injections of 1 ml of a solution of eosin in saline (11 mg eosin/injection) for 590 days (males) or 618 days (females). The maximum total amounts administered were 1.32 g (males) and 1.21 g (females) per animal. The median survival times were 770 days (males) and 465 days (females), and the observation period was up to 830 days. One female rat developed a mammary fibroadenoma. In the control groups, one female rat had a mammary fibrosarcoma (Hiller, 1962).

3.2 Other relevant biological data

(a) Experimental systems

The lowest lethal dose for eosin disodium salt given by i.p. or s.c. administration to rats was 500 or 1500 mg/kg bw, respectively (NIOSH, 1976).

Intravenously administered eosin was excreted unchanged in rats, with 50-70% in the bile and 2-6% in the urine (Webb et al., 1962). Similar results were obtained with eosin disodium salt (Iga et al., 1971). After an oral dose of 500 mg/kg bw, 94% was recovered as unchanged eosin in the urine and faeces (Webb et al., 1962).

Eosin disodium salt binds non-covalently to proteins to form protein-dye complexes (Gangolli et al., 1972).

No data on embryotoxicity or teratogenicity were available to the Working Group.

In the rec assay, which is believed to give an indication of reparable DNA damage, eosin disodium salt was not more toxic to *Bacillus subtilis* M45 (rec^-) than to H17 (rec^+), suggesting that this compound does not damage DNA (Kada, 1973).

(b) Man

No data were available to the Working Group.

3.3 Case reports and epidemiological studies

No data were available to the Working Group.

4. Comments on Data Reported and Evaluation

4.1 Animal data

Eosin has been tested only in rats by oral and subcutaneous administration, and eosin disodium salt has been administered to rats by subcutaneous injection; the data are insufficient for an evaluation of carcinogenicity of these compounds to be made.

4.2 Human data

No case reports or epidemiological studies were available to the Working Group.

5. References

Bowman, R.L. & Alexander, N. (1966) Ozone-induced chemiluminescence of organic compounds. Science, 154, 1454-1456

Camacho, I. & Duarte, M.I. (1971) Identification of dyes used in lipstick in Columbia. Rev. Colomb. Cienc. Quim.-Farm., 1, 5-32

Cesark, F.F. (1970) Xanthene dyes. In: Kirk, R.E. & Othmer, D.F., eds, Encyclopedia of Chemical Technology, 2nd ed., Vol. 22, New York, John Wiley and Sons, pp. 430-437

Dunn, H., Burachinsky, B.V., Ely, J.K. & Greubel, P.W. (1966) Inks. In: Kirk, R.E. & Othmer, D.F., eds, Encyclopedia of Chemical Technology, 2nd ed., Vol. 11, New York, John Wiley and Sons, p. 615

Gangolli, S.D., Grasso, P., Golberg, L. & Hooson, J. (1972) Protein binding by food colourings in relation to the production of subcutaneous sarcoma. Fd Cosmet. Toxicol., 10, 449-462

Grasselli, J.G., ed. (1973) CRC Atlas of Spectral Data and Physical Constants for Organic Compounds, Cleveland, Ohio, Chemical Rubber Co., p. B-493

Hiller, F.K. (1962) Prüfung des Tetrabromfluoresceins (Eosinsäure) auf Verträglichkeit und Cancerogenität. Arzneimittel-Forsch., 12, 587-588

Horwitz, W., ed. (1975) Official Methods of Analysis of the Association of Official Analytical Chemists, 12th ed., Washington DC, Association of Official Analytical Chemists, pp. 629-638

Iga, T., Awazu, S. & Nogami, H. (1971) Pharmacokinetic study of biliary excretion. III. Comparison of excretion behavior in xanthene dyes, fluorescein and bromsulphthalein. Chem. pharm. Bull., 19, 297-308

Kada, T. (1973) Mutagenicity testing of chemicals in microbial systems. In: Coulston, F. et al., eds, New Methods in Environmental Chemistry and Toxicology, Tokyo, Academic Scientific Books, pp. 127-133

Marshall, P.N. & Lewis, S.M. (1974) Batch variations in commercial dyes employed for Romanowsky-type staining: thin-layer chromatographic study. Stain Technol., 49, 351-358

Matsuyama, G. (1966) Indicators. In: Kirk, R.E. & Othmer, D.F., eds, Encyclopedia of Chemical Technology, 2nd ed., Vol. 11, New York, John Wiley and Sons, p. 558

Mizunoya, Y. & Omori, M. (1971) Polarography of coal tar food colors. II. Polarographic study of eosine and phloxine. Bunseki Kagaku, 20, 1172-1177

NIOSH (National Institute for Occupational Safety and Health) (1976) Registry of Toxic Effects of Chemical Substances, Rockville, Md, US Department of Health, Education and Welfare, p. 542

Onozaki, H. & Minami, K. (1971) Separate determinations of coal-tar dyes in candies by use of bakers' yeasts as an adsorbent. Nippon Shokuhin Kogyo Gakkai-Shi, 18, 346-350

Prager, B. & Jacobson, P., eds (1934) Beilsteins Handbuch der Organischen Chemie, 4th ed., Vol. 19, Syst. 2835, Berlin, Springer-Verlag, p. 228

The Society of Dyers and Colourists (1971a) Colour Index, 3rd ed., Vol. 4, Bradford, Yorks, p. 4426

The Society of Dyers and Colourists (1971b) Colour Index, 3rd ed., Vol. 3, Bradford, Yorks, pp. 3596-3597

The Society of Dyers and Colourists (1971c) Colour Index, 3rd ed., Vol. 1, Bradford, Yorks, p. 1153

Stenger, V.A. & Atchison, G.J. (1964) Bromine compounds. In: Kirk, R.E. & Othmer, D.F., eds, Encyclopedia of Chemical Technology, 2nd ed., Vol. 3, New York, John Wiley and Sons, p. 775

Takeshita, R., Yamashita, T. & Itoh, N. (1972) Separation and detection of water-soluble acid dyes on polyamide thin layers. J. Chromat., 73, 173-182

Tonogai, Y. (1973) Analysis of food additives. I. Determination of coal tar dyes in foods with liquid anion exchangers. Eisei Kagaku, 19, 231-235

Umeda, M. (1955) Rat sarcoma produced by the injection of eosine yellowish. Gann, 46, 367-368

Umeda, M. (1956) Experimental study of xanthene dyes as carcinogenic agents. Gann, 47, 51-78

US Food & Drug Administration (1976) Food and drugs. US Code of Federal Regulations, Title 21, part 9, pp. 171, 173, 175

US International Trade Commission (1976) Synthetic Organic Chemicals, US Production and Sales, 1974, ITC Publication 776, Washington DC, US Government Printing Office, pp. 61, 76

US Tariff Commission (1919) Part I. The Census of Dyes and Coal-Tar Chemicals, 1918, revised ed., Washington DC, US Government Printing Office

US Tariff Commission (1974) Imports of Benzenoid Chemicals and Products, 1973, TC Publication 688, Washington DC, US Government Printing Office, p. 37

Weast, R.C., ed. (1976) CRC Handbook of Chemistry and Physics, 57th ed., Cleveland, Ohio, Chemical Rubber Co., p. C-284

Webb, J.M., Fonda, M. & Brouwer, E.A. (1962) Metabolism and excretion patterns of fluorescein and certain halogenated fluorescein dyes in rats. J. Pharmacol. exp. Ther., 137, 141-147

Windholz, M., ed. (1976) The Merck Index, 9th ed., Rahway, NJ, Merck & Co., p. 471

Zuckerman, S. (1964) Colors for foods, drugs, and cosmetics. In: Kirk, R.E. & Othmer, D.F., eds, Encyclopedia of Chemical Technology, 2nd ed., Vol. 5, New York, John Wiley and Sons, pp. 865, 870, 872

ETHYLENE DIBROMIDE

1. Chemical and Physical Data

1.1 Synonyms and trade names

Chem. Abstr. Services Reg. No.: 106-93-4

Chem. Abstr. Name: 1,2-Dibromoethane

α,β-Dibromoethane; sym-dibromoethane; EDB; ethylene bromide; glycol bromide

Aadibrom; Dowfume W 85; Dowfume W-8; Iscobrome D; Nefis; Sanhyuum; Soilfume

1.2 Chemical formula and molecular weight

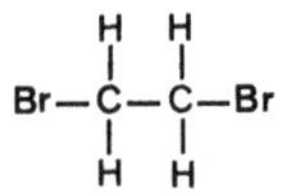

$$\text{Br}-\underset{\underset{H}{|}}{\overset{\overset{H}{|}}{C}}-\underset{\underset{H}{|}}{\overset{\overset{H}{|}}{C}}-\text{Br}$$

$C_2H_4Br_2$ Mol. wt: 187.9

1.3 Chemical and physical properties of the pure substance

From Spencer (1973), unless otherwise specified

(a) *Description*: Colourless liquid

(b) *Boiling-point*: 131.6°C

(c) *Melting-point*: 9.97°C

(d) *Density*: d_{25}^{25} 2.172

(e) *Refractive index*: n_D^{20} 1.53789

(f) *Spectroscopy data*: Infra-red, nuclear magnetic resonance and mass spectra have been tabulated by Grasselli (1973).

(g) *Solubility*: Slightly soluble in water (0.43 g/100 ml at 30°C); soluble in ethanol, ether and most organic solvents

(h) _Volatility_: Vapour pressure is 11 mm at 25°C.

(i) _Stability_: Turns brown on exposure to light

(j) _Reactivity_: Reacts as an alkylating agent, liberating bromide

1.4 _Technical products and impurities_

Ethylene dibromide is available in the US in tank-car and drum quantities (Anon., 1976a). Typical specifications are: d_{25}^{25} 2.165-2.185 and boiling range, such that the 5-95% fraction boils within a 2°C range, which includes 131.5°C (Spencer, 1973).

2. Production, Use, Occurrence and Analysis

For background information on this section, see preamble, p. 17.

2.1 _Production and use_

(a) Production

Ethylene dibromide was first made by Balard in 1826 by the reaction of ethylene with bromine (Prager & Jacobson, 1918) and this is the method currently used for its commercial production.

Production of ethylene dibromide was first reported in the US in 1923 (US Tariff Commission, 1924). In 1974, five US companies reported production of 150 million kg (US International Trade Commission, 1976), and imports were reported to be 1770 kg (US Department of Commerce, 1975); it has been estimated that 45 million kg were exported in 1973.

Ethylene dibromide is currently produced in the Benelux, France, Italy, Spain, Switzerland and the UK, and production in these countries has been estimated to be about 3-30 million kg annually. Another estimate of European production for 1974 was 40 million kg.

Ethylene dibromide was first produced commercially in Japan in 1960. In 1975, 1.4 million kg were produced by two companies, and 667 thousand kg were imported (Muto, 1976).

About 180,000 kg were imported into Australia in 1975-76.

(b) Use

The major uses of ethylene dibromide are as a lead scavenger in tetraalkyl lead petrol and antiknock preparations, as a soil and grain fumigant, as an intermediate in the synthesis of dyes and pharmaceuticals and as a solvent for resins, gums and waxes.

In 1974, approximately 97 million kg ethylene dibromide were formulated into tetraalkyl lead antiknock mixes in the US. Motor fuel antiknock mixes contain approximately 18% by weight ethylene dibromide (2.8 g/l), and aviation petrol antiknock mixes contain about 36% by weight. Its use in the US in these mixes has been declining since the early 1970's, in parallel with the decreased use of tetraalkyl lead (Anon., 1976b).

Use of ethylene dibromide as a fumigant was first reported in 1925 by Neifert (Spencer, 1973). In the US, it is registered for use as a soil fumigant on a variety of vegetable, fruit and grain crops (US Environmental Protection Agency, 1970). In 1971, an estimated 485 thousand kg were used by US farmers. In California in 1974, 106 thousand kg were used for insecticidal purposes (California Department of Food and Agriculture, 1975).

Tolerances for residues of inorganic bromides in or on raw agricultural commodities grown in soil treated with ethylene dibromide have been established at 10-50 mg/kg (US Environmental Protection Agency, 1976a); however, "The organic bromide residues are exempted from the requirement of a tolerance for residues when the insecticide ethylene dibromide is used as a fumigant after harvest for the following grains: barley, corn, oats, popcorn, rice, rye, sorghum (milo), and wheat" (US Environmental Protection Agency, 1976b).

Two notices of rebuttable presumption against registration are scheduled to be issued in 1977 (see 'General Remarks on Substances Considered', p. 28). One would affect its use as a grain fumigant and the other its use as a soil fungicide.

No acceptable daily intake for man was established for ethylene dibromide at the 1971 Joint Meeting of the FAO Working Party of Experts on Pesticide Residues and the WHO Expert Committee on Pesticide Residues (WHO, 1972).

The US Occupational Safety and Health Administration health standards for air contaminants require that an employee's exposure to ethylene dibromide shall not exceed an 8-hour time-weighted average of 150 mg/m^3 (20 ppm) in any 8-hour workshift of a 40-hour work week. The employee's exposure to ethylene dibromide "shall not exceed an acceptable ceiling concentration of 30 ppm [230 mg/m^3] except for a time period of 5 minutes and up to concentrations not exceeding 50 ppm [380 mg/m^3] (US Occupational Safety and Health Administration, 1976). An earlier threshold limit recommended by the American Conference of Governmental Industrial Hygienists was 190 mg/m^3 (25 ppm) (ILO, 1971).

In Australia, the time-weighted average concentration in the working atmosphere must not exceed 145 mg/m^3.

2.2 <u>Occurrence</u>

Ethylene dibromide is generally present in air in the US, according to the Environmental Protection Agency. Levels near groups of petrol stations and along well-travelled highways were around 11 µg/m^3 (Going & Long, 1975). Ethylene dibromide was found in concentrations of up to 96 µg/m^3 up to a mile away from a US Department of Agriculture fumigation centre (Newman, 1976).

When apples were fumigated with 12 or 24 mg/l ethylene dibromide at 13°C for 4 hours and stored at this temperature, the residues after one day were 36 and 75 mg/kg, which decreased after 6 days to 1.2 and 1.6 mg/kg (Dumas, 1973).

2.3 <u>Analysis</u>

An extensive review of analytical methods for the determination of ethylene dibromide and other fumigants in air and fumigated products has been published (Malone, 1971). Methods include determination of inorganic bromide after hydrolysis, X-ray fluorescence, electron and neutron activation techniques and gas chromatography. Reproducibility and limits of detection are given when available. The review also includes a discussion of methods of extraction and limitations in the determination of inorganic bromide.

Initially, analysis for residues on products fumigated with ethylene dibromide was based on the determination of total bromide, but this proved to be inadequate. More recently, both inorganic bromide and unreacted ethylene dibromide have been determined. Gas chromatography is the procedure most commonly used for determining unreacted ethylene dibromide (WHO, 1972).

The International Union of Pure and Applied Chemistry (IUPAC) has recognized a method for determining inorganic bromide by its reaction with ethylene oxide to form ethylene bromohydrin, followed by gas chromatography and electron capture; the method has a sensitivity of 0.5 mg/kg. Any residual ethylene dibromide remains intact and can be determined simultaneously if desired (Heuser & Scudamore, 1970).

Gas chromatography has been adopted by the Association of Official Analytical Chemists as the method of preference for the analysis of ethylene dibromide fumigant formulations (Horwitz, 1975).

A method using gas chromatography has been recommended by the US National Institute for Occupational Safety and Health for measuring concentrations of 110-470 mg/m^3 (±10%) ethylene dibromide in the working atmossphere; it involves adsorption on charcoal and subsequent extraction with carbon disulphide (NIOSH, 1975).

IUPAC (Abbott, 1970) has reviewed methods of analysis for fumigants and has evaluated the multidetection scheme of Heuser & Scudamore (1969). This was found to be reliable for the determination of the volatile residues of 17 fumigants, including ethylene dibromide. The method involves solvent extraction and gas chromatography with detection by flame ionization, electron capture or β-ionization.

Gas chromatography coupled with electron capture detection has also been used to determine ethylene dibromide in petrol, with an accuracy of ±3 mg/l at the 30 mg/l level (Perry, 1966), and in soils, with a sensitivity of 50 µg/kg (Tagawa & Tomaru, 1969).

A method involving steam distillation of ethylene dibromide residues on vegetables followed by extraction into toluene and X-ray fluorescence determination has a limit of detection of 0.2 mg/kg for a 100 g sample (Hargreaves et al., 1974).

Residual fumigant can be extracted from food samples by several methods, which were compared and reviewed by Malone (1969). One of these, which involved distillation from an acidified medium, has been further modified to provide a sensitivity level of 0.3 mg/kg (Malone, 1970).

The US Food and Drug Administration has recommended measurement of partition coefficients in several solvent systems, in conjunction with gas chromatographic retention times, in the identification of pesticide residues. Partition coefficients of ethylene dibromide and other pesticides are tabulated in the Pesticide Analytical Manual (US Food and Drug Administration, 1975).

3. Biological Data Relevant to the Evaluation of Carcinogenic Risk to Man

3.1 Carcinogenicity and related studies in animals[1]

Oral administration

Mouse: In a report of a study in progress, two groups of 50 male and 50 female (C57BlxC3H)F_1 mice had received ethylene dibromide (at least 96% pure) in corn oil by gavage 5 times per week for 42 weeks. The initial dose levels were 60 and 120 mg/kg bw/day, which were increased to 100 and 200 mg/kg bw between weeks 13 and 15. At week 15, the initial dose levels were again given, and at 42 weeks the dose level was adjusted to 60 mg/kg bw for all mice. By this time, 2/42 mice that had died following treatment with the high dose or had been killed, and 5/12 that had died or been killed following treatment with the low dose had developed squamous-cell carcinomas of the forestomach. No tumours were found in 20 male and 20 female controls (Olson et al., 1973). In a later report it was stated that such tumours

---

[1] The Working Group was aware of carcinogenicity studies in progress in rats involving oral administration, in mice with i.p. injection and in mice and rats with intragastric administration and exposure by inhalation (IARC, 1976).

developed in over 70% of treated animals after 62 weeks. The tumours were invasive and metastasized (Powers et al., 1975).

Rat: In a report of a study in progress, two groups of 50 male and 50 female Osborne-Mendel rats had received ethylene dibromide (at least 96% pure) dissolved in corn oil by gavage 5 times weekly for 54 weeks at two dose levels, originally 40 and 80 mg/kg bw/day. After 16 weeks, the higher dose level was discontinued for 14 weeks due to toxic effects, while administration of the lower dose was continued without interruption. From week 30 all rats received 40 mg/kg bw/day. At the time of reporting (54 weeks), 45/91 rats that had died or been killed following treatment with the higher dose and 73/91 that had died or been killed following treatment with the lower dose had developed squamous-cell carcinomas of the forestomach; the first tumour was found in a rat killed after 10 weeks of treatment. Among 20 male and 20 female controls, one mammary adenoma was observed in a female (Olson et al., 1973). In a later report, it was stated that more than 90% of treated rats developed such tumours after 62 weeks. The tumours were invasive and metastasized (Powers et al., 1975).

3.2 Other relevant biological data

(a) Experimental systems

The acute oral LD_{50} of ethylene dibromide is 110 mg/kg bw for guinea-pigs, 146 mg/kg bw for male rats, 117 mg/kg bw for female rats and 420 mg/kg bw for female mice (Rowe et al., 1952).

In the carcinogenicity experiments described above, rats tolerated daily doses of 40 mg/kg bw, and mice, 60 mg/kg bw, given 5 times weekly for up to 62 weeks; however, with doses of 80 and 100 mg/kg bw, rats and mice, respectively, developed toxic symptoms (Olson et al., 1973).

Rats tolerated exposure to 190 mg/m^3 (25 ppm) ethylene dibromide in air over 7 hours per day for 151 days, but 63 similar exposures to levels of 380 mg/m^3 (50 ppm) were lethal to 20-50% of animals. Deaths occurring from acute exposure to higher concentrations were usually due to lung congestion and haemorrhage, although liver and kidney damage, as well as corneal injury, were also observed. In rabbits, contact dermatitis was seen also (Rowe et al., 1952).

Ethylene dibromide given intraperitoneally at a dose of 10 mg/kg on 5 successive days to rats damaged spermatogenic cells; the effect was reversible (Edwards et al., 1970). Two to three weeks after the start of oral treatment of bulls with 4 mg/kg bw ethylene dibromide on alternate days, abnormal spermatozoa were observed, indicating an interference with spermatogenesis and with the maturation of spermatozoa in the epididymis (Amir, 1973); doses of 2 mg/kg bw/day had no effect on the reproductive capacity of cows and ewes (Alumot, 1972).

Adult hens maintained on feed containing 50-320 mg/kg ethylene dibromide laid smaller eggs; after 6 weeks on the diet containing the highest dose, egg laying ceased irreversibly (Bondi et al., 1955).

After i.p. administration of ^{14}C-ethylene dibromide to guinea-pigs (30 mg/kg), the greatest concentration of ^{14}C was found in those tissues in which pathological changes have been reported (kidneys, liver and adrenals). Sixty-five per cent of the dose was excreted as metabolites in the urine and 12% unchanged in the expired air (Plotnick & Conner, 1976).

Twenty-four hours after i.p. administration of 40 mg/kg bw ^{14}C-ethylene dibromide to mice, 40% was excreted as metabolites in the urine, and 15% could be accounted for in the body tissues, including 6% in the blood. The highest activity per gram of tissue, excepting the blood, was found in the kidney and stomach (including contents) (Edwards et al., 1970). The urinary metabolites in rats and mice after oral administration of ethylene dibromide were identified as *S*-(2-hydroxyethyl)cysteine and *N*-acetyl-*S*-(2-hydroxyethyl)cysteine; *N*-acetyl-*S*-(2-hydroxyethyl)cysteine-*S*-oxide was also identified after i.p. administration of the chemical (Edwards et al., 1970; Jones & Edwards, 1968).

Enzymic reaction with glutathione occurred *in vivo* and *in vitro* (Nachtomi, 1970). Glutathione levels were depleted in the liver after administration of toxic levels of ethylene dibromide. Further metabolism of the glutathione conjugate to *S*-(2-hydroxyethyl)cysteine and its sulphoxide occurred in the kidney (Nachtomi, 1970).

The antifertility effects of ethylene dibromide have been attributed to a direct alkylating effect of its primary metabolite, the glutathione conjugate of bromoethane, which is a more reactive alkylating agent than ethylene dibromide (Edwards et al., 1970).

No data on embryotoxicity or teratogenicity were available to the Working Group.

In the absence of a metabolic activation system, ethylene dibromide induced base-pair substitution reverse mutations in plate assays with *Salmonella typhimurium* G46, TA1530, TA1535 and TA100 (Ames, 1971; Brem et al., 1974; Buselmaier et al., 1972, 1973; McCann et al., 1975). It was positive in a host-mediated assay in mice (500 mg/kg, s.c.) with *S. typhimurium* G46 (Buselmaier et al., 1972). It did not increase deletion mutations in *S. typhimurium* gal E503 in a spot test (Alper & Ames, 1975). In a reverse mutation assay system with *Serratia marcescens* a21, ethylene dibromide was mutagenic neither in plate assays nor in the host-mediated assay in mice (Buselmaier et al., 1972). In the polymerase assay, which is believed to give an indication of reparable DNA damage, ethylene dibromide was more toxic to *Escherichia coli* p3478 ($polA_1^-$) than to *E. coli* W3110 ($polA^+$), suggesting that this compound can damage DNA (Brem et al., 1974).

Ethylene dibromide induced recessive lethal mutations in the ad-3 region of a two-component heterokaryon of *Neurospora crassa* (Malling, 1969; de Serres & Malling, 1970) and somatic visible mutations in mutable clones of *Tradescantia* (Nauman et al., 1974, 1975, 1976; Sparrow & Schairer, 1974, 1975; Sparrow et al., 1974; Villalobos-Pietrini et al., 1974).

It caused no chromosome breaking effects in *Allium* roots or in cultured human lymphocytes (Kristoffersson, 1974).

Treatment of 2-day old adult male *Drosophila melanogaster* for 3 days with 0.3 mM ethylene dibromide resulted in significant increases in the number of X-chromosomal recessive lethals for 3 consecutive breedings (Vogel & Chandler, 1974).

A concentration-dependent increase in ^{3}H-thymidine incorporation (unscheduled DNA repair synthesis) was obtained in opossum lymphocytes treated in culture with 10^{-5}-10^{-3}M ethylene dibromide (Meneghini, 1974).

Ethylene dibromide given orally (5 doses totalling 50 or 100 mg/kg bw) or by i.p. injection (18 or 90 mg/kg bw) caused no dominant lethal mutations in mice (Epstein et al., 1972).

(b) Man

One case of fatal poisoning has been reported in an adult female, after the ingestion of 4.5 ml ethylene dibromide. The patient vomited recurrently, had watery diarrhoea, became anuric and died 2 days later. Massive hepatic centrolobular necrosis and proximal tubular epithelial damage of the kidney were noted at autopsy (Olmstead, 1960). Prolonged contact with ethylene dibromide causes skin irritation (ILO, 1971).

3.3 Case reports and epidemiological studies

No data were available to the Working Group.

4. Comments on Data Reported and Evaluation[1]

4.1 Animal data

Ethylene dibromide is carcinogenic in mice and rats after its oral administration, the only route tested; it produced squamous-cell carcinomas of the forestomach.

4.2 Human data

No case reports or epidemiological studies were available to the Working Group.

---

[1]See also the section, 'Animal Data in Relation to the Evaluation of Risk to Man' in the introduction to this volume, p. 15.

5. References

Abbott, D.C. (1970) IUPAC commission on the development, improvement, and standardization of methods of pesticide residue analysis. J. Ass. off. analyt. Chem., 53, 1004-1009

Alper, M.D. & Ames, B.N. (1975) Positive selection of mutants with deletions of the *gal-chl* region of the *Salmonella* chromosome as a screening procedure for mutagens that cause deletions. J. Bacteriol., 121, 259-266

Alumot, E. (1972) The mechanism of ethylene dibromide action on laying hens. Res. Rev., 41, 1-11

Ames, B.N. (1971) The detection of chemical mutagens with enteric bacteria. In: Holländer, A., ed., Chemical Mutagens: Principles and Methods for Their Detection, Vol. 1, New York, Plenum Press, pp. 267-282

Amir, D. (1973) The sites of the spermicidal action of ethylene dibromide in bulls. J. Reprod. Fert., 35, 519-525

Anon. (1976a) Current prices of chemicals and related products. Chemical Marketing Reporter, 210, 47

Anon. (1976b) Industry/Business. Chem. Eng. News, 54, 9

Bondi, A., Olomucki, E. & Calderon, M. (1955) Problems connected with ethylene dibromide fumigation of cereals. II. Feeding experiments with laying hens. J. Sci. Fd Agric., 6, 600-602

Brem, H., Stein, A.B. & Rosenkranz, H.S. (1974) The mutagenicity and DNA-modifying effect of haloalkanes. Cancer Res., 34, 2576-2579

Buselmaier, W., Röhrborn, G. & Propping, P. (1972) Mutagenitäts-Untersuchungen mit Pestiziden im Host-mediated assay und mit dem Dominanten Letaltest an der Maus. Biol. Zbl., 91, 311-325

Buselmaier, W., Röhrborn, G. & Propping, P. (1973) Comparative investigations on the mutagenicity of pesticides in mammalian test systems. Mutation Res., 21, 25-26

California Department of Food and Agriculture (1975) Pesticide Use Report 1974, Sacramento, pp. 77-78

Dumas, T. (1973) Inorganic and organic bromide residues in foodstuffs fumigated with methyl bromide and ethylene dibromide at low temperatures. J. agric. Fd Chem., 21, 433-436

Edwards, K., Jackson, H. & Jones, A.R. (1970) Studies with alkylating esters. II. A chemical interpretation through metabolic studies of the antifertility effects of ethylene dimethanesulphonate and ethylene dibromide. Biochem. Pharmacol., 19, 1783-1789

Epstein, S.S., Arnold, E., Andrea, J., Bass, W. & Bishop, Y. (1972) Detection of chemical mutagens by the dominant lethal assay in the mouse. *Toxicol. appl. Pharmacol.*, 23, 288-325

Going, J. & Long, S. (1975) Sampling and analysis of selected toxic substances: Task II - ethylene dibromide. EPA/560/6-75/001. Washington DC, Environmental Protection Agency

Grasselli, J.G., ed. (1973) *CRC Atlas of Spectral Data and Physical Constants for Organic Compounds*, Cleveland, Ohio, Chemical Rubber Co., p. B-504

Hargreaves, P.A., Wainwright, D.H. & Hamilton, D.J. (1974) A method for the estimation of 1,2-dibromoethane in vegetables. *Pest. Sci.*, 5, 225-229

Heuser, S.G. & Scudamore, K.A. (1969) Determination of fumigant residues in cereals and other foodstuffs: a multi-detection scheme for gas chromatography of solvent extracts. *J. Sci. Fd Agric.*, 20, 566-572

Heuser, S.G. & Scudamore, K.A. (1970) Selective determination of ionised bromide and organic bromides in foodstuffs by gas-liquid chromatography with special reference to fumigant residues. *Pest. Sci.*, 1, 244-249

Horwitz, W., ed. (1975) *Official Methods of Analysis of the Association of Official Analytical Chemists*, 12th ed., Washington DC, Association of Official Analytical Chemists, p. 91

IARC (1976) *IARC Information Bulletin on the Survey of Chemicals Being Tested for Carcinogenicity*, No. 6, Lyon, pp. 127, 199, 269

ILO (International Labour Office) (1971) *Encyclopaedia of Occupational Health and Safety*, Vol. 1, Geneva, pp. 384-385

Jones, A.R. & Edwards, K. (1968) The comparative metabolism of ethylene dimethanesulphonate and ethylene dibromide. *Experientia*, 24, 1100-1101

Kristoffersson, U. (1974) Genetic effects of some gasoline additives. *Hereditas*, 78, 319

Malling, H.V. (1969) Ethylene dibromide: a potent pesticide with high mutagenic activity. *Genetics*, 61, s39

Malone, B. (1969) Analysis of grains for multiple residues of organic fumigants. *J. Ass. off. analyt. Chem.*, 52, 800-805

Malone, B. (1970) Method for determining multiple residues of organic fumigants in cereal grains. *J. Ass. off. analyt. Chem.*, 53, 742-746

Malone, B. (1971) Analytical methods for the determination of fumigants. *Res. Rev.*, 38, 21-80

McCann, J., Choi, E., Yamasaki, E. & Ames, B.N. (1975) Detection of carcinogens as mutagens in the *Salmonella*/microsome test: assay of 300 chemicals. Proc. nat. Acad. Sci. (Wash.), 72, 5135-5139

Meneghini, R. (1974) Repair replication of opossum lymphocyte DNA: effect of compounds that bind to DNA. Chem.-biol. Interact., 8, 113-126

Muto, T. (1976) Noyaku Yoran, Tokyo, Nippon Plant Boeki Association, p. 35

Nachtomi, E. (1970) The metabolism of ethylene dibromide in the rat. The enzymic reaction with glutathione *in vitro* and *in vivo*. Biochem. Pharmacol., 19, 2853-2860

Nauman, C.H., Villalobos-Pietrini, R. & Sautkulis, R.C. (1974) Response of a mutable clone of *Tradescantia* to gaseous chemical mutagens and to ionizing radiation. Mutation Res., 26, 444

Nauman, C.H., Sparrow, A.H., Schairer, L.A. & Sautkulis, R.C. (1975) Influences of temperature, ionizing radiation and chemical mutagens on somatic mutation rate in *Tradescantia*. Mutation Res., 31, 318-319

Nauman, C.H., Sparrow, A.H. & Schairer, L.A. (1976) Comparative effects of ionizing radiation and two gaseous chemical mutagens on somatic mutation induction in one mutable and two non-mutable clones of *Tradescantia*. Mutation Res., 38, 53-70

Newman, D.R., ed. (1976) Ethylene dibromide 'ubiquitous' in air, EPA report says. Toxic Materials News, 18 August, p. 12

NIOSH (National Institute for Occupational Safety and Health) (1975) Ethylene dibromide, Method No. S104, Set H, Springfield, Virginia, National Technical Information Service

Olmstead, E.V. (1960) Pathological changes in ethylene dibromide poisoning. Arch. industr. Hlth, 21, 525-529

Olson, W.A., Habermann, R.T., Weisburger, E.K., Ward, J.M. & Weisburger, J.H. (1973) Induction of stomach cancer in rats and mice by halogenated aliphatic fumigants. J. nat. Cancer Inst., 51, 1993-1995

Perry, S.G. (1966) Application of an electron capture detector to the determination of dibromoethane in gasolines. J. Chromat., 24, 32-38

Plotnick, H.B. & Conner, W.L. (1976) Tissue distribution of ^{14}C-labeled ethylene dibromide in the guinea pig. Res. Commun. chem. Path. Pharmacol., 13, 251-258

Powers, M.B., Voelker, R.W., Page, N.P., Weisburger, E.K. & Kraybill, H.F. (1975) Carcinogenicity of ethylene dibromide (EDB) and 1,2-dibromo-3-chloropropane (DBCP) after oral administration in rats and mice. Toxicol. appl. Pharmacol., 33, 171-172

Prager, B. & Jacobson, P., eds (1918) Beilsteins Handbuch der Organischen Chemie, 4th ed., Vol. 1, Syst. 8, Berlin, Springer-Verlag, p. 90

Rowe, V.K., Spencer, H.C., McCollister, D.D., Hollingsworth, R.L. & Adams, E.M. (1952) Toxicity of ethylene dibromide determined on experimental animals. Arch. industr. Hyg., 6, 158-173

de Serres, F.J. & Malling, H.V. (1970) Genetic analysis of *ad*-3 mutants of *Neurospora crassa* induced by ethylene dibromide - a commonly used pesticide. Environm. Mut. Soc. Newslett., 3, 36-37

Sparrow, A.H. & Schairer, L.A. (1974) Mutagenic response of *Tradescantia* to treatment with X-rays, EMS, DBE, ozone, SO_2, N_2O and several insecticides. Mutation Res., 26, 445

Sparrow, A.H. & Schairer, L.A. (1975) Interaction of exposure time and gaseous mutagen concentration on somatic mutation frequency in *Tradescantia*. Mutation Res., 31, 318

Sparrow, A.H., Schairer, L.A. & Villalobos-Pietrini, R. (1974) Comparison of somatic mutation rates induced in *Tradescantia* by chemical and physical mutagens. Mutation Res., 26, 265-276

Spencer, E.Y. (1973) Guide to the Chemicals Used in Crop Protection, Publication 1093, 6th ed., London, Ontario, University of Western Ontario, Research Branch, Agriculture Canada, p. 263

Tagawa, H. & Tomaru, K. (1969) Soil sterilization with fumigants. I. Determination of soil fumigants in soil by electron-capture gas chromatography. Hatano Tabako Shikenjo Hokoku, 65, 77-83

US Department of Commerce (1975) US Imports for Consumption and General Imports, FT 246/Annual 1974, Bureau of the Census, Washington DC, US Government Printing Office, p. 206

US Environmental Protection Agency (1970) EPA Compendium of Registered Pesticides, Washington DC, US Government Printing Office, pp. III-E-9.1-III-E-9.5

US Environmental Protection Agency (1976a) Inorganic bromides or total combined bromide resulting from fumigation with ethylene dibromide; tolerances for residues. US Code of Federal Regulations, Title 40, part 180.146, p. 175

US Environmental Protection Agency (1976b) Organic bromide residues for ethylene dibromide; exemption for the requirement of a tolerance. US Code of Federal Regulations, Title 40, part 180.1006, p. 222

US Food and Drug Administration (1975) Pesticide Analytical Manual, Vol. I, Methods Which Detect Multiple Residues, Section 621, Rockville, Maryland, US Department of Health, Education and Welfare

US International Trade Commission (1976) Synthetic Organic Chemicals, US Production and Sales, 1974, ITC Publication 776, Washington DC, US Government Printing Office, pp. 203, 229

US Occupational Safety and Health Administration (1976) Air contaminants. US Code of Federal Regulations, Title 29, part 1910.1000(e), p. 30

US Tariff Commission (1924) Census of Dyes and Other Synthetic Organic Chemicals, 1923, Tariff Information Series No. 32, Washington DC, US Government Printing Office

Villalobos-Pietrini, R., Sparrow, A.H., Schairer, L.A. & Sparrow, R.C. (1974) Variation in somatic mutation rates induced by X-rays, DBE and EMS in several *Tradescantia* species and hybrids. Radiation Res., 59, 153

Vogel, E. & Chandler, J.L.R. (1974) Mutagenicity testing of cyclamate and some pesticides in *Drosophila melanogaster*. Experientia, 30, 621-623

WHO (1972) 1971 Evaluations of some pesticide residues in food. Wld Hlth Org. Pest. Res. Ser., No. 1, pp. 266-275

HEXAMETHYLPHOSPHORAMIDE

1. Chemical and Physical Data

1.1 Synonyms and trade names

Chem. Abstr. Services Reg. No.: 680-31-9

Chem. Abstr. Name: Hexamethylphosphoric triamide

Hexametapol; hexamethylphosphamide; hexamethylphosphoric acid triamide; N,N,N,N,N,N-hexamethylphosphoric triamide; hexamethylphosphorotriamide; hexamethylphosphotriamide; hexmethylphosphoramide; HMPA; HMPT; HPT; phosphoric tris(dimethylamide); phosphoryl hexamethyltriamide; tris(dimethylamino)phosphine oxide; tris(dimethylamino)phosphorus oxide

ENT 50,882; Hempa

1.2 Chemical formula and molecular weight

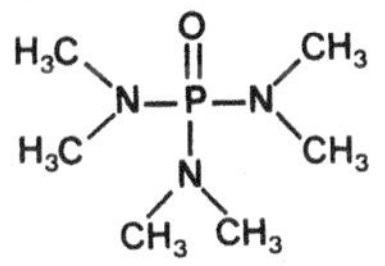

$$\begin{array}{c} H_3C \\ \end{array} \!\!\! N - \overset{\overset{O}{\|}}{\underset{\underset{CH_3\ CH_3}{N}}{P}} - N \!\!\! \begin{array}{c} CH_3 \\ CH_3 \end{array}$$

$C_6H_{18}N_3OP$ Mol. wt: 179.2

1.3 Chemical and physical properties of the pure substance

From Robert (1967)

(a) Description: Colourless, mobile liquid with aromatic odour

(b) Boiling-point: 233°C at 760 mm

(c) Freezing-point: 5-7°C

(d) Density: d^{20} 1.027

(e) Refractive index: n_D^{20} 1.459

(f) Solubility: Miscible with water and with organic liquids, except high-boiling saturated hydrocarbons

(g) Volatility: Vapour pressure is 0.03 mm at room temperature.

(h) Stability: Does not hydrolyse in alkaline media but hydrolyses slowly in acids

(i) Reactivity: Reacts upon heating with organic acids to form the dimethylamide of the organic acid

1.4 Technical products and impurities

The specifications for the technical grade of hexamethylphosphoramide in the US and Japan appear to be essentially identical to the properties of the pure substance.

2. Production, Use, Occurrence and Analysis

For background information on this section, see preamble, p. 17. Two reviews on hexamethylphosphoramide have been published (NIOSH, 1975; Robert, 1967).

2.1 Production and use

(a) Production

Hexamethylphosphoramide was first prepared in 1903 by Michaelis. It is reported to be produced commercially by the reaction of an excess of dimethylamine with phosphorus oxychloride (Robert, 1967).

The chemical is made in the US by one major producer, which uses it all internally. There are two minor producers, and there were two others in the past (NIOSH, 1975). In 1974, only one US company reported commercial production of this chemical (see preamble, p. 17) (US International Trade Commission, 1976). Certain US distributors have been reported to sell hexamethylphosphoramide that has been imported (NIOSH, 1975).

Annual production of hexamethylphosphoramide in western Europe is estimated to be less than 100,000 kg; the Federal Republic of Germany is the major producing country; France, Italy and the UK also make it.

Production of hexamethylphosphoramide was started by one company in Japan in 1968 and continued until October 1975, when a warning of its toxic properties was published. Japanese annual production reached a maximum in 1975 of 50 thousand kg.

(b) Use

Hexamethylphosphoramide is used as a solvent for polymers, as a selective solvent for gases, as a polymerization catalyst, as a stabilizer against thermal degradation in polystyrene, as an additive to polyvinyl and polyolefin resins to protect against degradation by ultra-violet light, and as a solvent in organic and organometallic reactions in research laboratories (NIOSH, 1975; Robert, 1967).

In the US, the major producer uses the chemical only as a processing solvent for aromatic polyamide fibre. Its use as a solvent in research laboratories may result in the exposure of 90% of an estimated 5000 people who are occupationally exposed to hexamethylphosphoramide in the US (NIOSH, 1975). No US standard has been established for the limits of occupational exposure to this chemical (NIOSH, 1975).

Hexamethylphosphoramide has been tested as a chemosterilant for insects and, to some extent, as an antistatic agent, a flame retardant and a de-icing additive for jet fuels (NIOSH, 1975).

In Japan, 90% of the chemical produced is reported to be used for solvent purposes and 10% as a catalyst and as an additive for synthetic resins.

2.2 Occurrence

Hexamethylphosphoramide is not known to occur as a natural product.

2.3 Analysis

A gas chromatographic method involving a flame-photometric detector has been used for determining 0.1 ng hexamethylphosphoramide in insect tissues (Bowman & Beroza, 1966). Gas chromatography with flame photometric detection, using four separate silicone-type stationary phases, has been used to separate 138 pesticides and metabolites containing phosphorus and sulphur. Identification of individual compounds was made by comparison of the relative retention data from the four columns (Bowman & Beroza,

1970). Thin-layer and gas chromatographic techniques have been used for the purification and analysis of hexamethylphosphoramide (Terranova & Schmidt, 1967).

Phosphoramide derivatives, including hexamethylphosphoramide, have been separated by thin-layer chromatography using chloroform-methanol and chloroform-methanol-ammonium hydroxide systems, with a sensitivity of 2 µg (Reissbrodt et al., 1973).

A method of separating twelve phosphorus compounds, including hexamethylphosphoramide, involves gel chromatography (Woelke et al., 1973). A polarographic method for testing the degradation of hexamethylphosphoramide during storage has been described (Gal & Yvernault, 1971).

3. Biological Data Relevant to the Evaluation of Carcinogenic Risk to Man

3.1 Carcinogenicity and related studies in animals

(a) *Oral administration*

Rat: Groups of 15 6-week old male Sherman rats were fed diets containing hexamethylphosphoramide at concentrations resulting in daily intakes of 0.78, 1.56, 3.12 and 6.25 mg/kg bw for 2 years. Two groups of 15 control rats were fed the basal diet alone. At 2 years, 8, 5, 3 and 5 rats in the treated groups, respectively, and 11 controls were still alive. A low incidence of tumours (5 in treated animals and 4 in controls) was observed. The tumours were mainly reticulum-cell sarcomas or lymphosarcomas of the lung (Kimbrough & Gaines, 1973) [The Working Group noted the small number of animals used, the insufficient number of animals at termination and that no indication of time or cause of death of individual animals was given].

(b) *Inhalation and/or intratracheal administration*

Rat: In a preliminary note, it was reported that groups of 120 male and 120 female Charles River CD rats were exposed to concentrations of 0, 50, 400 or 4000 ppb (0, 0.366, 2.93 or 29.3 mg/m^3) hexamethylphosphoramide (by volume) in air 6 hours a day for 5 days each week. At the time of reporting (8 months after the start of the experiment), 7/8 rats receiving 400 ppb and 12/15 receiving 4000 ppb that had died or been killed, had squamous-cell carcinomas of the nasal cavity. No such tumours were found in 6 rats randomly selected from the group receiving 50 ppb (Zapp, 1975a).

3.2 Other relevant biological data

(a) Experimental systems

The acute oral LD_{50} in male rats is 2650 mg/kg bw and that in female rats, 3360 mg/kg bw (Kimbrough & Gaines, 1966); by i.v. injection in mice it is 800 mg/kg bw (Kopecky & Smejkal, 1966). The dermal LD_{50} in rabbits is 2600 mg/kg bw (Shott et al., 1971).

In the carcinogenicity experiment in rats reported above, the cause of death of animals exposed to hexamethylphosphoramide in air at levels of up to 4000 ppb (29.3 mg/m^3) was degenerative changes in the convoluted tubules of the kidney (Zapp, 1975b).

Severe bronchiectasis and bronchopneumonia with areas of squamous metaplasia were observed in rats given hexamethylphosphoramide in the diet at concentrations resulting in daily intakes of 106-127 mg/kg bw over a period of 52-72 days (Kimbrough & Sedlak, 1968).

Rats receiving 6 consecutive oral daily doses of 500 mg/kg bw remained sterile for up to 23 weeks after treatment, with a reduction in weight of testes and destruction of gonadal cells (Jackson et al., 1969).

Seventy per cent of ^{32}P-labelled hexamethylphosphoramide given intraperitoneally was excreted within 20 hours by rats and mice as ^{32}P (Jackson & Craig, 1966).

Hexamethylphosphoramide is excreted in the milk of cows following its oral administration (Godfrain et al., 1971).

When rats were given daily doses of 200 mg/kg bw from day 7-20 of pregnancy, no abnormalities were detected in offspring (Kimbrough & Gaines, 1966). No adverse effects could be detected in a fertility test in rats performed over a period of 169 days when 10 mg/kg bw/day were given by gavage (Shott et al., 1971).

In rats and mice, hexamethylphosphoramide undergoes a sequence of N-demethylation reactions to yield pentamethylphosphoramide, N',N',N'',N'''-tetramethylphosphoramide and N',N'',N'''-trimethylphosphoramide. *In vitro* studies with rat liver slices indicated oxidative demethylation, with the simultaneous formation of formaldehyde (Jones & Jackson, 1968).

Concentrations of up to 2.3×10^{-2} M hexamethylphosphoramide did not induce *Escherichia coli* K12 and K39 lysogenic for the temperate bacteriophage λ to release λ repression and produce bacteriophage (Zetterberg, 1971).

Hexamethylphosphoramide was ineffective as a chemosterilant in *Oncopeltus fasciatis* (Dallas) (Economopoulos & Gordon, 1969), *Ostrinia nubilalis* (Hübner) (Jackson & Brindley, 1971), *Circulifer tenellus* (Baker) (Ameresekere & Georghiou, 1971) and male *Pectinophora gossypiella* (Saunders) (Wolfenbarger et al., 1972).

It is an effective chemosterilant for *Musca domestica* L. (the common housefly) (Chang et al., 1964; LaChance & Leopold, 1969; LaChance et al., 1969; Matolín, 1969; Pausch, 1971; Zakharova, 1972), *Musca autumnalis* De Geer (Kaur & Wentworth, 1972), *Dacus oleae* (GMEL), *Ceratitis capitata* Wiedemann (Orphanidis & Patsakos, 1970), *Culex pipiens fatigans* Wiedemann (Grover & Pillai, 1972; Grover et al., 1971, 1972, 1973), *Culex pipiens* L. (Sacca et al., 1971), *Culex pipiens molestus* (Amirkhanian, 1973), *Diparopsis castanea* (HMPS) (Campion & Lewis, 1971) and *Drosophila melanogaster* (Šrám, 1972). The mechanism of action was by death of the germ cells and/or dominant lethal mutations.

No increases in chromosomal aberrations were observed in Chinese hamster lung cells treated in culture with 0.05 M hexamethylphosphoramide for 2 hours or in *Vicia faba* seedlings treated for 24 hours with 0.1 M solutions (Sturelid, 1971). These results are in contrast to the observations of chromosome aberrations in insects (Grover et al., 1973; LaChance & Leopold, 1969).

I.p. injection of 15 mg/kg bw to mice did not increase the frequency of aberrations in chromosomes taken from bone marrow at intervals from 15 minutes to 144 hours after injection (Manna & Das, 1973).

Hexamethylphosphoramide induced dominant lethality in male inbred mice of the A/L and C57Bl/6J strains, injected intraperitoneally with two doses of 50 and 125 mg/kg bw, 12 hours apart; 25 mg/kg bw had no effect. With 50 mg/kg bw, total lethality and preimplantation losses (judged by corpora lutea) were increased, indicating an equal effect throughout the entire spermatogenic cycle; while with 125 mg/kg bw, the increase in pre- and postimplantation lethality was most pronounced during the second week, i.e., when late spermatids were the most sensitive (Šrám et al., 1970).

In contrast, Epstein et al. (1972), using ICR/Ha Swiss mice, found no reproducible dominant lethality when the animals were injected intraperitoneally with 7 different dose levels of between 168 and 2000 mg/kg bw.

(b) Man

Chang & Klassen (1968) reported no significant increase in chromosome aberrations when cultured human leucocytes were treated with 5×10^{-3} M hexamethylphosphoramide.

3.3 Case reports and epidemiological studies

No data were available to the Working Group.

4. Comments on Data Reported and Evaluation[1]

4.1 Animal data

Hexamethylphosphoramide is carcinogenic in rats, the only species tested, following its administration by inhalation; in this study, which was reported as a preliminary note, it produced squamous-cell carcinomas of the nasal cavity. It has also been inadequately tested in rats by oral administration.

---

[1] See also the section, 'Animal Data in Relation to the Evaluation of Risk to Man' in the introduction to this volume, p. 15.

4.2 Human data

No case reports or epidemiological studies were available to the Working Group.

5. References

Ameresekere, R.V.W.E. & Georghiou, G.P. (1971) Sterilization of the beet leafhopper: induction of sterility and evaluation of biotic effects with a model sterilant (OM-53139) and ^{60}Co irradiation. J. econ. Entomol., 64, 1074-1080

Amirkhanian, J.D. (1973) *Culex pipiens molestus* as a convenient test system for the evaluation of mutagenic agents: based on dominant lethal assays, inheritable semi-sterility and cytogenetical studies. Genetics, 74, s6

Bowman, M.C. & Beroza, M. (1966) Gas chromatographic determination of trace amounts of the insect chemosterilants tepa, metepa, methiotepa, hempa, and apholate and the analysis of tepa in insect tissue. J. Ass. off. analyt. Chem., 49, 1046-1052

Bowman, M.C. & Beroza, M. (1970) GLC retention times of pesticides and metabolites containing phosphorus and sulfur on four thermally stable columns. J. Ass. off. analyt. Chem., 53, 499-508

Campion, D.G. & Lewis, C.T. (1971) Studies of competitiveness, chemosterilant persistence and sperm structure in treated red bollworms, *Diparopsis castanea* (HMPS). In: Proceedings of a Symposium on Sterility Principle for Insect Control or Eradication, Athens, 1970, Vienna, International Atomic Energy Agency, pp. 183-202

Chang, S.C., Terry, P.H. & Borkovec, A.B. (1964) Insect chemosterilants with low toxicity for mammals. Science, 144, 57-58

Chang, T.-H. & Klassen, W. (1968) Comparative effects of tretamine, tepa, apholate and their structural analogs on human chromosomes *in vitro*. Chromosoma (Berl.), 24, 314-323

Economopoulos, A.P. & Gordon, H.T. (1969) Action of certain chemosterilants on males of the large milkweed bug. J. econ. Entomol., 62, 1326-1330

Epstein, A.S., Arnold, E., Andrea, J., Bass, W. & Bishop, Y. (1972) Detection of chemical mutagens by the dominant lethal assay in the mouse. Toxicol. appl. Pharmacol., 23, 288-325

Gal, J.Y. & Yvernault, T. (1971) Polarographic method for testing the degradation of purified hexametapol during its storage. C.R. Acad. Sci. (Paris), Ser. C, 272, 42-44

Godfrain, J.-C., Rico, A.G., Lorgue, G., Burgat, V., Sy, M., Maillet, M., Megemont, C., Felix, C., Borrel, A. & Dumas, G. (1971) Contribution à l'étude, à l'aide de phosphore radioactif, du métabolisme de l'hexamétapol ^{32}P (H.M.P.T.) chez les ovins et les bovins. Rev. Méd. vét., 122, 371-390

Grover, K.K. & Pillai, M.K.K. (1972) Chemosterilization of *Culex pipiens fatigans* Wiedemann by exposure of aquatic stages. III. Induction of dominant lethal mutations in the F_1 generation by certain aziridines, phosphoramides and S-triazines. Bull. Wld Hlth Org., 47, 305-308

Grover, K.K., Pillai, M.K.K. & Dass, C.M.S. (1971) Cytogenetic basis of chemically induced sterility in *Culex pipiens fatigans* Wiedemann. III. Effect of apholate and hempa on DNA synthesis in the gonads. Ind. J. exp. Biol., 9, 150-152

Grover, K.K., Pillai, M.K.K. & Dass, C.M.S. (1972) Cytogenetic basis of chemically induced sterility in *Culex pipiens fatigans* Wiedemann. II. Cytopathological effects of certain chemosterilants on the gonadal and embryonic tissues. J. med. Entomol., 9, 451-460

Grover, K.K., Pillai, M.K.K. & Dass, C.M.S. (1973) Cytogenetic basis of chemically induced sterility in *Culex pipiens fatigans* Wiedemann. I. Chemosterilant-induced damage in the somatic chromosomes. Cytologia, 38, 21-28

Jackson, H. & Craig, A.W. (1966) Antifertility action and metabolism of hexamethylphosphoramide. Nature (Lond.), 212, 86-87

Jackson, H., Jones, A.R. & Cooper, E.R.A. (1969) Effects of hexamethylphosphoramide on rat spermatogenesis and fertility. J. Reprod. Fert., 20, 263-269

Jackson, R.D. & Brindley, T.A. (1971) Hempa and metepa as chemosterilants of imagos of the European corn borer. J. econ. Entomol., 64, 1065-1068

Jones, A.R. & Jackson, H. (1968) The metabolism of hexamethylphosphoramide and related compounds. Biochem. Pharmacol., 17, 2247-2252

Kaur, D. & Wentworth, B.C. (1972) Studies on the chemosterilization of the face fly. J. econ. Entomol., 65, 21-23

Kimbrough, R.D. & Gaines, T.B. (1966) Toxicity of hexamethylphosphoramide in rats. Nature (Lond.), 211, 146-147

Kimbrough, R.D. & Gaines, T.B. (1973) The chronic toxicity of hexamethylphosphoramide in rats. Bull. environm. Contam. Toxicol., 10, 225-226

Kimbrough, R.D. & Sedlak, V.A. (1968) Lung morphology in rats treated with hexamethylphosphoramide. Toxicol. appl. Pharmacol., 12, 60-67

Kopecký, J. & Šmejkal, J. (1966) Hexamethylphosphoramide as an amidating reagent. Chem. & Industr., Sept. 3, 1529-1530

LaChance, L.E. & Leopold, R.A. (1969) Cytogenetic effect of chemosterilants in house fly sperm: incidence of polyspermy and expression of dominant lethal mutations in early cleavage divisions. Canad. J. Genet. Cytol., 11, 648-659

LaChance, L.E., Degrugillier, M. & Leverich, A.P. (1969) Comparative effects of chemosterilants on spermatogenic stages in the house fly. I. Induction of dominant lethal mutations in mature sperm and gonial cell death. Mutation Res., 7, 63-74

Manna, G.K. & Das, P.K. (1973) Effect of two chemosterilants apholate and hempa on the bone-marrow chromosomes of mice. Canad. J. Genet. Cytol., 15, 451-459

Matolín, S. (1969) The effect of chemosterilants on the embryonic development of *Musca domestica* L. Acta ent. bohemoslov., 66, 65-69

NIOSH (National Institute for Occupational Safety and Health) (1975) Background Information on Hexamethylphosphoric Triamide, 24 October, Rockville, Maryland, US Department of Health, Education and Welfare

Orphanidis, P.S. & Patsakos, P.G. (1970) Chimiostérilisation des *Dacus oleae* (GMEL) et *Ceratitis capitata* Wied. au moyen de substances chimiques avec ou sans propriétés d'alkylation. Ann. Inst. phytopath. Benaki, N.S., 9, 134-146

Pausch, R.D. (1971) Local house fly control with baited chemosterilants. I. Preliminary laboratory studies. J. econ. Entomol., 64, 1462-1465

Reissbrodt, R., Fleischer, R. & Fiedler, H.J. (1973) Thin-layer chromatographic method for analytical determination of covalent nitrogen-phosphorus compounds. Arch. Acker-Pflanzenbau Bodenk., 17, 567-572

Robert, L. (1967) Propriétes et emploi de l'hexaméthylphosphorotriamide. Chim. Industr. Gén. chim., 97, 337-345

Saccá, G., Scirocchi, A. & Mastrilli, M.L. (1971) Studi sulla chemosterilizzazione di *Culex pipiens* L. Riv. Parassitol., 32, 219-227

Shott, L.D., Borkovec, A.B. & Knapp, W.A., Jr (1971) Toxicology of hexamethylphosphoric triamide in rats and rabbits. Toxicol. appl. Pharmacol., 18, 499-506

Šrám, R.J. (1972) The differences in the spectra of genetic changes in *Drosophila melanogaster* induced by chemosterilants TEPA and HEMPA. Folia biol. (Prague), 18, 139-148

Šrám, R.J., Beneš, V. & Zudová, Z. (1970) Induction of dominant lethals in mice by TEPA and HEMPA. Folia biol. (Prague), 16, 407-416

Sturelid, S. (1971) Chromosome-breaking capacity of tepa and analogues in *Vicia faba* and Chinese hamster cells. Hereditas, 68, 255-276

Terranova, A.C. & Schmidt, C.H. (1967) Purification and analysis of hempa by chromatographic techniques. J. econ. Entomol., 60, 1659-1663

US International Trade Commission (1976) Synthetic Organic Chemicals, US Production and Sales, 1974, ITC Publication 776, Washington DC, US Government Printing Office, p. 214

Woelke, M., Toepelmann, W. & Lehmann, H.A. (1973) Gel-chromatographic behavior of alkyl phosphates, phosphoramidates, phosphorodiamidates, and phosphoric triamides. Z. anorg. allg. Chem., 397, 157-161

Wolfenbarger, D.A., Nosky, J.B., Gonzalez, N.C., Mangum, C.L. & Borkovec, A.B. (1972) Sterilization of pink bollworms with aziridine chemosterilants and with hempa. J. econ. Entomol., 65, 962-965

Zakharova, N.F. (1972) Action of the chemosterilant hexamethylphosphoramide on male and female *Musca domestica*. Med. Parasit. (Mosk.), 77, 583-587

Zapp, J.A., Jr (1975a) HMPA: a possible carcinogen. Science, 190 422

Zapp, J.A., Jr (1975b) Inhalation toxicity of hexamethylphosphoramide. Amer. industr. Hyg. Ass. J., 36, 916

Zetterberg, G. (1971) Bacteriophage development in lysogenic *Escherichia coli* and mutations in fungi induced with analogs of tris(1-aziridinyl)-phosphine oxide, TEPA. Hereditas, 68, 245-254

ISOPROPYL ALCOHOL AND ISOPROPYL OILS

1. Chemical and Physical Data

1.1 Synonyms and trade names

Isopropyl alcohol

Chem. Abstr. Services Reg. No.: 67-63-0

Chem. Abstr. Name: 2-Propanol

Dimethyl carbinol; dimethylcarbinol; IPA; isohol; isopropanol; petrohol; PRO; propan-2-ol; iso-propanol; sec-propyl alcohol; secondary propyl alcohol

Alcosolve 2; Avantine; Lutosol

Isopropyl oils

Not applicable

1.2 Chemical formula and molecular weight

Isopropyl alcohol

$$CH_3-CHOH-CH_3$$

C_3H_8O Mol. wt: 60.1

Isopropyl oils

Not applicable

1.3 Chemical and physical properties of the pure substance

Isopropyl alcohol

From Weast (1976), unless otherwise specified

(a) Description: Colourless liquid (Wickson, 1968)

(b) Boiling-point: 82.4°C

(c) Melting-point: -89.5°C

(d) Density: d_4^{20} 0.7855

(e) _Refractive index_: n_D^{20} 1.3776

(f) _Spectroscopy data_: λ_{max} 181 nm (E_1^1 = 103) (gaseous form); infra-red, ultra-violet, nuclear magnetic resonance and mass spectra have been tabulated by Grasselli (1973).

(g) _Solubility_: Soluble in acetone, very soluble in benzene; miscible with water, ethanol and ether

(h) _Volatility_: Vapour pressure is 32.4 mm at 20°C (Wickson, 1968).

Isopropyl oils

Not applicable

1.4 Technical products and impurities

Isopropyl alcohol

Three commercial grades of isopropyl alcohol available in the US, which differ mainly in water content, are 91 by volume %, 95 by volume %, and anhydrous (Wickson, 1968). A typical specification for anhydrous isopropyl alcohol is: purity, 99.8 by volume %, min.; water, 0.1 wt %, max.; acidity (as acetic acid), 0.002 wt %, max.; colour, Pt-Co, 5 max.; distillation range, 1°C; initial boiling-point, 81.3°C min.; dry-point, 83.0°C max.; nonvolatile matter, 0.002 g/100 ml max.; water miscibility at 20°C, 10 volumes; density, 0.786-0.787; and appearance, bright and clear.

Isopropyl alcohol is also available as a National Formulary grade containing 99-100.5% of the pure chemical for solvent use. Isopropyl rubbing alcohol contains 68-72 by volume % of the pure chemical, water, possibly perfume oils, and colour additives certified by the US Food and Drug Administration for use in drugs (National Formulary Board, 1970).

Isopropyl alcohol is also available in the US as a cosmetic grade (91 by volume % and anhydrous), which contains perfume as a masking agent, as an electronic grade, with low conductivity, and as reagent grades for use in analytical laboratory methods (Wickson, 1968).

In Japan, product specifications for commercial grade isopropyl alcohol are similar to those for the anhydrous grade in the US.

Isopropyl oils

Isopropyl oils are a by-product of isopropyl alcohol manufacture. Gas chromatograpic and mass spectrometric analysis of isopropyl oils produced by the older, strong-acid process [see section 2.1(a)] showed it to be a mixture composed primarily of trimeric and tetrameric polypropylene, with small amounts (less than 1% each) of benzene, toluene, alkyl benzenes, polyaromatic ring compounds, hexane, heptane, acetone, ethanol, isopropyl alcohol and isopropyl ether. Fluorescence of the residue after successive distillations of the isopropyl oils yielded spectra characteristic of benzanthracene. Chromatographic fractions of the residue from isopropyl oil distillation contained 86.8% carbon and 12.0% hydrogen (depending on the method of determination) (Weil *et al.*, 1952).

The isopropyl oils produced in the newer, weak-acid process [see section 2.1(a)] may contain polymers of lower molecular weight than those produced by the strong-acid method (NIOSH, 1976).

2. Production, Use, Occurrence and Analysis

For background information on this section, see preamble, p. 17. A review on isopropyl alcohol has been published (Wickson, 1968).

2.1 Production and use

Isopropyl alcohol

(a) Production

The reaction of propylene and sulphuric acid was used to prepare isopropyl alcohol by Berthelot in 1855; however, the product was first recognized as isopropyl alcohol in 1862, when Kolbe identified and named it (Wickson, 1968).

Isopropyl alcohol is manufactured in the US by an indirect hydration technique in which a fraction containing 40-60% propylene that is isolated from refinery exhaust gases is reacted with sulphuric acid

(Lowenheim & Moran, 1975). In an older process (strong-acid), 88-93% sulphuric acid was reacted with propylene gas at 25-60°C for a long time. In a newer process (weak-acid), which has replaced the strong-acid process, propylene gas is absorbed in 60% sulphuric acid at 85°C for a short reaction time (NIOSH, 1976).

In Europe and Japan, the indirect hydration process is being replaced by a direct hydration process in which propylene reacts directly with water in the presence of a catalyst. In Japan, 66% of the isopropyl alcohol is produced by the newer direct hydration process.

Commercial production of isopropyl alcohol was begun in the US in 1921, when three companies manufactured a total of 84 thousand kg (US Tariff Commission, 1922). In 1974, five US companies reported a total production of 880 million kg isopropyl alcohol (US International Trade Commission, 1976a). Preliminary data for 1975 indicate a total US production of 700 million kg (US International Trade Commission, 1976b). In 1975, the US exported 56 million kg isopropyl alcohol to the following countries (% of total exports received): Australia (2.5), Belgium (8.2), Brazil (3.8), Canada (2.5), Colombia (4.6), the Federal Republic of Germany (9.3), Italy (3.7), Mexico (8.6), The Netherlands (26.7), Venezuela (17.8) and at least fourteen other countries (12.3) (US Department of Commerce, 1976). US imports are negligible.

Six countries in western Europe produced an estimated 360 million kg isopropyl alcohol in 1975, as follows (% of total production): the Federal Republic of Germany (19.3), France (15.2), Italy (2.5), The Netherlands (29.0), Spain (8.3) and the UK (25.7). About 85 million kg were imported and about 90 million kg exported in these countries in that year.

Isopropyl alcohol has been produced commercially in Japan for over thirty years. In 1975, three Japanese companies produced a combined total of 58 million kg isopropyl alcohol. About 10 million kg were exported to east Asia (Korea, Taiwan, and Philippines) in that same year (The Chemical Daily Co. Ltd, 1976; Ministry of International Trade and Industry, 1976).

About 2 million kg were imported into Australia in 1975-76.

(b) Use

Estimated use of isopropyl alcohol in the US in 1975 was as follows: for acetone manufacture, 40%, as a solvent, 35%, in the manufacture of other chemicals, 10%, in drug and cosmetic formulations, 5%, miscellaneous uses, 7%, and exports, 3% (Anon., 1975).

In the production of acetone, isopropyl alcohol may be dehydrogenated catalytically at 400°C to give acetone and hydrogen (major process) or oxidized at high pressure to give acetone and hydrogen peroxide.

The second main use of isopropyl alcohol is as a solvent: it is used to extract and/or purify numerous natural products, such as oils, gums, shellacs, waxes, kelp and pectin. One potential use is as a solvent in the manufacture of fish protein concentrate. Isopropyl alcohol is used as a solvent for synthetic resins, e.g., coatings such as phenolic varnishes and nitrocellulose lacquers (Lowenheim & Moran, 1975; Wickson, 1968).

The third principal use is in the manufacture of other chemicals, such as isopropyl acetate, isopropylamine, di-isopropylamine, herbicidal esters, isopropyl xanthate, isopropyl myristate, isopropyl palmitate, isopropyl oleate, aluminium isopropoxide and isopropyl ether (Wickson, 1968).

Isopropyl alcohol is also used as a solvent in drug and cosmetic formulations and is the major component of rubbing compounds used as solvents and rubefacients (National Formulary Board, 1970). Its use in cosmetics has generally been limited to highly scented or relatively inexpensive products (Wickson, 1968).

Other reported applications of isopropyl alcohol include its use as a denaturant in special industrial solvents; in windshield-wiper concentrates, aerosol windshield de-icers and automobile petrol antifreeze mixtures; in aerosol home and garden insecticides, glass cleaners and other household specialities; as a coolant in beer manufacture; as a cleaning and drying agent in the manufacture of electronic tubes; as a de-icer for aircraft propellers; and as a fuel ingredient in refrigerator-car heaters (Wickson, 1968).

Use of isopropyl alcohol in western Europe in 1975 has been estimated as follows: as a source for acetone production, 46%; as a solvent in surface coatings, 20%; in other solvent usage, 15%; and for other miscellaneous uses, 19%.

In Japan, isopropyl alcohol is used as a solvent in surface coatings (25-30%) and inks (20%) and for other uses (50-55%).

The US Occupational Safety and Health Administration's health standards for exposure to air contaminants require that an employee's exposure to isopropyl alcohol does not exceed an eight-hour time-weighted average of 400 ppm (980 mg/m^3) in the working atmosphere in any eight-hour work shift of a forty-hour work week (US Occupational Safety & Health Administration, 1976); a ceiling of 800 ppm (1960 mg/m^3) was determined during a sampling time of 15 minutes (NIOSH, 1976). An estimated 141,000 employees may be exposed occupationally to isopropyl alcohol in the US (NIOSH, 1976).

In Australia, 980 mg/m^3 has also been recommended as the maximum in the working atmosphere.

The US Food and Drug Administration requires that isopropyl alcohol residue levels, after its use as an extractant, may not exceed 50 mg/kg in spice oleoresins, paprika oleoresin or annatto extract, 6 mg/kg in lemon oil, and 2.0% by weight in hops. The use of isopropyl alcohol as a defoaming agent is limited to the processing of beet sugar and yeast. When it is used as a synthetic flavouring substance and adjuvant, isopropyl alcohol must be used in the minimum quantity required to produce the intended effect. When it is used as a diluent in colour additive mixtures for marking foods, no residues may remain on the food (US Food & Drug Administration, 1976b).

<u>Isopropyl oils</u>

(a) <u>Production</u>

Isopropyl oils are produced as by-products in the reaction of propylene and sulphuric acid during the manufacture of isopropyl alcohol and consist of the residue after distillation. The older, indirect hydration, or strong-acid, process utilized concentrated sulphuric acid (88-93%) as a reactant. The reaction with propylene took place in a mixture of isopropyl sulphates at 25-60°C. The reaction time was long and produced isopropyl oils containing compounds with high molecular weight [see section 1.4] (NIOSH, 1976). One US factory which began production in 1943 utilized a concentration of 85-86% sulphuric acid (Anon., 1976).

A direct catalytic hydration, or weak-acid, process has replaced the strong-acid process in the US; with this method, a concentration of 60% sulphuric acid is used as a catalyst to absorb and react with the propylene gas. The reaction is maintained at 85°C, and reaction time is reported to be very short, thus producing isopropyl oils that may contain polymer oils of low molecular weight, although an analysis of the material has not been reported [see section 1.4] (NIOSH, 1976). One US company currently uses a concentration of 67-70% sulphuric acid in its weak-acid process (Anon., 1976).

No information was available on the quantities of isopropyl oils formed per kg of isopropyl alcohol produced by either process.

(b) Use

No evidence has been found that isopropyl oils have ever been used commercially.

2.2 Occurrence

Isopropyl alcohol

Isopropyl alcohol has been detected in air samples from polypropylene production plants at concentrations of up to 340 mg/m^3 (Shvedchenko, 1969), and as 2.7% of the total gaseous emission from streptomycin production (Kondakova et al., 1973).

It has been detected in trace quantities in some samples of drinking-water in the US (US Environmental Protection Agency, 1975) and as a constituent of tar-water resulting from the distillation of shale tar (Eizen et al., 1966).

Isopropyl alcohol has been detected in the volatiles of the following products: grapefruit essence oil (Coleman et al., 1972), roasted filbert nuts (Kinlin et al., 1972), lime essence (Moshonas & Shaw, 1972), Reunion geranium oil (*Pelargonium roseum* Bourbon) (Timmer et al., 1971), *Pinus densiflora* logs (Oda, 1974) and milk products (Palo & Ilková, 1970).

Isopropyl oils

Isopropyl oils are not known to occur naturally; they are found only as a by-product in factories manufacturing isopropyl alcohol.

2.3 Analysis

Isopropyl alcohol

A review of methods for sampling and analysing isopropyl alcohol in air has been published (NIOSH, 1976).

The Association of Official Analytical Chemists (AOAC) has published an Official Final Action for the determination of isopropyl alcohol in a variety of flavour extracts, using a titrimetric method in the absence of acetone and a colorimetric method if acetone is present. The AOAC has also published official methods for determining isopropyl alcohol in drugs and flavours by gas chromatography using a flame ionization detector (Horwitz, 1975). The gas chromatographic method for drugs was studied collaboratively, and a standard deviation of 0.142-1.079 was found among 9 laboratories (Falcone, 1973).

The majority of methods for determining isopropyl alcohol use gas chromatography with flame ionization detection. In the determination of residual isopropyl alcohol in oilseed meals and flours, there is a simple volatilization procedure for preparing samples for gas chromatography (Fore *et al.*, 1971). Head-space analysis using gas chromatography has been employed for its determination in cosmetics at concentrations of more than 0.5% (Grant, 1974). Concentrations of more than 10 mg/l have been determined in blood by direct injection into the gas chromatograph (Jain, 1971), and 0.2 mg/l has been found in milk and milk products by direct injection onto porous polymer bead columns (Palo & Ilková, 1970). Direct injection into gas chromatographs using flame ionization detection has been used for the analysis of environmental pollutants, including isopropyl alcohol, with a sensitivity of 0.2 µg/l (Dmitriev & Kitrosskii, 1969). Gas chromatography has also been used for the analysis of fruits dewaxed with isopropyl alcohol (Calhoun & Dellamonica, 1974).

Concentrations of 505-1890 mg/m^3 in the working atmosphere have been determined by gas chromatography (NIOSH, 1976), and the limit of detection of gas chromatographic-mass spectrometric analysis of the ambient air was 20 ppm (49 mg/m^3) (Cooper et al., 1971).

Infra-red spectrophotometry of the ester formed by reaction with nitrous acid has been used to determine as little as 4 µl isopropyl alcohol in foods (Coppini & Albasini, 1969).

Isopropyl oils

Isopropyl oils formed as by-products of the indirect hydration (strong-acid) process have also been analysed by mass spectroscopy combined with chromatography (Weil et al., 1952).

3. Biological Data Relevant to the Evaluation of Carcinogenic Risk to Man

3.1 Carcinogenicity and related studies in animals[1]

(a) Skin application

Mouse: A group of 30 Rockland mice were treated thrice weekly for 1 year with isopropyl alcohol. No skin tumours were detected (NIOSH, 1976) [The Working Group noted that the sex, dose and observation period were not specified].

Five groups of 30 Rockland mice were treated with isopropyl oils, made either by the strong-acid or weak-acid process, or with distilled water thrice weekly for 1 year. Of animals in the 3 groups treated with isopropyl oils made by the strong-acid process, 9/90 mice developed skin papillomas; no skin tumours occurred among 30 mice treated with isopropyl oils made by the weak-acid process. One skin papilloma and 1 skin carcinoma occurred in 1/30 mice that had been treated with distilled water (NIOSH, 1976) [The Working Group noted that the sex, dose and observation period were not specified].

---

[1] The Working Group was aware of a carcinogenicity study in progress in rats involving oral administration of isopropyl alcohol (IARC, 1976).

(b) Inhalation and/or intratracheal administration

Mouse: Groups of 3-month old male C3H, ABC or C57BL mice were exposed for 3-7 hours/day on 5 days/week for 5-8 months to a concentration of 7700 mg/m^3 isopropyl alcohol in air. The animals were killed at 8-12 months of age. The incidence of lung tumours was not increased, compared with that in controls (Weil *et al.*, 1952).

Groups of 3-month old male mice of various strains were exposed for 3-7 hours/day on 5 days/week for 5-8 months to 2-8 mg/l air of different samples of isopropyl oils produced by the strong-acid process in two different factories. The mice were then killed and examined for lung tumours. Of C3H mice exposed to 4 or 8 mg/l of a mixed sample from the first factory, 5/41 and 6/41 animals had lung tumours, compared with 2/69 controls (P<0.05). No increased incidences of tumours were found in C57BL or ABC mice exposed in the same way. Of ABCT mice exposed to 2 or 4 mg/l isopropyl oils from a second factory, 4/39 and 6/34 survivors developed lung tumours, compared with 0/21 controls (P<0.05). No increases in the incidences of lung tumours were observed in CFW and CF1 mice exposed to 2 or 4 mg/l isopropyl oils from either the first or the second factory, compared with controls (Weil *et al.*, 1952).

Dog: Four groups, each of 5 mongrel dogs, were exposed for 1 hour once weekly for 2 years to aerosols of isopropyl oils prepared by the strong-acid process in two factories (about 0.012 ml/l air). The dogs were left untreated for 1 year, and thereafter the treatment was given every third week for another 2 years. Another group of 4 dogs received direct instillations into the sinuses of 1 ml isopropyl oils once a month for 4 years. At autopsy, when the dogs were 9-12 years of age, no sinus tumours were detected, but some benign thyroid adenomas were reported (NIOSH, 1976; Weil *et al.*, 1952).

(c) Subcutaneous and/or intramuscular administration

Mouse: Groups of 3-month old male C3H, ABC and C57BL mice were treated by s.c. injection with 0.025 ml isopropyl alcohol once weekly for 20-40 weeks, at which time the animals were killed. No increases in the incidence of lung tumours were found (Weil *et al.*, 1952).

Groups of 3-month old male C3H, C57BL and ABC mice were treated once weekly for 20-40 weeks with 0.025 ml isopropyl oils produced by the strong-acid process in two factories. With one of the samples, 27/47 surviving ABC mice developed lung tumours, compared with 22/59 untreated controls ($P<0.05$). No increase in lung tumours was found in two other groups of ABC mice treated with the same sample (Weil et al., 1952).

Groups of 20-40 3-month old mice of the C3H, CFW, CF_1, dba or A/He strains were treated once weekly with 0.025 ml isopropyl oils made by the strong- or weak-acid processes or with a mixture of both. The animals were killed at the age of 8 months. An increased incidence of lung tumours was seen only in CF1 mice injected with the mixture of isopropyl oils (13/27 *versus* 6/30) (NIOSH, 1976).

3.2 Other relevant biological data

The biological properties of isopropyl alcohol have been reviewed by Browning (1965), NIOSH (1976), Treon (1963) and WHO (1971).

(a) Experimental systems

The oral LD_{50} of isopropyl alcohol in rats, rabbits and dogs is about 5 g/kg bw (Lehman & Chase, 1944). The dermal LD_{50} in rabbits is about 13 g/kg bw, and inhalation of 16,000 ppm (39.2 g/m^3) for 8 hours was lethal for 4/6 rats (Smyth & Carpenter, 1948).

The signs of intoxication after application of isopropyl alcohol are similar to those with ethanol, although it is 1.5-2 times as toxic as ethanol. Death is usually preceded by dizziness, narcosis, deep coma and shock (Lehman et al., 1945; Morris & Lightbody, 1938). An orally administered dose of 2 g/kg bw produced narcotic effects in rabbits for about 8 hours (Morris & Lightbody, 1938). Accumulation of liver triglycerides was observed in rats following a single oral dose of 6 g/kg bw (Nordmann et al., 1973). After a single oral dose of 2 g/kg bw to mice, augmented hepatotoxicity to various chlorinated hydrocarbons was noted (Traiger & Plaa, 1974).

When rats were exposed continuously for 86 days to air concentrations of 8.14 ppm (20 mg/m^3) isopropyl alcohol, they showed changes in reflex behaviour and increase in retention of bromosulphophthalein. The post-mortem findings included enlarged spleen, some evidence of liver parenchymal-cell dystrophy and degenerative changes in the cerebral motor cortex. A concentration of 0.6 mg/m^3 (0.24 ppm) had no effect on rats exposed continuously for 86 days (Baikov et *al.*, 1974).

Addition of 10% isopropyl alcohol to the diet of young rats (60 g) for 30 days had no effect on growth, liver weight or lipid content (Miyazaki, 1955). A daily dose of 1.3 g/kg bw isopropyl alcohol administered in the drinking-water to 3 dogs for 1 hour daily over 6 months led to no consistent pathological changes; the clinical signs were restricted to drunkenness 3-5 hours after intake (Lehman et *al.*, 1945).

Ingested isopropyl alcohol is most rapidly absorbed by the intestine as a whole and least by the stomach (Wax et *al.*, 1949). After increasing oral administration of 4-72 g isopropyl alcohol to 3 dogs, about 4% of the dose was excreted unchanged in the urine and 2% as acetone; less than 0.1% of the dose was found in the faeces (Kemal, 1937). After a single oral dose of 3 g/kg bw isopropyl alcohol to rabbits, 10% was excreted in the urine conjugated with glucuronic acid (Kamil et *al.*, 1953).

The disappearance rate of isopropyl alcohol in blood is half that of ethanol but 5 times that of methanol. The metabolite acetone is mainly oxidized (Neymark, 1938). The elimination of isopropyl alcohol in rats is decreased by simultaneous ingestion of ethanol or 1-propanol, but not with methanol or tertiary butanol. These results suggest that isopropyl alcohol is oxidized by alcohol dehydrogenase (Abshagen & Rietbrock, 1970).

Isopropyl alcohol was given continuously in the drinking-water in doses of 1.5, 1.4 and 1.3 g/kg bw/day to parents and to two successive generations of rats, respectively. Neither growth, reproductive function nor embryonic nor postnatal development were affected, except for some retardation of growth early in the life of first-generation rats (Lehman et *al.*, 1945).

No data on the mutagenicity of isopropyl alcohol or oils were available to the Working Group.

(b) Man

Ten volunteers exposed for 3-5 minutes to air concentrations of 200, 400 and 800 ppm (490, 980 and 1960 mg/m^3) isopropyl alcohol reported mild to moderate irritation of the eyes, nose and throat with the two higher doses (Nelson et al., 1943). The odour threshold ranged from 40 ppm (98 mg/m^3) (May, 1966) to 200 ppm (490 mg/m^3) (Scherberger et al., 1958).

Isopropyl alcohol is not a dermal irritant (Nixon et al., 1975), although several cases of allergic contact dermatitis have been reported (Fregert et al., 1971; McInnes, 1973; Richardson et al., 1969; Wasilewski, 1968).

Several lethal cases have been described as a result of ingestion of about 1 pint (0.47 l) of 70% isopropyl alcohol. Death was preceded by deep coma and shock and resulted from respiratory arrest (Adelson, 1962). Other persons survived after ingesting similar amounts (Chapin, 1949; Juncos & Taguchi, 1968). Treatment with haemodialysis was successful in 2 patients who had each ingested 1 litre of 70% isopropyl alcohol (Freireich et al., 1967; King et al., 1970).

Daily oral intake of low doses (2.6 or 6.4 mg/kg bw) of isopropyl alcohol by groups of 8 men for 6 weeks had no effect on blood cells, serum or urine and produced no subjective symptoms (Wills et al., 1969).

After oral intake of 0.1-20 g isopropyl alcohol, none was excreted in the urine of the volunteers during the following 48 hours, and no formic acid was detected (Kemal, 1927). About 47% of an oral dose of 720 mg isopropyl alcohol was exhaled unchanged over 3 hours; less than 3% was eliminated in the breath as acetone (Hahn, 1937).

3.3 Case reports and epidemiological studies

Among 71 men who had worked for more than 5 years between 1928 and 1950 in a US isopropyl alcohol manufacturing unit, in which isopropyl oils were formed as by-products, 7 neoplasms of the respiratory tract were found: 4 cancers of the paranasal sinuses, 1 carcinoma of the lung, 1 malignant tumour of the vocal cords and 1 non-malignant tumour (papilloma) of the vocal cords. The periods of exposure for these 7 patients ranged from 6-16 years. A total of 182 men worked in the suspected unit, 25 being generally employed at any one time (Hueper, 1966; Weil *et al.*, 1952) [At a conservative estimate, based on figures from the Connecticut Tumor Registry, the incidence of paranasal sinus cancer in this group of workers is more than 3 times that expected in the general population].

In another isopropyl alcohol manufacturing factory, in operation in the US since 1927, 2 sinus cancers and 2 intrinsic laryngeal cancers occurred among a total of 11 cancers in 779 employees. All cancer cases occurred in subjects who had worked in the factory for more than 9 years. The incidence of sinus and laryngeal cancers in this group (134.5/100,000) was reported to be 21 times that expected in the general population aged 45-54 years (Eckardt, 1974; Hueper, 1966).

Both studies were made in factories using the strong-acid process for manufacturing isopropyl alcohol. No epidemiological data are available from factories using the weak-acid or other processes.

4. Comments on Data Reported and Evaluation

4.1 Animal data

Isopropyl alcohol has been inadequately tested in mice by skin application, inhalation exposure and subcutaneous injection. Due to various limitations of these studies, no evaluation of the carcinogenicity of this compound can be made.

Isopropyl oils formed during the strong-acid process for synthesis of isopropyl alcohol were tested in mice by skin application, inhalation exposure and subcutaneous injection, and isopropyl oils formed during the weak-acid process were tested in mice by skin application and subcutaneous injection. Although an increased incidence of lung tumours was observed following inhalation or subcutaneous injection of isopropyl oils formed during the strong-acid process, all of these studies had some limitations due to short duration or incomplete reporting and to the unknown or variable composition of the materials tested. The available data thus do not provide sufficient evidence on which to base an evaluation of the carcinogenicity of isopropyl oils in experimental animals.

4.2 Human data

In two factories manufacturing isopropyl alcohol by the strong-acid process, involving the formation of isopropyl oils as by-products, an excess risk of cancers of the paranasal sinuses was found. An excess risk of laryngeal cancer may also have been present.

5. References

Abshagen, U. & Rietbrock, N. (1970) Zum Mechanismus der 2-Propanoloxydation. Interferenzversuche mit niederen aliphatischen Alkoholen *in vivo* und an der isolient perfundierten Rattenleber. Naunyn-Schmiedeberg's Arch. exp. Path. Pharmakol., 265, 411-424

Adelson, L. (1962) Fatal intoxication with isopropyl alcohol (rubbing alcohol). Amer. J. clin. Path., 38, 144-151

Anon. (1975) Chemical profile - isopropanol. Chemical Marketing Reporter, August 4, p. 9

Anon. (1976) Shell Oil reports 14 cases of cancer at its Texas facilities. Occupational Health and Safety Letter, 8 July

Baikov, B.K., Gorlova, O.E., Gusev, M.I., Novikov, Y.V., Yudina, T.V. & Sergeev, A.N. (1974) Hygienic standardization of the daily average maximal permissible concentrations of propyl and isopropyl alcohols in the atmosphere. Gig. i Sanit., 4, 6-13

Browning, E. (1965) Toxicity and Metabolism of Industrial Solvents, Amsterdam, Elsevier, pp. 335-341

Calhoun, M.J. & Dellamonica, E.S. (1974) Determination of 2-propanol residue in some fruits dewaxed with alcohol vapors. J. Ass. off. analyt. Chem., 57, 1342-1345

Chapin, M.A. (1949) Isopropyl alcohol poisoning with acute renal insufficiency. J. Maine med. Ass., 40, 288-290

The Chemical Daily Co., Ltd (1976) 6376-Chemicals, Tokyo, pp. 231-232

Coleman, R.L., Lund, E.D. & Shaw, P.E. (1972) Analysis of grapefruit essence and aroma oils. J. agric. Fd Chem., 20, 100-103

Cooper, C.V., White, L.D. & Kupel, R.E. (1971) Qualitative detection limits for specific compounds utilizing gas chromatographic fractions, activated charcoal and a mass spectrometer. Amer. industr. Hyg. Ass. J., 32, 383-386

Coppini, D. & Albasini, A. (1969) Determinazione di alcoli monovalenti inferiori mediante spettrofotometria infrarossa. Mitt. Lebensmitt. Hyg., 60, 460-465

Dmitriev, M.T. & Kitrosskii, N.A. (1969) Concerning determination of certain organic substances by ionization chromatography. Gig. i Sanit., 34, 80-87

Eckardt, R.E. (1974) Annals of industry - noncasualties of the work place. J. occup. Med., 16, 472-477

Eizen, O.G., Khallik, A. & Klesment, I.R. (1966) Composition of water-soluble, neutral oxygen compounds of shale tar. Proc. Eston. Acad. Sci. Ser., 2, 230-238

Falcone, N. (1973) Gas chromatographic determination of ethanol and isopropanol or acetone in drugs. J. Ass. off. analyt. Chem., 56, 684-688

Fore, S.P., Rayner, E.T. & Dupuy, H.P. (1971) Determination of residual solvent in oilseed meals and flours. III. Isopropanol. J. Amer. Oil chem. Soc., 48, 140-142

Fregert, S., Groth, O., Gruvberger, B., Magnusson, B., Mobacken, H. & Rorsman, H. (1971) Hypersensitivity to secondary alcohols. Acta derm.-venereol. (Stockh.), 51, 271-272

Freireich, A.W., Cinque, T.J., Xanthaky, G. & Landau, D. (1967) Hemodialysis for isopropanol poisoning. New Engl. J. Med., 277, 699-700

Grant, G.L.P. (1974) Gas-liquid chromatographic determination of methanol, ethanol, and isopropanol in cosmetics, using the headspace analytical technique. J. Ass. off. analyt. Chem., 57, 565-567

Grasselli, J.G., ed. (1973) CRC Atlas of Spectral Data and Physical Constants for Organic Compounds, Cleveland, Ohio, Chemical Rubber Co., p. B-818

Hahn, E. (1937) Beitrag zur Bestimmung von Isopropylalkohol in der Atemluft. Biochem Z., 292, 148-151

Horwitz, W., ed. (1975) Official Methods of Analysis of the Association of Official Analytical Chemists, 12th ed., Washington DC, Association of Official Analytical Chemists, pp. 328, 337-338, 343, 656-658

Hueper, W.C. (1966) Occupational and environmental cancers of the respiratory system. Recent Results Cancer Res., 3, 105-107, 183

IARC (1976) IARC Information Bulletin on the Survey of Chemicals Being Tested for Carcinogenicity, No. 6, Lyon, p. 145

Jain, N.C. (1971) Direct blood-injection method for gas chromatographic determination of alcohols and other volatile compounds. Clin. Chem., 17, 82-85

Juncos, L. & Taguchi, J.T. (1968) Isopropyl alcohol intoxication: report of a case associated with myopathy, renal failure, and hemolytic anemia. J. Amer. med. Ass., 204, 732-734

Kamil, I.A., Smith, J.N. & Williams, R.T. (1953) The metabolism of aliphatic alcohols: the glucuronic acid conjugation of acyclic aliphatic alcohols. Biochem. J., 53, 129-136

Kemal, H. (1927) Beitrag zur Kenntnis der Schicksale des Isopropylalkohols im menschlichen Organismus. Biochem. Z., 187, 461-466

Kemal, H. (1937) Über den Gehalt von Aceton in Harn, Kot und Organen von Hunden nach Zufuhr von Isopropylalkohol. Hoppe-Seylers Z. physiol. Chem., 246, 59-63

King, L.H., Jr, Bradley, K.P. & Shires, D.L., Jr (1970) Hemodialysis for isopropyl alcohol poisoning. J. Amer. med. Ass., 211, 1855

Kinlin, T.E., Muralidhara, R., Pittet, A.O., Sanderson, A. & Walradt, J.P. (1972) Volatile components of roasted filberts. J. agric. Fd Chem., 20, 1021-1028

Kondakova, L.V., Krasnov, V.N. & Shaposhnikov, Y.K. (1973) Analysis of gaseous emissions from streptomycin production. Gig. i Sanit., 8, 89

Lehman, A.J. & Chase, H.F. (1944) The acute and chronic toxicity of isopropyl alcohol. J. Lab. clin. Med., 29, 561-567

Lehman, A.J., Schwerma, H. & Rickards, E. (1945) Isopropyl alcohol: acquired tolerance in dogs, rate of disappearance from the blood stream in various species, and effects on successive generation of rats. J. Pharmacol. exp. Ther., 85, 61-69

Lowenheim, F.A. & Moran, M.K. (1975) Faith, Keyes, and Clark's Industrial Chemicals, 4th ed., New York, John Wiley and Sons, pp. 496-501

May, J. (1966) Geruchsschwellen von Lösemitteln zur Bewertung von Lösemittelgerüchen in der Luft. Staub-Reinhalt. Luft, 26, 385-389

McInnes, A. (1973) Skin reaction to isopropyl alcohol. Brit. med. J., i, 357

Ministry of International Trade and Industry (1976) Year Book of Chemical Industries Statistics, Tokyo, Research and Statistics Department, p. 86

Miyazaki, M. (1955) Studies on the nutritive value of aliphatic alcohols. I. The nutritive value of C_1~C_5 saturated alcohols. J. agric. chem. Soc. Japan, 29, 497-501

Morris, H.J. & Lightbody, H.D. (1938) The toxicity of isopropanol. J. industr. Hyg. Toxicol., 20, 428-434

Moshonas, M.G. & Shaw, P.E. (1972) Analysis of flavor constituents from lemon and lime essence. J. agric. Fd Chem., 20, 1029-1030

National Formulary Board (1970) *National Formulary XIII*, Washington DC, American Pharmaceutical Association, pp. 382-383

Nelson, K.W., Ege, J.F., Jr, Ross, M., Woodman, L.E. & Silverman, L. (1943) Sensory response to certain industrial solvent vapors. *J. industr. Hyg. Toxicol.*, 25, 282-285

Neymark, M. (1938) Die Kinetik beim Umsatz von Normalpropyl- und Isopropylalkohol. *Skand. Arch. Physiol.*, 78, 242-248

NIOSH (National Institute for Occupational Safety and Health) (1976) *Criteria for a Recommended Standard ... Occupational Exposure to Isopropyl Alcohol*, HEW Publication No. 76-142, Washington DC, US Department of Health, Education and Welfare

Nixon, G.A., Tyson, C.A. & Wertz, W.C. (1975) Interspecies comparisons of skin irritancy. *Toxicol. appl. Pharmacol.*, 31, 481-490

Nordmann, R., Grudicelli, Y., Beaugé, F., Clément, M., Ribière, C., Rouach, H. & Nordmann, J. (1973) Studies on the mechanisms involved in the isopropanol-induced fatty liver. *Biochim. biophys. acta*, 326, 1-11

Oda, K. (1974) Volatile compounds from felled logs of *Pinus densiflora*. *Ringyo Shikenjo Kenkyu Hokoku*, 266, 1-11

Palo, V. & Ilková, H. (1970) Direct gas chromatographic estimation of lower alcohols, acetaldehyde, acetone and diacetyl in milk products. *J. Chromat.*, 53, 363-367

Richardson, D.R., Caravati, C.M., Jr & Weary, P.E. (1969) Allergic contact dermatitis to 'alcohol' swabs. *Cutis*, 5, 1115-1118

Scherberger, R.F., Happ, G.P., Miller, F.A. & Fassett, D.W. (1958) A dynamic apparatus for preparing air-vapor mixtures of known concentrations. *Amer. industr. Hyg. Ass. J.*, 19, 494-498

Shvedchenko, V.S. (1969) *Hygienic characteristics of working conditions in polypropylene production.* In: *Proceedings of a Conference on the Hygienic Problems of the Production Using Polymer Materials*, Moscow, Research Institute of Hygiene, pp. 5-9

Smyth, H.F., Jr & Carpenter, C.P. (1948) Further experience with the range-finding test in the industrial toxicology laboratory. *J. industr. Hyg. Toxicol.*, 30, 63-68

Timmer, R., ter Heide, R., de Valois, P.J. & Wobben, H.J. (1971) Qualitative analysis of the most volatile neutral components of Reunion geranium oil (*Pelargonium roseum* Bourbon). *J. agric. Fd Chem.*, 19, 1066-1068

Traiger, G.J. & Plaa, G.L. (1974) Chlorinated hydrocarbon toxicity: potentiation by isopropyl alcohol and acetone. Arch. environm. Hlth, 28, 276-278

Treon, J.F. (1963) Alcohols. In: Patty, F.A., ed., Industrial Hygiene and Toxicology, Vol. II, Toxicology, New York, Interscience, pp. 1436-1440

US Department of Commerce (1976) US Exports, Schedule B Commodity by Groupings, Schedule B Commodity by Country, FT410/December 1975, Washington DC, Bureau of the Census, US Government Printing Office, pp. 2-78-2-79

US Environmental Protection Agency (1975) Preliminary Assessment of Suspected Carcinogens in Drinking Water. Report to Congress, Washington DC, US Government Printing Office, p. II-5

US Food and Drug Administration (1976) Food and drugs. US Code of Federal Regulations, Title 21, parts 8.300, 8.305, 8.308, 121.1403, 121.1099, 121.1164

US International Trade Commission (1976a) Synthetic Organic Chemicals, US Production and Sales, 1974, ITC Publication 776, Washington DC, US Government Printing Office, pp. 201, 222

US International Trade Commission (1976b) Synthetic Organic Chemicals, US Production and Sales of Miscellaneous Chemicals, 1975 Preliminary, Washington DC, US Government Printing Office, p. 9

US Occupational Safety and Health Administration (1976) Air contaminants. US Code of Federal Regulations, Title 29, part 1910.1000, p. 29

US Tariff Commission (1922) Census of Dyes and Other Synthetic Organic Chemicals, 1921, Tariff Information Series No. 26, Washington DC, US Government Printing Office, p. 150

Wasilewski, C., Jr (1968) Allergic contact dermatitis from isopropyl alcohol. Arch. Dermatol., 98, 502-504

Wax, J., Ellis, F.W. & Lehman, A.J. (1949) Absorption and distribution of isopropyl alcohol. J. Pharmacol. exp. Ther., 97, 229-237

Weast, R.C., ed. (1976) CRC Handbook of Chemistry and Physics, 57th ed., Cleveland, Ohio, Chemical Rubber Co., p. C-459

Weil, C.S., Smyth, H.F., Jr & Nale, T.W. (1952) Quest for a suspected industrial carcinogen. Arch. industr. Hyg. occup. Med., 5, 535-547

WHO (1971) Toxicological evaluation of some extraction solvents and certain other substances. Wld Hlth Org. Fd Add./70.39, pp. 140-142

Wickson, E.J. (1968) Propyl alcohols (iso). In: Kirk, R.E. & Othmer, D.F., eds, *Encyclopedia of Chemical Technology*, 2nd ed., Vol. 16, New York, John Wiley and Sons, pp. 564-578

Wills, J.H., Jameson, E.M. & Coulston, F. (1969) Effects on man of daily ingestion of small doses of isopropyl alcohol. *Toxicol. appl. Pharmacol.*, 15, 560-565

METHYL IODIDE

1. Chemical and Physical Data

1.1 Synonyms and trade names

Chem. Abstr. Services Reg. No.: 74-88-4

Chem. Abstr. Name: Iodomethane

1.2 Chemical formula and molecular weight

CH_3I Mol. wt: 141.95

1.3 Chemical and physical properties of the pure substance

From Weast (1976), unless otherwise specified

(a) Description: Colourless liquid with a pungent odour (Hart et al., 1966)

(b) Boiling-point: 42.4°C

(c) Melting-point: -66.45°C

(d) Density: d_4^{20} 2.279

(e) Refractive index: n_D^{20} 1.5380

(f) Spectroscopy data: Infra-red, nuclear magnetic resonance and mass spectra have been tabulated by Grasselli (1973).

(g) Solubility: Slightly soluble in water (1.4 g/100 ml at 20°C); soluble in acetone, benzene and carbon tetrachloride; miscible with ethanol and ether (Hart et al., 1966; Weast, 1976)

(h) Volatility: Vapour pressure is 400 mm at 25°C (Irish, 1963).

(i) Stability: Turns brown on exposure to light, due to decomposition and liberation of free iodine (Hart et al., 1966; Windholz, 1976); decomposes at 270°C

(j) Reactivity: Reacts with many compounds as an alkylating agent (Hart et al., 1966)

1.4 Technical products and impurities

Methyl iodide is available in the US and Japan in a grade containing at least 99% of the pure chemical, with a boiling range of 41-43°C. Iodine may be present as an impurity.

2. Production, Use, Occurrence and Analysis

For background information on this section, see preamble, p. 17.

2.1 Production and use

(a) Production

Methyl iodide was prepared in 1909 by Kaufler & Herzog by electrolysis of an aqueous solution of potassium acetate in the presence of iodine or potassium iodide (Prager & Jacobson, 1918).

It is prepared commercially by the reaction of methanol with iodine and phosphorus, or by the reaction of dimethyl sulphate with an aqueous iodine slurry which contains a reducing agent such as powdered iron or sodium bisulphite. Methyl iodide can also be prepared by reacting methanol with hydriodic acid, by reacting methyl-*para*-toluenesulphonate with potassium iodide or by reacting methyl phenyl ether with iodine and aluminium (Hart *et al.*, 1966).

Commercial production of methyl iodide in the US was first reported in 1943, when about 1400 kg were manufactured (US Tariff Commission, 1945). In 1973, three companies reported a combined production of 8600 kg (US International Trade Commission, 1975), and in 1974, two companies reported its manufacture (see preamble, p. 17) (US International Trade Commission, 1976).

Methyl iodide is reported to be produced in the Federal Republic of Germany, Spain and the UK, with a total annual production in the range of 1-10 million kg.

Commercial production of methyl iodide in Japan first began in 1960, and one company is currently producing it (another stopped manufacture in 1975). About 60-80 thousand kg methyl iodide were produced in 1975, and a negligible amount was exported to the US.

(b) Use

Methyl iodide is used as a methylating agent in the preparation of pharmaceutical intermediates and in organic synthesis (Hart *et al.*, 1966). It is also used in microscopy, due to its high refractive index, as a reagent in testing for pyridine and as embedding material used to examine diatoms (Windholz, 1976).

In India, methyl iodide has been investigated for use as a fumigant to control internal fungi of grain sorghum (Ragunathan *et al.*, 1974).

The US Occupational Safety and Health Administration's health standards for exposure to air contaminants require that an employee's exposure to methyl iodide does not exceed an eight-hour time-weighted average of 28 mg/m^3 (5 ppm) in the working atmosphere in any eight-hour work shift of a forty-hour work week (US Occupational Safety and Health Administration, 1976).

2.2 Occurrence

Methyl iodide occurs in the sea as a natural product of marine algae. The mean concentration of this chemical in the air over the Atlantic Ocean has been reported to be 1.2×10^{-12} parts by volume (7 µg/l), implying an annual world production by algae of 4×10^{10} kg. It appears to be a natural carrier of iodine between the seas and the land (Lovelock *et al.*, 1973).

An ambient concentration of 80×10^{-12} parts by volume (460 µg/l) methyl iodide has been detected in the air over New Brunswick, New Jersey (Lillian & Singh, 1974). It can be formed in the environment of nuclear reactors (Barnes *et al.*, 1966) and is found in exhaust gases (Apple *et al.*, 1974).

2.3 Analysis

A method for sampling and analysis recommended by the US National Institute for Occupational Safety and Health for determining methyl iodide in working atmospheres is based on adsorption of methyl iodide from the air on activated charcoal, subsequent desorption with toluene, and analysis by gas chromatography with flame ionization detection. The precision of the method is about ±10% (NIOSH, 1975). Gas chromatography with flame ionization detection has also been used to measure methyl iodide, methyl nitrate and methanol in exhaust gases from nuclear reactors (Apple et al., 1974). Gas chromatography coupled with mass spectrometry has been used to determine methyl iodide as an impurity in hydrogen iodide at levels of 0.005%, with a relative experimental error of 10-12% (Dudorov et al., 1974). Gas chromatography with electron capture detection has been used to separate and identify the presence in hydrocarbons of several alkyl iodides, including methyl iodide, in the range of 10^{-12} parts by volume (6 µg/l) (Castello et al., 1969). Gas chromatography with an electron capture detector operated coulometrically was used to measure methyl iodide in air in the range of 10^{-12} parts by volume (6 µg/l) (Lillian & Singh, 1974; Lovelock et al., 1973).

A method for detecting methyl iodide in air in concentrations as low as 4 ng/l involves infra-red emission by laser excitation (Robinson et al., 1969).

Far ultra-violet (160-220 nm) spectroscopy has been proposed as a method for the analysis of 388 compounds, including methyl iodide; their far ultra-violet spectra are given, with corresponding references (Kaye, 1961).

A chemiluminescence method for determination of organic halides, including methyl iodide, has a limit of detection of 0.01×10^{-6} parts by volume (0.06 mg/m^3) (Crider, 1969).

A portable instrument for continuous monitoring of methyl iodide contains a pyrolyser and a microcoulomb detector; the method has a lower limit of detection of 2 ppb (1.2 µg/m^3) (McFee & Bechtold, 1971).

A colorimetric method for determining the methyl iodide residue on rice has been described, in which potassium iodide, produced from the methyl iodide, is used as the catalyst for the oxidation of As(III) by Ce(IV). The applicable range was 0.01-0.1 µg/3 ml aliquot (Rangaswamy et al., 1972).

3. Biological Data Relevant to the Evaluation of Carcinogenic Risk to Man

3.1 Carcinogenicity and related studies in animals

(a) Subcutaneous and/or intramuscular administration

Rat: Groups of BD rats, about 100-days old (sex unspecified), received weekly s.c. injections of 10 or 20 mg/kg bw methyl iodide in a vegetable oil for one year, or a single s.c. injection of 50 mg/kg bw, and were observed for life. S.c. sarcomas occurred in 9/16 rats injected with 10 mg/kg bw, in 6/8 rats injected with 20 mg/kg bw and in 4/14 rats given single injections of 50 mg/kg bw. Local tumours occurred between 500-700 days after the first injection. In most cases, pulmonary metastases were observed. No tumours were reported to have occurred in control rats (number unspecified) injected with the vegetable oil alone (Druckrey et al., 1970; Preussmann, 1968)

(b) Intraperitoneal administration

Mouse: Groups of 10 male and 10 female A/He 6-8-week old mice were injected intraperitoneally thrice weekly with methyl iodide in tricaprylin, for a total of 24 doses. Three dose levels were given, to provide total doses of 8.5, 21.3 and 44.0 mg/kg bw. All survivors were killed 24 weeks after the first injection. Survivors in the three groups were 19/20, 20/20 and 11/20, respectively. The numbers of mice with lung tumours were 4, 6 and 5 in the respective groups, and the average numbers of lung tumours per mouse were 0.21, 0.3 and 0.55. The incidence of lung tumours in untreated mice was 0.21/animal (6/29 mice), and that in tricaprylin-treated control mice was 0.22/animal (34/154). The only group in which the lung tumour incidence was significantly different ($P<0.05$) from that in controls was the group receiving the highest dose level (Poirier et al., 1975) [The Working Group noted the small number of animals used in this screening test].

3.2 **Other relevant biological data**

(a) Experimental systems

The s.c. LD_{50} of methyl iodide in mice is 110 mg/kg bw (Kutob & Plaa, 1962). In female white rats (Porton strain), the acute oral LD_{50} was found to be 76 mg/kg bw when methyl iodide was applied in a glycerol formol vehicle. Oral doses of 50 mg/kg bw on 5 days per week for one month produced no toxic effects (Johnson, 1966). When mice were given 5 mg/l (860 ppm) by inhalation for varying times, a linear relationship was obtained when the probit of the percentage mortality was plotted against the log of time. Under these conditions, 20 minutes' exposure resulted in 0%, 57 minutes in 50%, and 80 minutes in 100% mortality (Buckell, 1950).

Orally administered methyl iodide was rapidly converted in the liver to S-methylglutathione, which was shown to be excreted in the bile (22-28% of a 50 mg/kg bw dose) (Johnson, 1966). Barnsley & Young (1965) reported that following s.c. injection of 50 mg/kg bw in male rats, small amounts of S-methyl-L-cysteine, N-(methylthioacetyl)glycine, methylmercapturic acid and methylthioacetic acid were identified in the urine.

No data on embryotoxicity or teratogenicity were available to the Working Group.

Methyl iodide did not increase the back mutation frequency in *Aspergillus nidulans* to methionine independence when applied at concentrations of 0.01-0.1 M for 5-40 minutes; survival was 100% under these conditions (Moura Duarte, 1971). McCann *et al.* (1975) found that methyl iodide is mutagenic to *Salmonella typhimurium* TA100 when plates are exposed to vapours of this chemical.

(b) Man

Two cases of human poisoning after industrial exposure to vapours of methyl iodide have been reported (Garland & Camps, 1945; ILO, 1971). The first, described by Jaquet in 1901, showed symptoms of vertigo, diplopia, ataxia, delirium and serious mental disturbances. The second case, observed by Garland & Camps, was found to be drowsy, unable to walk and with slurred, incoherent speech. Death occurred 7-8 days after exposure, and autopsy revealed bronchopneumonia and congestion of all organs. The similarity to methyl bromide poisoning has been recorded.

Application of 1 ml methyl iodide under a gauze dressing to the skin of a volunteer for half-an-hour produced an erythematous reaction with vesicles 19 hours after application (Buckell, 1950).

Retention of inhaled ^{132}I-methyl iodide in 18 volunteers ranged from 43-92%, with a mean of 72% of the amount inhaled; the level was highly dependent on respiratory rate, low rates being associated with high retention and *vice versa* (Morgan & Morgan, 1967). Inhaled ^{132}I-methyl iodide was rapidly cleared from the lungs of 4 volunteers and broken down to release iodide ion. Between 30 and 40% of iodine introduced as methyl iodide appears to be accumulated in the thyroid (Morgan *et al.*, 1967).

3.3 Case reports and epidemiological studies

No data were available to the Working Group.

4. Comments on Data Reported and Evaluation[1]

4.1 Animal data

Methyl iodide is carcinogenic in rats, inducing local sarcomas after single or repeated subcutaneous injections. In a study in which only a few mice were used, it caused an increased incidence of lung tumours after its intraperitoneal injection.

4.2 Human data

No case reports or epidemiological studies were available to the Working Group.

---

[1] See also the section, 'Animal Data in Relation to the Evaluation of Risk to Man' in the introduction to this volume, p. 15.

5. References

Apple, R.F., Davis, H.G. & Meyer, A.S. (1974) Analysis of methyl iodide, methyl nitrate and methyl alcohol in 20 M nitric acid by gas chromatography. *Analyt. Lett.*, 7, 671-674

Barnes, R.H., Kircher, J.F. & Townley, C.W. (1966) Chemical-equilibrium studies of organic-iodide formation under nuclear-reactor-accident conditions. AEC Accession No. 43166, *Report No. BMI-1781*, Washington DC, US Energy Research and Development Administration

Barnsley, E.A. & Young, L. (1965) The metabolism of iodomethane. *Biochem. J.*, 95, 77-81

Buckell, M. (1950) The toxicity of methyl iodide. I. Preliminary survey. *Brit. J. industr. Med.*, 7, 122-124

Castello, G., D'Amato, G. & Biagini, E. (1969) The gas chromatography of alkyl iodides. *J. Chromat.*, 41, 313-324

Crider, W.L. (1969) Hydrogen-air flame chemiluminescence of some organic halides. *Analyt. Chem.*, 41, 534-537

Druckrey, H., Kruse, H., Preussmann, R., Ivankovic, S. & Landschütz, C. (1970) Cancerogene alkylierende Substanzen. III. Alkyl-halogenide, -sulfate, -sulfonate und ringgespannte Heterocyclen. *Z. Krebsforsch.*, 74, 241-270

Dudorov, V., Agliulov, N.K. & Faerman, V.I. (1974) Mass-spectrometric and gas-chromatographic analysis of hydrogen iodide. *Zh. analyt. Khim.*, 29, 361-364

Garland, A. & Camps, F.E. (1945) Methyl iodide poisoning. *Brit. J. industr. Med.*, 2, 209-211

Grasselli, J.G., ed. (1973) *CRC Atlas of Spectral Data and Physical Constants for Organic Compounds*, Cleveland, Ohio, Chemical Rubber Co., p. B-653

Hart, A.W., Gergel, M.G. & Clarke, J. (1966) *Iodine compounds (organic)*. In: Kirk, R.E. & Othmer, D.F., eds, *Encyclopedia of Chemical Technology*, 2nd ed., Vol. 11, New York, John Wiley and Sons, pp. 862-863

ILO (International Labour Office) (1971) *Encyclopedia of Occupational Health and Safety*, Vol. 1, Geneva, pp. 689-691

Irish, D.D. (1963) *Halogenated hydrocarbons: I. Aliphatic*. In: Patty, F.A., ed., *Industrial Hygiene and Toxicology*, Vol. II, *Toxicology*, New York, Interscience, 1255-1256

Johnson, M.K. (1966) Metabolism of iodomethane in the rat. Biochem. J., 98, 38-43

Kaye, W.I. (1961) Far ultraviolet spectroscopy. II. Analytical applications. Appl. Spectr., 15, 130-144

Kutob, S.D. & Plaa, G.L. (1962) A procedure for estimating the hepatotoxic potential of certain industrial solvents. Toxicol. appl. Pharmacol., 4, 354-361

Lillian, D. & Singh, H.B. (1974) Absolute determination of atmospheric halocarbons by gas phase coulometry. Analyt. Chem., 46, 1060-1063

Lovelock, J.E., Maggs, R.J. & Wade, R.J. (1973) Halogenated hydrocarbons in and over the Atlantic. Nature (Lond.), 241, 194-196

McCann, J., Choi, E., Yamasaki, E. & Ames, B.N. (1975) Detection of carcinogens as mutagens in the *Salmonella*/microsome test: assay of 300 chemicals. Proc. nat. Acad. Sci. (Wash.), 72, 5135-5139

McFee, D.R. & Bechtold, R.R. (1971) Pyrolyzer-microcoulomb detector system for measurement of toxicants. Amer. industr. Hyg. Ass. J., 32, 766-770

Morgan, A., Morgan, D.J., Evans, J.C. & Lister, B.A.J. (1967) Studies on the retention and metabolism of inhaled methyl iodide. II. Metabolism of methyl iodide. Hlth Phys., 13, 1067-1074

Morgan, D.J. & Morgan, A. (1967) Studies on the retention and metabolism of inhaled methyl iodide. I. Retention of inhaled methyl iodide. Hlth Phys., 13, 1055-1065

Moura Duarte, F.A. (1971) Efeitos mutagênicos de alguns ésteres de acidos inorgânicos em *Aspergillus nidulans* (Eidam) Winter. Cienc. Cult., 24, 42-52

NIOSH (National Institute for Occupational Safety and Health) (1975) Methyl Iodide, Method No. S98, Set H., Springfield, Virginia, National Technical Information Service

Poirier, L.A., Stoner, G.D. & Shimkin, M.B. (1975) Bioassay of alkyl halides and nucleotide base analogs by pulmonary tumor response in strain A mice. Cancer Res., 35, 1411-1415

Prager, B. & Jacobson, P. (1918) Beilsteins Handbuch der Organischen Chemie, 4th ed., Vol. 1, Syst. 5, Berlin, Springer-Verlag, pp. 69-70

Preussmann, R. (1968) Direct alkylating agents as carcinogens. Fd Cosmet. Toxicol., 6, 576-577

Ragunathan, A.N., Muthu, M. & Majumder, S.K. (1974) Further studies on the control of internal fungi of sorghum by fumigation. *J. Fd Sci. Technol. (India)*, 11, 80-81

Rangaswamy, J.R., Majumder, S.K. & Poornima, P. (1972) Colorimetric method for estimation of methyl iodide residues on jowar (sorghum) and rice. *J. Ass. off. analyt. Chem.*, 55, 800-801

Robinson, J.W., Hailey, D.M. & Barnes, H.M. (1969) Infrared emission of organic compounds stimulated by a laser beam. *Talanta*, 16, 1109-1111

US International Trade Commssion (1975) *Synthetic Organic Chemicals, US Production and Sales, 1973*, ITC Publication 728, Washington DC, US Government Printing Office, pp. 205, 231

US International Trade Commission (1976) *Synthetic Organic Chemicals, US Production and Sales, 1974*, ITC Publication 776, Washington DC, US Government Printing Office, p. 229

US Occupational Safety and Health Administration (1976) Air contaminants. *US Code of Federal Regulations*, Title 29, part 1910.1000, p. 29

US Tariff Commission (1945) *Synthetic Organic Chemicals, US Production and Sales, 1941-43*, Report No. 153, Second Series, Washington DC, US Government Printing Office, p. 64

Weast, R.C., ed. (1976) *CRC Handbook of Chemistry and Physics*, 57th ed., Cleveland, Ohio, Chemical Rubber Co., p. C-374

Windholz, M., ed. (1976) *The Merck Index*, 9th ed., Rahway, NJ, Merck & Co., p. 794

para-QUINONE

1. Chemical and Physical Data

1.1 Synonyms and trade names

Chem. Abstr. Reg. Services No.: 106-51-4

Chem. Abstr. Name: 2,5-Cyclohexadiene-1,4-dione

Benzoquine; benzoquinone; 1,4-benzoquinone; *para*-benzoquinone; chinone; cyclohexadienedione; 1,4-cyclohexadienedione; 1,4-cyclohexadiene dioxide; quinone

1.2 Chemical formula and molecular weight

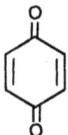

$C_6H_4O_2$ Mol. wt: 108.1

1.3 Chemical and physical properties of the pure substance

From Windholz (1976), unless otherwise specified

(a) *Description*: Yellow monoclinic prisms with a penetrating odour resembling that of chlorine

(b) *Melting-point*: 115.7°C

(c) *Spectroscopy data*: Infra-red, ultra-violet, nuclear magnetic resonance and mass spectra have been tabulated by Grasselli (1973).

(d) *Solubility*: Slightly soluble in water; soluble in ethanol, ether and hot petroleum ether

(e) *Volatility*: Sublimes; volatile with steam

(f) *Reactivity*: Acts as an oxidizing agent and is reduced to hydroquinone (Thirtle, 1968)

1.4 *Technical products and impurities*

para-Quinone is available in the US as a technical grade with a melting-point of 112°C. The grade available in Japan has a purity of over 99%.

2. Production, Use, Occurrence and Analysis

For background information on this section, see preamble, p. 17.

2.1 *Production and use*

(a) *Production*

para-Quinone was prepared in 1838 by Woskresensky by the oxidation of quinic acid obtained by extraction of cinchona bark (Thirtle, 1968). Although it can be prepared by the oxidation of benzene or of numerous benzene derivatives, oxidation of aniline has been the preferred method for commercial production in both the US and Japan. An older process used sodium dichromate and sulphuric acid, but the most widely-used process uses manganese dioxide and sulphuric acid (Thirtle, 1968).

Commercial production of *para*-quinone in the US was first reported in 1919 (US Tariff Commission, 1921); only one US company reported production of *para*-quinone in 1974 (see preamble, p. 17) (US International Trade Commission, 1976a). US imports of *para*-quinone through the principal customs districts in 1974 amounted to 2.72 thousand kg (US International Trade Commission, 1976b).

para-Quinone has been produced in the UK by one company since 1972 (Anon., 1972), and it is produced in the Federal Republic of Germany and France. Annual production in these countries is estimated to be 3-30 million kg.

para-Quinone was first produced in Japan in 1938 or 1939. Annual production in recent years was approximately 1,000 kg, but the factories of both producing companies were closed down in 1975.

(b) Use

The major use for *para*-quinone is as an intermediate in the production of hydroquinone[1]. It is used as a polymerization inhibitor (Nowak & Rubens, 1969), as an intermediate for the production of a variety of derivatives (e.g., rubber accelerators, oxidizing agents), as an oxidizing agent, a photographic chemical and a tanning agent, and as a chemical reagent (Windholz, 1976).

para-Quinone is also used as a chemical intermediate to make: (i) its dioxime and the dibenzoate of the dioxime, both of which are rubber accelerators; (ii) quinhydrone, a complex of *para*-quinone and hydroquinone used in electrodes for pH determinations; and (iii) 2,3-dichloro-5,6-dicyanobenzoquinone, a selective oxidizing agent used in steroid synthesis.

The US Occupational Safety and Health Administration's health standards for exposure to air contaminants require that an employee's exposure to *para*-quinone does not exceed an eight-hour time-weighted average of 0.1 ppm (0.4 mg/m^3) in the working atmosphere in any eight-hour work shift of a forty-hour work week (US Occupational Safety and Health Administration, 1976). The corresponding standard in the Federal Republic of Germany and in Australia is also 0.4 mg/m^3, and the acceptable ceiling concentration of *para*-quinone in the USSR is 0.05 mg/m^3 (Winell, 1975).

2.2 Occurrence

para-Quinone occurs naturally in a variety of arthropods (Harrison & Weatherston, 1967). It has been found as a pollutant in filtered surface and ground water at a water treatment plant (Thielemann, 1969).

2.3 Analysis

Paper and thin-layer chromatography have been used for the detection of quinones, including *para*-quinone (Simatupang & Hausen, 1970), and thin-layer chromatography has been applied for determining its purity (Thielemann, 1971).

---

[1] See also monograph on hydroquinone, p. 155.

Thin-layer chromatography using several different spray reagents has been used for the detection and semi-quantitative determination of *para*-quinone. The limits of detection were 0.4-10 µg (Thielemann, 1974). Thin-layer chromatography systems have been investigated for use in the separation and identification of naturally occurring benzoquinones, including *para*-quinone (Harrison & Weatherston, 1967). Polyamide layers on thin-layer plates have been used to separate the chemical, which was then detected under ultra-violet light (254 nm) as a quenched spot after treatment with ammonia (Wang *et al.*, 1969).

A colorimetric method for the determination of concentrations of 2 mg/l or more *para*-quinone in air and urine was based on the absorbance at 410 nm of its complex with *para*-dimethylaminobenzaldehyde (Kulik, 1969). In another colorimetric method used to measure concentrations of 5-50 µg/l, the absorbance of its complex with 1-phenyl-2,3-dimethyl-4-amino-5-pyrazolone was measured at 530 nm (Thielemann, 1972).

Nuclear magnetic resonance spectra have been reported to be suitable for the quantitative analysis of pharmaceutical preparations of a wide range of chemicals, including *para*-quinone (Bowen *et al.*, 1974).

3. Biological Data Relevant to the Evaluation of Carcinogenic Risk to Man

3.1 Carcinogenicity and related studies in animals

(a) Skin application

Mouse: A group of mice were painted with a 0.25% solution of *para*-quinone in benzene every one or two days. Of 44 mice that survived more than 200 days, 3 developed skin papillomas, 1 developed a skin carcinoma and 5 developed lung adenocarcinomas. When a 0.1% solution was used, 41 mice survived more than 200 days, and 6 developed skin papillomas, 2 developed skin carcinomas and 10 developed lung adenocarcinomas [$P<0.05$]. Of 46 surviving controls treated with benzene, 1 developed a skin papilloma, and 2 developed lung adenocarcinomas (Takizawa, 1940) [The Working Group noted that the sex and strain of the animals and the duration of the experiment were not specified].

(b) Inhalation and/or intratracheal administration

Mouse: A group of 25 mice (sex and strain unspecified) were exposed to 5 mg para-quinone in a 130-l chamber for 1 hour, 6 times per week; 25 mice were untreated and served as controls. In 11 treated mice that survived more than 100 days, 2 lung adenocarcinomas were observed. Among 12 controls that died after more than 100 days, 2 lung adenomas were observed (Kishizawa, 1954). In another experiment carried out under the same conditions of exposure, 2 lung adenocarcinomas were found in 25 treated mice, compared with 1 lung adenoma among 25 controls (Kishizawa, 1955). The same experiment was repeated, and 2 lung adenocarcinomas were observed in 25 mice and 1 lung adenoma in 25 controls (Kishizawa, 1956).

(c) Subcutaneous and/or intramuscular administration

Rat: A group of 24 rats (15 Wistar strain and 9 hybrids), weighing about 200 g each, were injected subcutaneously with 0.5 ml of a solution of para-quinone in propylene glycol at weekly intervals. The concentration given during the first 53 days was 1%; this was reduced to 0.2% from days 54-173, and again increased to 0.4% after 173 days. Seventeen rats survived the injection period of 394 days and received a total of 32 injections (para-quinone 81 mg, propylene glycol 16.5 ml) during this period. Injection-site fibrosarcomas developed in 2 rats. No local tumours were observed among 11 rats of a Saitama mixed strain injected weekly with 1 ml propylene glycol for 15 months, then 0.5 ml, and surviving 300 or more days [$P>0.05$] (Umeda, 1957).

3.2 Other relevant biological data

(a) Experimental systems

The oral LD_{50} in rats is 130 mg/kg bw, and the i.v. LD_{50} is 25 mg/kg bw (Woodard et al., 1949). Administration of large doses of para-quinone induced local irritation, clonic convulsions, respiratory difficulties, drop in blood pressure and death due to paralysis of the medullary centres. Asphyxia plays an important role, due to pulmonary damage and effects on haemoglobin. Signs of kidney damage were observed in severely poisoned animals (Deichmann & Keplinger, 1963).

para-Quinone depresses respiration in tissue preparations (Hirai & Takizawa, 1951; Miller *et al.*, 1973). It also causes local greying of hair of coloured mice (Boyland & Sargent, 1951).

para-Quinone is readily absorbed from the gastrointestinal tract and s.c. tissue (species not specified). It is excreted partly unchanged, and partly as hydroquinone, of which the major proportion is eliminated as conjugates with hexuronic, sulphuric and other acids (Deichmann & Keplinger, 1963).

No data on embryotoxicity or teratogenicity were available to the Working Group.

Toxic concentrations of *para*-quinone were not mutagenic to *Neurospora* tested for forward *pyr* mutations (requirement for pyrimidines) or reverse mutations to arginine independence (Reissig, 1963).

A single i.p. injection of 6.25 mg/kg bw *para*-quinone did not induce dominant lethal mutations in male mice (Röhrborn & Vogel, 1967).

(b) Man

Following local exposure to *para*-quinone, skin changes include discolouration, erythema, swelling and the formation of papules and vesicles; prolonged contact may lead to necrosis. Exposure to vapours induces serious disturbances of vision; the injury extends through the entire layer of the conjunctiva and is characterized by a deposit of pigment. All layers of the cornea are also involved (Deichmann & Keplinger, 1963).

3.3 Case reports and epidemiological studies

No data were available to the Working Group.

4. Comments on Data Reported and Evaluation

4.1 Animal data

para-Quinone has been tested in mice by skin application and inhalation and in rats by subcutaneous injection. The available data are insufficient to evaluate the carcinogenicity of this compound.

4.2 **Human data**

No case reports or epidemiological studies were available to the Working Group.

5. References

Anon. (1972) *p*-Benzoquinone plant opens. <u>Chemical Marketing Reporter</u>, 28 August, p. 5

Bowen, M.H., O'Neill, I.K. & Pringuer, M.A. (1974) Quantitative applications of nuclear magnetic resonance in pharmaceutical analysis. <u>Proc. Soc. analyt. Chem.</u>, <u>11</u>, 294-297

Boyland, E. & Sargent, S. (1951) The local greying of hair in mice treated with X-rays and radiomimetic drugs. <u>Brit. J. Cancer</u>, <u>5</u>, 433-440

Deichmann, W.B. & Keplinger, M.L. (1963) <u>Phenols and phenolic compounds</u>. In: Patty, F.A., ed., <u>Industrial Hygiene and Toxicology</u>, Vol. 2, <u>Toxicology</u>, New York, Interscience, pp. 1383-1385

Grasselli, J.G., ed. (1973) <u>CRC Atlas of Spectral Data and Physical Constants for Organic Compounds</u>, Cleveland, Ohio, Chemical Rubber Co., p. B-324

Harrison, V.J. & Weatherston, J. (1967) Thin-layer chromatography of simple naturally occurring benzoquinones. <u>J. Chromat.</u>, <u>31</u>, 258-259

Hirai, Y. & Takizawa, N. (1951) Experimental studies on the mechanism of quinone carcinogenesis. First report: changes in tissue respiration due to quinone influence. <u>Gann</u>, <u>42</u>, 91-94

Kishizawa, F. (1954) Carcinogenic action of *para*-benzoquinone on the lung of mice by the experimental inhalation (1). <u>Gann</u>, <u>45</u>, 389-391

Kishizawa, F. (1955) Carcinogenic action of benzoquinone on the lung of mice by the experimental inhalation (report 2). <u>Gann</u>, <u>46</u>, 359-361

Kishizawa, F. (1956) Carcinogenic action of *para*-benzoquinone on the lung of mice by the experimental inhalation (report 3). <u>Gann</u>, <u>47</u>, 601-603

Kulik, V.A. (1969) <u>Determination of some quinones in air and in urine</u>. In: Murav'eva, S.I., ed., <u>News of Industrial and Sanitary Chemistry of the District</u>, Moscow, Meditsina, pp. 249-253

Miller, J.J., Powell, G.M., Olavesen, A.H. & Curtis, C.G. (1973) Metabolism and toxicity of phenols in cats. <u>Biochem. Soc. Trans.</u>, <u>1</u>, 1163-1165

Nowak, R.M. & Rubens, L.C. (1969) <u>Unsaturated polyesters</u>. In: Kirk, R.E. & Othmer, D.F., eds, <u>Encyclopedia of Chemical Technology</u>, 2nd ed., Vol. 20, New York, John Wiley and Sons, pp. 822-825

Reissig, J.L. (1963) Induction of forward mutants in the *pyr*-3 region of *Neurospora*. <u>J. gen. Microbiol.</u>, <u>30</u>, 317-325

Röhrborn, G. & Vogel, F. (1967) Mutationen durch chemische Einwirkung bei Säuger und Mensch. 2. Genetische Untersuchungen an der Maus. Dtsch. med. Wschr., 92, 2315-2321

Simatupang, M.H. & Hausen, B.M. (1970) Chromatographische Nachweisreaktionen von chinoiden Verbindungen. J. Chromat., 52, 180-183

Takizawa, N. (1940) Über die experimentelle Erzeugung der Haut- und Lungenkrebse bei der Maus durch Bepinselung mit Chinone. Gann, 34, 158-160

Thielemann, H. (1969) Thin-layer chromatographic results for identification of organic pollution components of shore-filtered surface and ground water (Halle-Beesen waterworks). Z. Chem., 9, 189-190

Thielemann, H. (1971) Thin-layer chromatographic determination of the purity of 1,4-benzoquinone or 1,4-dihydroxybenzene. Mikrochim. acta, 3, 522-523

Thielemann, H. (1972) Quantitative determination of 1,4-benzoquinone, 1,4-naphthoquinone, 2-methyl-3-phytyl-1,4-naphthoquinone (vitamin K_1), 2-methyl-3-difarnesyl-1,4-naphthoquinone (vitamin K_2), 2-methyl-1,4-naphthoquinone (vitamin K_3), and 5-hydroxy-1,4-naphthoquinone (Juglone) by reactions with 4-aminophenazone. Sci. Pharm., 40, 134-135

Thielemann, H. (1974) Detection and semiquantitative thin-layer chromatographic determination of 1,4-benzoquinone on finished foils and silica gel G sorption layers with different spray reagents. Z. Chem., 14, 28-29

Thirtle, J.R. (1968) Quinones. In: Kirk, R.E. & Othmer, D.F., eds, Encyclopedia of Chemical Technology, 2nd ed., Vol. 16, New York, John Wiley and Sons, pp. 899-913

Umeda, M. (1957) Production of rat sarcoma by injections of propylene glycol solution of p-quinone. Gann, 48, 139-144

US International Trade Commission (1976a) Synthetic Organic Chemicals, US Production and Sales, 1974, ITC Publication 776, Washington DC, US Government Printing Office, p. 205

US International Trade Commission (1976b) Imports of Benzenoid Chemicals and Products, 1974, ITC Publication 762, Washington DC, US Government Printing Office, p. 12

US Occupational Safety and Health Administration (1976) Air contaminants. US Code of Federal Regulations, Title 29, part 1910.1000, p. 31

US Tariff Commission (1921) Census of Dyes and Coal-Tar Chemicals, 1919, Tariff Information Series No. 22, Washington DC, US Government Printing Office, p. 25

Wang, K.-T., Wu, P.-H. & Shih, T.-B. (1969) Polyamide layer chromatography. XXII. Separation of quinones. J. Chromat., 44, 635-637

Windholz, M., ed. (1976) The Merck Index, 9th ed., Rahway, NJ, Merck & Co., p. 1051

Winell, M.A. (1975) An international comparison of hygienic standards for chemicals in the work environment. Ambio, 4, 34-36

Woodard, G., Hagan, E.C. & Radomski, J.L. (1949) Toxicity of hydroquinone for laboratory animals. Fed. Proc., 8, 348

SUCCINIC ANHYDRIDE

1. Chemical and Physical Data

1.1 Synonyms and trade names

Chem. Abstr. Services Reg. No.: 108-30-5

Chem. Abstr. Name: Dihydro-2,5-furandione

Butanedioic anhydride; 2,5-diketotetrahydrofuran; succinic acid anhydride; succinyl oxide; tetrahydro-2,5-dioxofuran

1.2 Chemical formula and molecular weight

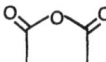

$C_4H_4O_3$ Mol. wt: 100.1

1.3 Chemical and physical properties of the pure substance

From Windholz (1976), unless otherwise specified

(a) Description: Orthorhombic prisms from ethanol

(b) Boiling-point: 261°C; sublimes at 115°C and 5 mm

(c) Melting-point: 119.6°C

(d) Spectroscopy data: λ_{max} 278 nm (E_1^1 = 141.3) in benzene (Weast, 1975); infra-red and mass spectra have been tabulated by Grasselli (1973).

(e) Solubility: Soluble in chloroform, carbon tetrachloride and ethanol; very slightly soluble in ether and water

(f) Reactivity: Reacts with the sulphydryl group of cysteine in neutral aqueous solution (Dickens & Cooke, 1965)

1.4 Technical products and impurities

Succinic anhydride is available in the US as a commercial grade containing at least 99.5% of the pure chemical, with maximums of 0.5% unsaturated compounds (as maleic anhydride), 0.15% chlorides, 0.04% sulphates (as SO_4) and 20 mg/kg heavy metals (Turi, 1969).

2. Production, Use, Occurrence and Analysis

For background information on this section, see preamble, p. 17. A review on succinic anhydride has been published (Turi, 1969).

2.1 Production and use

(a) Production

Succinic anhydride was prepared by Gerhardt & Chiozza in 1853 by reacting succinic acid with phosphorus pentachloride (Prager & Jacobson, 1933). It can also be prepared by the dry distillation of maleic acid, by the dehydration of succinic acid at high temperatures, by treating succinic acid with diketene, succinyl chloride or acetic anhydride, or by reacting the diethyl ester with boron chloride. It is reported to be produced commercially by the hydrogenation of maleic anhydride (Turi, 1969).

Succinic anhydride has been produced commercially in the US for more than 50 years (US Tariff Commission, 1922); two companies produced it in 1974 (see preamble, p. 17) (US International Trade Commission, 1976a). US imports of succinic anhydride through the principal customs districts were 4500 kg in 1972 (US Tariff Commission, 1973), 5000 kg in 1973 (US Tariff Commission, 1974) and 2700 kg in 1974 (US International Trade Commission, 1976b).

(b) Use

Succinic anhydride and succinic acid appear to be used interchangeably as chemical intermediates for a wide variety of industrial applications. Succinic anhydride is used in the manufacture of polymeric materials, pharmaceuticals, agricultural chemicals, dyestuffs, photographic chemicals, surface-active agents, lubricant additives, fire-retardants for paper and in the food industry. It is also used in the manufacture of certain adhesive resins, alkyd resins used in coating compositions and reinforced and non-reinforced casting, and molding and laminating resins. It is used as a cross-linking agent in ion-exchange membranes, as a curing agent for epoxy resins and in the manufacture of elastomers for specialty applications (Turi, 1969).

Succinic anhydride is also used in the manufacture of pharmaceutical products such as chemotherapeutic agents, vitamins, steroids, antihemorrhagic drugs, anticonvulsants and muscle relaxants (Turi, 1969).

It is used in the manufacture of N-dimethylaminosuccinamic acid, a plant growth regulator (Spencer, 1973) and may also be used in the manufacture of insect repellants and herbicides (Turi, 1969).

Succinic anhydride is used in the manufacture of silver halide photographic emulsions; anthraquinone dyes which can be applied to nylon or acetate rayons; drying oils; lubricant additives; fire-retardants for paper and other cellulose products; components of surfactants (e.g., succinylated monoglycerides, used as food emulsifiers) and demulsifying agents; fabric-treatment chemicals; and many other miscellaneous uses (Turi, 1969).

It is also used as a food starch modifier; not more than 4% succinic anhydride may be used in the US for esterifying food starches such as corn starch (US Food & Drug Administration, 1975).

2.2 Occurrence

Succinic anhydride is not known to occur as a natural product.

2.3 Analysis

A titration method based on the reaction of succinic anhydride with morpholine has been used for determining its purity, with an accuracy of ±0.1% (Critchfield & Johnson, 1956).

A colorimetric determination is based on the reaction of succinic anhydride with 2-nitrophenylhydrazine in a basic medium (Munson, 1974). A general analytical method based on the reaction of an anhydride with hydroxylamine, followed by treatment with a ferric ion to yield a highly coloured chelate complex, has been reported. The method applies to a concentration range of 10^{-3}-10^{-2}M and has an accuracy of ±2% (Goddu et al., 1955).

A method for determining anhydrides, including succinic anhydride, is based on the fluorescence of the condensation product of succinic anhydride and 2-carboxy-isonitrosoacetanilide. The limits of detection are 5×10^{-10}-5×10^{-9}M/l, with an error of 15-25% (Dziomko et al., 1969).

3. Biological Data Relevant to the Evaluation of Carcinogenic Risk to Man

3.1 Carcinogenicity and related studies in animals

Subcutaneous and/or intramuscular administration

Rat: Six male rats, weighing about 100 g, were treated twice weekly with 2 mg/animal succinic anhydride in 0.5 ml arachis oil for 65 weeks (total dose, 260 mg). Subcutaneous sarcomas developed at the injection site in all of 3 rats that survived 93-106 weeks. No tumours occurred in 24 controls injected with arachis oil alone that survived 45-106 weeks (Dickens & Jones, 1964, 1965).

3.2 Other relevant biological data

(a) Experimental systems

Succinic anhydride did not induce reverse mutations in *Salmonella typhimurium* TA1535, TA1537, TA98 and TA100 either in the presence or absence of a rat liver post-mitochondrial supernatant (McCann et al., 1975).

(b) Man

No data were available to the Working Group.

3.3 Case reports and epidemiological studies

No data were available to the Working Group.

4. Comments on Data Reported and Evaluation

4.1 Animal data

In the only study available, which involved few rats, succinic anhydride produced local sarcomas after its subcutaneous injection. Further studies are required before an evaluation of the carcinogenicity of this compound can be made.

4.2 Human data

No case reports or epidemiological studies were available to the Working Group.

5. References

Critchfield, F.E. & Johnson, J.B. (1956) Reaction of carbon disulfide with primary and secondary aliphatic amines as an analytical tool. Analyt. Chem., 28, 430-436

Dickens, F. & Cooke, J. (1965) Rates of hydrolysis and interaction with cysteine of some carcinogenic lactones and related substances. Brit. J. Cancer, 19, 404-410

Dickens, F. & Jones, H.E.H. (1964) Further studies on carcinogenesis by lactones and related substances. A.R. Brit. Emp. Cancer Campgn, 42, 141-142

Dickens, F. & Jones, H.E.H. (1965) Further studies on the carcinogenic action of certain lactones and related substances in the rat and mouse. Brit. J. Cancer, 19, 392-403

Dziomko, V.M., Ivanov, O.V. & Kremenskaya, I.N. (1969) New luminescent method for the determination of acylating agents. Zh. analyt. Khim., 24, 927-930

Goddu, R.F., LeBlanc, N.F. & Wright, C.M. (1955) Spectrophotometric determination of esters and anhydrides by hydroxamic acid reaction. Analyt. Chem., 27, 1251-1255

Grasselli, J.G., ed. (1973) CRC Atlas of Spectral Data and Physical Constants for Organic Compounds, Cleveland, Ohio, Chemical Rubber Co., p. B-905

McCann, J., Choi, E., Yamasaki, E. & Ames, B.N. (1975) Detection of carcinogens as mutagens in the *Salmonella*/microsome test: assay of 300 chemicals. Proc. nat. Acad. Sci. (Wash.), 72, 5135-5139

Munson, J.W. (1974) 2-Nitrophenylhydrazine: a selective reagent for colorimetric determination of carboxylic acid anhydrides and chlorides. J. pharm. Sci., 63, 252-256

Prager, B. & Jacobson, P., eds (1933) Beilsteins Handbuch der Organischen Chemie, 4th ed., Vol. 17, Syst. 2475, Berlin, Springer-Verlag, p. 407

Spencer, E.Y. (1973) Guide to the Chemicals Used in Crop Protection, Publication 1093, 6th ed., London, Ontario, University of Western Ontario, Research Branch, Agriculture Canada, p. 469

Turi, P. (1969) Succinic acid and succinic anhydride. In: Kirk, R.E. & Othmer, D.F., eds, Encyclopedia of Chemical Technology, 2nd ed., Vol. 19, New York, John Wiley and Sons, pp. 134-150

US Food and Drug Administration (1975) Food starch-modified. US Code of Federal Regulations, Title 21, part 121.1031

US International Trade Commission (1976a) *Synthetic Organic Chemicals, US Production and Sales, 1974*, ITC Publication 776, Washington DC, US Government Printing Office, p. 218

US International Trade Commission (1976b) *Imports of Benzenoid Chemicals and Products, 1974*, ITC Publication 762, Washington DC, US Government Printing Office, p. 27

US Tariff Commission (1922) *Census of Dyes and Other Synthetic Organic Chemicals, 1921*, Tariff Information Series No. 26, Washington DC, US Government Printing Office, p. 15L

US Tariff Commission (1973) *Imports of Benzenoid Chemicals and Products, 1972*, TC Publication 601, Washington DC, US Government Printing Office, p. 23

US Tariff Commission (1974) *Imports of Benzenoid Chemicals and Products, 1973*, TC Publication 688, Washington DC, US Government Printing Office, p. 23

Weast, R.C., ed. (1975) *CRC Handbook of Chemistry and Physics*, 56th ed., Cleveland, Ohio, Chemical Rubber Co., p. C-495

Windholz, M., ed. (1976) *The Merck Index*, 9th ed., Rahway, NJ, Merck & Co., p. 1148

2,4,5-T AND ESTERS

1. Chemical and Physical Data

1.1 Synonyms and trade names

Chem. Abstr. Services Reg. No.: 93-76-5

Chem. Abstr. Name: (2,4,5-trichlorophenoxy)acetic acid

2,4,5-Trichlorophenoxyacetic acid

For a representative list of other synonyms and trade names of products containing 2,4,5-T, its salts or esters, either as the sole active ingredient or as mixtures with other compounds, see Appendix A.

1.2 Chemical formula and molecular weight

$C_8H_5Cl_3O_3$ Mol. wt: 255.5

1.3 Chemical and physical properties of the pure substance

From Weed Science Society of America (1974), unless otherwise specified

(a) *Description*: White solid

(b) *Melting-point*: 158°C (Martin, 1968)

(c) *Spectroscopy data*: λ_{max} 206, 289, 297 nm (E_1^1 = 1872, 99, 91) (Grasselli & Ritchey, 1975); ultra-violet and infra-red absorption spectra have been tabulated by Gore *et al.* (1971).

(d) *Solubility*: Soluble (590 mg/kg) in ethanol or isopropyl alcohol and in water (238 mg/l) at 50°C

(e) *Stability*: Stable at its melting-point

(<u>f</u>) <u>Reactivity</u>: Reacts with organic and inorganic bases to form salts and with alcohols to form esters

1.4 Technical products and impurities

Technical grade 2,4,5-T must have a melting-point of approximately 150-151°C; a typical batch from one producer was found to have the following composition: >95% of the pure chemical, 2.9% dichloromethoxyphenoxyacetic acids, 0.6% related trichlorophenoxyacetic acids, 0.5% dichlorophenoxyacetic acids, 0.4% bis(2,4,5-trichlorophenoxy)acetic acid and less than 0.5 mg/kg 2,3,7,8-tetrachlorodibenzo-*para*-dioxin (TCDD) [See also monograph on chlorinated dibenzodioxins, p. 41]. In another sample of commercially produced 2,4,5-T, TCDD was found to be present at concentrations of about 27 mg/kg (WHO, 1971), and chlorodioxins have been reported in other batches of 2,4,5-T (US Department of Agriculture, 1971).

2,4,5-T produced prior to 1965 contained 30 mg/kg or more TCDD (Anon., 1970). 2,4,5-T with a dioxin content of less than 0.05 mg/kg is presently produced in several countries and is available in commercial quantities. Furthermore, techniques are available for producing 2,4,5-T with a TCDD content below detectable levels (0.02 mg/kg)(Neubert & Dillmann, 1972).

In Japan, technical grade 2,4,5-T has a melting-point of 154-157°C and a purity of more than 99%.

2,4,5-T is available in the US as the triethylamine salt and as esters of the following alcohols: 2-butoxyethyl, butoxypolypropyleneglycol, sec-butyl and iso-octyl (US International Trade Commission, 1976a). Typical formulations include emulsifiable concentrates containing the esters and water-soluble concentrates of the amine salt (Martin, 1968).

2. Production, Use, Occurrence and Analysis

For background information on this section, see preamble, p. 17.

2.1 Production and use

(a) Production

2,4,5-T was prepared in 1941 by the interaction of 2,4,5-trichlorophenol, monochloroacetic acid and sodium hydroxide (Pokorny, 1941), and a similar process is believed to be used in its commercial production.

It was first produced commercially in the US in 1944 (US Tariff Commission, 1946). The quantity of 2,4,5-T acid produced increased steadily between 1960 and 1968, when it reached a maximum of 7.9 million kg; production decreased to 2.3 million kg in 1969 (US Department of Agriculture, 1972, 1976). In 1975, three US companies reported commercial production of this chemical (see preamble, p. 17) (US International Trade Commission, 1976a). In 1974, 70.3 thousand kg 2,4,5-T were imported through the principal US customs districts (US International Trade Commission, 1976b). In 1975, combined US exports to Canada, Colombia, Dominican Republic, Malaysia, Turkey and Venezuela of the various forms of 2,4-D and 2,4,5-T, expressed as free acid, amounted to 5.7 million kg (US Department of Commerce, 1975).

Combined production of 2,4,5-T in the Federal Republic of Germany, Spain and the UK is estimated to be 2-20 million kg annually. Another estimate of the total annual production of 2,4,5-T in the Federal Republic of Germany and the UK is 4.5 million kg.

2,4,5-T was first produced commercially in Japan in 1965, and two companies are believed to have produced it until 1973-1974, when production was discontinued. The only significant Japanese exports were in 1972, when 162 thousand kg of emulsifiable concentrates were exported, probably because of restrictions on the use of 2,4,5-T in Japan.

About 15,000 kg were imported into Australia in 1975-1976.

(b) Use

2,4,5-T is a systemic herbicide used for control of woody and herbaceous weeds by air or ground spray applications (Weed Science Society of America, 1974). It was used to defoliate jungle areas in south Vietnam, where it was a component of 'Agent Orange' (a 50:50 mixture of the n-butyl esters of 2,4-D and 2,4,5-T, containing up to 30 mg/kg or more TCDD), and of 'Agent Purple' (a 50:30:20 mixture of the n-butyl esters of 2,4-D and the n-butyl and isobutyl esters of 2,4,5-T). About 40 million litres of 'Agent Orange' were sprayed in south Vietnam between 1965-1971 for defoliation or crop destruction. 'Agent Purple' was used until 1964, but no information about the quantity sprayed are available (Committee on the Effects of Herbicides in Vietnam, 1974).

In April 1970, the Surgeon General of the US reported that the use of 2,4,5-T might be hazardous to human health. On 15 April 1970, the Secretaries of the US Departments of Health, Education and Welfare and of Agriculture issued a joint order calling for an immediate cessation of all uses of 2,4,5-T on or around lakes, ponds and ditch banks and of all uses of liquid formulations around homes and recreation areas. Another order was issued by these two Departments on 1 May 1970 which cancelled all uses of granular formulations of 2,4,5-T around homes, recreation areas, etc. and all uses of 2,4,5-T on crops intended for human consumption. Cancellation of its use on rice was appealed, leading to its continued use in this way.

On 23 July 1971, a report of a Scientific Advisory Committee recommended restoration of registration of 2,4,5-T to the status existing prior to April 1970, with the following conditions: (1) a 0.1 mg/kg tolerance of 2,4,5-T on edible food crops; (2) a limit of 0.5 mg/kg TCDD in existing 2,4,5-T and 0.1 mg/kg in 2,4,5-T produced in the future, with certified analyses being furnished by the manufacturers to the Environmental Protection Agency (EPA); and (3) provisions for warnings on labels of formulations used around the home, for additional research on possible soil accumulation and food chain magnification of TCDD and for the establishment of monitoring programmes for detection of adverse effects.

On 13 April 1972, a new order was issued by the EPA, continuing the suspension of 2,4,5-T use around homes, recreational sites and aquatic areas and the cancellation of uses in crops used for human food (Southwick, 1974).

In June 1974, the EPA dropped proceedings to ban most uses of 2,4,5-T and cancelled the scheduled hearings. The Department of Agriculture decision made in 1970 to cancel use of 2,4,5-T in homes, gardens and recreational areas is not affected by this action. Therefore, currently allowed uses in the US are only on rice, pastures, rangelands and rights-of-way (Anon., 1974). In 1975, an estimated 2 million kg of the chemical were used for commercial and industrial (non-crop) weed control and 1 million kg on pasture and rangeland. A decision regarding the possible issuance of a notice of a rebuttable presumption against renewal of registration (see 'General Remarks on Substances Considered', p. 28) is schedule to be made on 15 June 1977.

Use of 2,4,5-T was banned in Italy in 1970; its use is also banned in The Netherlands and in Sweden.

The US Occupational Safety and Health Administration health standards for exposure to air contaminants require that an employee's exposure to 2,4,5-T does not exceed an eight-hour time-weighted average of 10 mg/m^3 in the working atmosphere in any eight-hour work shift of a forty-hour work week (US Occupational Safety and Health Administration, 1976).

No acceptable daily intake for man was established for 2,4,5-T at the Joint Meeting of the FAO Working Party of Experts on Pesticide Residues and the WHO Expert Committee on Pesticide Residues (WHO, 1971).

2.2 Occurrence

2,4,5-T is not known to occur as a natural product.

In Europe, residues of 0.05 mg/kg 2,4,5-T have been found on the grain and 1 mg/kg on the straw of wheat, barley, oats and rye (WHO, 1971).

2,4,5-T is broken down more slowly than 2,4-D by soil organisms, and there is reportedly no accumulation in soil as a result of annual applications (Weed Science Society of America, 1974).

Air samples were collected near wheat-growing areas around Pullman and Kennewick Highlands, Washington, USA, between April and August 1964 after applications of 2,4,5-T. An average concentration of 0.045 $\mu g/m^3$ and a maximum concentration of 3.38 $\mu g/m^3$ of an aerosol of 2,4,5-T methyl ester were found in 24-hour samples near Pullman. A sample of dust collected in Cincinnati, Ohio, USA in January 1965, which had its origin in a dust storm in New Mexico and Texas, contained 0.04 mg/kg 2,4,5-T (Finkelstein, 1969).

People in the Federal Republic of Germany have been exposed by gathering berries and mushrooms in forests treated with aerial applications of 2,4,5-T (Wellenstein, 1975).

Soil samples from areas sprayed in 1964-65 in connection with military defoliation operations in south Vietnam were collected in 1971 and analysed for herbicide persistence. Where the highest amounts had been sprayed (1075 kg/ha), in order to calibrate aerial spray equipment, concentrations of up to 1.5 kg/ha were recovered after 6-7 years. When 88.5 kg/ha 2,4,5-T had been applied between 1965-68, levels of between 0.022 and 0.27 kg/ha were recovered in 1971-72 in 2/3 of the samples (Committee on the Effects of Herbicides in Vietnam, 1974).

2.3 Analysis

The Association of Official Analytical Chemists (AOAC) has published an Official Final Action for the determination of 2,4,5-T in formulations by measurement of total chlorine (Horwitz, 1975). A method for determining 2,4,5-T in formulations by gas chromatography of its trimethylsilyl derivative has been described (Collier & Grimes, 1974; Zweig, 1972). Recoveries of 100.5 ± 1.0% compare favourably with those obtained using an AOAC infra-red spectroscopy method (Collier & Grimes, 1974).

Several methods for determining 2,4,5-T residues are summarized in the Pesticide Analytical Manual (US Food and Drug Administration, 1975). A general method for extraction and cleanup of chlorophenoxy acids in fatty and nonfatty foods is given. Suitable methods for detection of the methyl derivative by gas chromatography are also included.

A gas chromatographic procedure has been used to separate mixtures of herbicidal acids as their pentafluorobenzyl derivatives, which give better separation and better responses in the electron capture detector than do the methyl or silyl derivatives; the method has a sensitivity of 0.5 µg/kg for 2,4,5-T (Chau & Terry, 1976). An automated, gel permeation chromatographic procedure permits cleanup of pesticide residues in lipid-containing plant and animal extracts prior to their determination by gas chromatography with electron capture detection (Johnson et al., 1976).

3. Biological Data Relevant to the Evaluation of Carcinogenic Risk to Man

3.1 Carcinogenicity and related studies in animals[1]

(a) Oral administration

Mouse: Groups of 18 male and 18 female (C57BL/6xC3H/Anf)F_1 mice and 18 male and 18 female (C57BL/6xAKR)F_1 mice received commercial 2,4,5-T (98% pure, m.p. 149-151°C) according to the following dose schedule: 21.5 mg/kg bw in 0.5% gelatine by stomach tube at 7 days of age and the same amount (not adjusted for increasing body weight) daily up to 28 days of age; subsequently, the mice were given 60 mg/kg of diet. The dose was the maximum tolerated dose for infant and young mice. The experiment was terminated when the mice were 78 weeks of age, at which time 15, 17, 14 and 14 mice in the four groups, respectively, were still alive. The numbers of mice with tumours in each of the groups were 6 (4 of which had hepatomas), 1, 3 and 2, respectively. The tumour incidences in treated mice were not increased (P>0.05) for any type of tumour in any group or combination of groups compared with those in groups of 79, 87, 90 and 82 mice of each sex and strain which were either untreated or had received gelatine only (Innes et al., 1969; NTIS, 1968a).

A group of 20 male and 19 female 6-week old inbred XVII/G mice were given 100 mg/l 2,4,5-T (containing less than 0.05 mg/kg chlorinated dibenzodioxins) in the drinking-water for 2 months. Subsequently, 2,4,5-T was mixed directly with the diet at a concentration of 80 mg/kg of diet for lifespan. Average survival times were 555 days in treated males and 632 days in treated females, compared with 516 and 553 days in 32 male and 40

---

[1]The Working Group was aware of carcinogenicity studies in progress in mice involving i.p. injection and in rats with oral administration (IARC, 1976).

female controls. No significant increase in the incidence of tumours was noted. A group of 22 male and 25 female C3Hf mice were treated similarly. Average survival times were 523 days in treated males and 621 days in treated females, compared with 641 and 661 days in 43 male and 44 female controls. The total numbers of tumours were 13/22 in treated males and 13/25 in treated females, which were significantly different from that in female controls, 9/44 ($P<0.01$) but not from that in males, 22/43. One osteosarcoma, 2 squamous-cell carcinomas of the skin, 4 hepatomas, 3 leukaemias, 2 sarcomas and 1 tumour of the cervix occurred in treated females; in control females, 5 lung tumours, 3 hepatomas and 1 leukaemia were observed (Muranyi-Kovacs et al., 1976).

(b) Subcutaneous and/or intramuscular administration

Mouse: Groups of 18 male and 18 female (C57BL/6xC3H/Anf)F_1 mice and 18 male and 18 female (C57BL/6xAKR)F_1 mice were given single s.c. injections of 215 mg/kg bw 2,4,5-T (98% pure, m.p. 149-151°C) in dimethyl sulphoxide at 28 days of age and observed up to 78 weeks of age, at which time 11, 17, 17 and 18 mice, in the four groups, respectively, were still alive. Tumour incidences were compared with those in groups of 141, 154, 161 and 157 controls that were either untreated or were injected with dimethyl sulphoxide, 0.5% aqueous gelatin or corn oil. The tumour incidence in any group or combination of groups was not significantly different from that in controls ($P>0.05$) (NTIS, 1968a).

3.2 Other relevant biological data

(a) Experimental systems

Acute and short-term toxicity

There are species differences in the acute oral toxicity of 2,4,5-T and of its derivatives (Table 1).

Single oral doses of 100 mg/kg bw 2,4,5-T fed to pigs caused anorexia, vomiting, diarrhoea and ataxia. At autopsy, haemorrhagic enteritis and congestion of the liver and kidney were found (Björklund & Erne, 1966).

TABLE 1

Acute oral toxicity of 2,4,5-T and esters[a]

Compound of 2,4,5-T	Species	Sex	LD_{50} (mg/kg bw)
Acid	Mice	M	389
	Rats	M	500
	Guinea-pigs	M&F	381
	Dogs		100
	Chicks	M&F	310
Isopropyl ester	Mice	F	551
	Rats	M&F	495
	Guinea-pigs	F	449
Mixed butyl esters	Mice	F	940
	Rats	F	481
	Guinea-pigs	F	750
	Rabbit	M	712
Mixed amyl esters	Rats	F	750

[a] From Rowe & Hymas, 1954

Sub-acute and chronic toxicity

Groups of male and female rats were maintained for 90 days on diets with added 2,4,5-T (containing less than 1 mg/kg TCDD); animals received 3, 10, 30 or 100 mg/kg bw daily. Changes were found only in animals of both sexes fed 100 mg/kg bw/day; these included depression in body weight gain and slight decrease in food intake. Elevated serum alkaline phosphatase levels were observed in both sexes, and male rats had slightly increased serum glutamic-pyruvic transaminase levels (Dow, 1970, cited in WHO, 1971).

No adverse effects were noted in rats of both sexes maintained for 90 days on diets containing 100 or 300 mg/kg of diet of a standardized mixture of mono-, di- and tripropylene glycol butyl ether esters of 2,4,5-T (equivalent to 6.2 and 18.6 mg/kg bw free acid). A small number (2/10) of animals fed 1000 mg/kg of diet of the mixture (equivalent to 62 mg/kg bw free acid) exhibited central lobular necrosis in the liver; a significant increase was noted in the average weight of the kidney in male rats fed this level. Animals fed 3000 mg/kg of diet of the mixture (equivalent to 186 mg/kg bw free acid) displayed growth retardation, and kidney:body weight ratios were increased in male animals. The livers of animals of both sexes were enlarged and had slight central lobular necrosis; in females, some kidney necrosis was also evident. Serum alkaline phosphatase levels were elevated in males given this dose (Dow, 1961, cited in WHO, 1971).

Dogs fed 2,4,5-T (98.9% pure) 5 times per week for 90 days at dosage levels of 2, 5 or 10 mg/kg bw exhibited no adverse effects. Daily doses of 20 mg/kg bw resulted in deaths 11-75 days after the beginning of dosing (Drill & Hiratzka, 1953).

Absorption, distribution and excretion

After single s.c. administration of 100 mg/kg bw 2,4,5-T to mice, 23% of the dose was recovered in the body over 24 hours (Zielinski & Fishbein, 1967). In rats, 85.8% of a single i.v. dose of 100 mg/kg bw was found in the urine within 6 days (Sauerhoff et al., 1976).

Single oral doses to rats of 100 mg/kg bw of the triethanolamine salt of 2,4,5-T were readily absorbed, distributed and eliminated; excretion was primarily via the kidneys (Erne, 1966). Seven days after oral administration of 50 mg/kg bw 2,4,5-T (99.6% pure) to rats, 56-69% of the dose was recovered in the urine: 70-85% of the recovered dose was unchanged 2,4,5-T, and approximately 15-30% was found as the glycine and taurine conjugates and as 2,4,5-trichlorophenol; the two conjugates were excreted in nearly equal amounts (Böhme & Grunow, 1974; Grunow et al., 1971). Similar results were obtained in mice, except that the quantity of the taurine conjugate was greater (Grunow & Böhme, 1974).

The biological half-life of 5 mg/kg bw 2,4,5-T administered orally to dogs (77 hours) was longer than that in rats (4.7 hours). When the dose of 2,4,5-T to rats was increased to 200 mg/kg bw, the biological half-life was prolonged to 25 hours, indicating that the excretory capacity of the animals could be exceeded (Piper et al., 1973).

Similar results were obtained with single i.v. injections of 5 or 100 mg/kg bw ^{14}C-2,4,5-T in rats, where 2.3 and 7.6% of the radioactivity were excreted in the faeces, respectively, suggesting that at the higher dose biliary excretion of 2,4,5-T and/or its degradation products is involved in the overall elimination of 2,4,5-T from the body (Sauerhoff et al., 1976).

Marked differences in the pharmacokinetics of 2,4,5-T are seen with different species, ages and doses: clearance of 2,4,5-T from the plasma and body of dogs, mice and man is slower than that in rats. The volume of distribution after a single oral dose of 5 mg/kg bw also differs: in man, 0.079; in rats, 0.14; and in dogs, 0.22 l/kg (Gehring et al., 1973; Piper et al., 1973).

A single dose of 100 mg/kg bw 2,4,5-T to pregnant mice was almost entirely eliminated by 72 hours; however, after 4 daily administrations of the same dose, 2,4,5-T accumulated in maternal tissues and foetuses, and by 48 hours 2,4,5-T was still detectable throughout the foetuses (Ebron & Courtney, 1976).

No radioactivity was found in NMRI strain mouse embryos in an early stage of gestation after administration of ^{14}C-2,4,5-T to the dams. When given in late gestation, the foetal tissue had a level similar to that in maternal tissue (Lindquist & Ullberg, 1971). Selective uptake of 2,4,5-T into the yolk sac epithelium and absence of placental transfer in early pregnancy are effects similar to those seen with trypan blue in mouse embryos (Lloyd & Beck, 1969).

No radioactivity was detected in hamster embryos in a late stage of gestation after similar administration of 2,4,5-T to the dams (Dencker, 1976).

The biological half-life of ^{14}C-2,4,5-T was significantly longer in newborn than in adult rats (Fang et al., 1973; Hook et al., 1974).

Radioactivity was found in all tissues examined as well as in milk and foetuses after a single oral administration of 0.17-41 mg/kg bw ^{14}C-2,4,5-T to pregnant rats (Fang et al., 1973).

Embryotoxicity and teratogenicity

Doses of more than 20 mg/kg bw 2,4,5-T (containing less than 0.1 mg/kg TCDD) can increase the frequency of cleft palates in some strains of mice. Foetal growth retardation may also be observed when such doses are administered on days 6-15 of pregnancy (NTIS 1968b). No clearcut teratogenic effects have been reported in rats, rabbits, sheep or monkeys. Few data are available concerning possible postnatal changes after prenatal exposure.

2,4,5-T (later found to contain 30 mg/kg TCDD) was teratogenic and foetocidal in two strains of mice (C57BL/6 and AKR) when given orally at a dose of 113 mg/kg bw/day in honey or s.c. in dimethyl sulphoxide on days 6-14 or 9-17 of gestation. Cleft palates and cystic kidneys were seen in C57BL/6 mice and only cleft palates in AKR mice. No teratogenic effect was observed in C57BL/6 mice given lower doses (21.5 mg/kg bw), but with a dose of 46.4 mg/kg bw cystic kidneys occurred. A dose-response relationship has been suggested for the foetocidal and teratogenic properties of 2,4,5-T given by either route (Courtney et al., 1970).

The effects of two samples of 2,4,5-T (technical grade, containing 0.5 mg/kg TCDD, and analytical grade, containing less than 0.05 mg/kg TCDD) were compared with those of TCDD in studies with 3 strains of mice, random-bred CD-1, inbred DBA/2J and inbred C57BL/6J. Compounds were administered subcutaneously from days 6-15 of pregnancy as solutions in 100% dimethyl sulphoxide in a volume of 100 µl/animal/injection. Both samples of 2,4,5-T produced cleft palate in all three strains of mice when administered at levels of 100 mg/kg bw, and both produced kidney malformations in CD-1 mice. When 100 mg/kg bw 2,4,5-T and 1 µg/kg bw TCDD were administered in combination to CD-1 mice, the activity was not potentiated at the doses employed (Courtney & Moore, 1971).

Significant increases in the frequency of cleft palate and of embryotoxic effects were found in NMRI mice following oral administration of 35-130 mg/kg bw 2,4,5-T (containing less than 0.1 or 0.05 mg/kg TCDD) from days 6-15 of pregnancy. A dose of 20 mg/kg bw/day 2,4,5-T was established as the 'teratogenic no-effect level' (Roll, 1971).

The purest sample of 2,4,5-T available (containing less than 0.02 mg/kg TCDD) produced embryotoxic effects in NMRI mice when given orally on days 6-15 of gestation. The frequency of cleft palate exceeded that in controls when doses higher than 20 mg/kg bw (about 1/16 the LD_{50}) were administered. While reductions in foetal weight were found with 10-15 mg/kg bw, there was no definite increase in embryolethality over that seen in controls. Cleft palates were produced with a single oral dose of 150-300 mg/kg bw 2,4,5-T; the maximal teratogenic effect was obtained when the compound was administered on day 12 or 13 of gestation. When a dose of 60 mg/kg bw was given on days 6-15 of pregnancy, 5% of the foetuses had cleft palates, as compared with about 0.7% of control animals ($P<0.01$). With doses of 30 mg/kg bw, no significant increase was observed. 2,4,5-T butyl ester was shown to have embryotoxic effects on mice analogous to those found after administration of 2,4,5-T during days 6-15 of gestation (Neubert & Dillmann, 1972).

2,4,5-T (technical grade, containing 0.5 mg/kg TCDD) was neither teratogenic nor foetotoxic when administered orally to CD rats at levels of 10, 21.5, 46.4 and 80.0 mg/kg bw (Courtney & Moore, 1971) or to Sprague-Dawley rats at levels of 1, 3, 6, 12 or 24 mg/kg bw (Emerson et al., 1971) on days 6-15 of gestation. No cleft palates were observed in foetuses from control or experimental CD rats, and prenatal administration of 2,4,5-T did not affect postnatal growth and development (Courtney & Moore, 1971). Doses of up to 24 mg/kg bw 2,4,5-T (containing 1 mg/kg TCDD) had no teratogenic effect in rats when given on days 6-15 of gestation (Emerson et al., 1970).

2,4,5-T (containing less than 0.5 mg/kg TCDD) induced some foetopathy and increased the incidence of skeletal anomalies in Wistar rats following single daily oral doses of 100-150 mg/kg bw on days 6-15 of gestation. The butyl ester of 2,4,5-T had no evident effect when given at 50 or 150 mg/kg bw dose levels. Postnatal parameters were found not to be related to the teratogenic potential of the chemicals (Khera & McKinley, 1972).

However, more recent data (Sjöden & Söderberg, 1977) may indicate that a prenatal exposure to 2,4,5-T (single oral doses of 100 mg/kg bw on days 7, 8 or 9 of pregnancy) leads to behavioural abnormalities and changes in thyroid activity and brain serotonin levels in the progeny.

In order to examine the possibility that the most sensitive teratological test would be one involving a single treatment during organogenesis, groups of pregnant Wistar rats were treated by gavage on day 9 of gestation (a highly sensitive time in rat embryogenesis) with doses of 100, 200 or 400 mg/kg bw 2,4,5-T (containing 0.5 mg/kg TCDD) in 0.2% carboxymethylcellulose. A single dose of 100 mg/kg bw caused no increase in abnormal development or decrease in intrauterine growth but caused a slight increase in intrauterine deaths. This effect was accentuated at higher doses, and a moderate increase in malformations above control levels was also noted. Intrauterine growth was affected only with 400 mg/kg bw, a dose sufficient to cause severe embryotoxicity (Wilson *et al.*, 1971).

Studies on pregnant rats and their progeny of the effects of adequate or low-protein diets containing 250 and 1000 mg/kg of diet 2,4,5-T showed that, of mothers receiving 20% casein diets, only those fed high levels of 2,4,5-T showed a decrease in food intake, weight gain and feed efficiency ratio. The progeny of this group were taken on day 22 of gestation, and placenta, body, brain, liver and kidney weights were found to be significantly reduced (Hall, 1972).

Commercial samples of 2,4,5-T (containing 0.1, 0.5, 2.9 or 45 mg/kg TCDD) were foeticidal and teratogenic in Syrian golden hamsters when administered orally on days 6-10 of pregnancy at levels of 20, 40, 80 or 100 mg/kg bw; the incidence of effects increased with both the 2,4,5-T dosage and the content of TCDD. No malformations were produced by doses of less than 100 mg/kg bw 2,4,5-T containing no detectable TCDD. Bulging eyes (absence of eyelid) and delayed head ossification accounted for the majority of the terata caused by 2,4,5-T containing TCDD. TCDD contamination increased the incidence of haemorrhages in liveborn hamsters and also produced marked oedema (Collins & Williams, 1971).

No congenital malformations and no increase in the frequency of developmental variations were observed when New Zealand white rabbits were treated orally with 10, 20 or 40 mg/kg bw/day 2,4,5-T (containing 0.5 mg/kg TCDD) on days 6-18 of gestation. No deaths occurred among pregnant females, and maternal weight gain and foetal mortality and weight were unaffected (Emerson et al., 1971).

2,4,5-T did not appear to be teratogenic in rhesus monkeys (*Macaca mulatta*), nor did it interfere with normal development of the young, when groups of 10 pregnant females were treated with 0.05, 1.0 and 10.0 mg/kg bw 2,4,5-T (containing less than 0.05 mg/kg TCDD) in gelatin capsules by stomach tube daily from days 22-38 of pregnancy (Dougherty et al., 1973). Pregnant rhesus monkeys were also treated with 2,4,5-T (containing 0.5 mg/kg TCDD) at doses of 5, 10, 20 and 40 mg/kg bw thrice weekly for 4 weeks between days 20-48 of pregnancy. Twelve foetuses removed by hysterectomy after 100 days of gestation were developmentally normal and were within the range of weight for untreated foetuses of that age (J.G. Wilson, cited in Wilson et al., 1971).

Mutagenicity

2,4,5-T was not mutagenic *in vitro* in assays with *Salmonella typhimurium* G46, TA1535, TA1536, TA1537 or TA1538, *Escherichia coli* WP2 (hcr^+ or hcr^-), *Serratia marcescens* a21 and *Saccharomyces cerevisiae* D4 (Andersen et al., 1972; Buselmaier et al., 1972; Fahrig, 1974; Shirasu et al., 1976; Siebert & Lemperle, 1974). However, it has been reported that 2,4,5-T increases the reversion of a histidine-requiring strain of *S. cerevisiae* RAD18 when tested in suspension (35 µg/ml, pH 4.3) (Zetterberg, 1977). When 2,4,5-T was tested in the rec assay, which is believed to give an indication of reparable DNA damage, it was not more toxic to *Bacillus subtilis* M45 (rec^-) than to H17 (rec^+), suggesting that this compound does not damage DNA (Shirasu et al., 1976) [Metabolic activation systems were not included in any of these tests].

2,4,5-T administered subcutaneously to mice at a dose of 500 mg/kg bw was not mutagenic in host-mediated assays with *S. typhimurium* G46 or *S. marcescens* a21 (Buselmaier et al., 1972).

Adult *Drosophila melanogaster* receiving 250 mg/kg of diet 2,4,5-T (containing less than 0.1 mg/kg TCDD) for 5-6 days exhibited disturbances in somatic pairing between homologous chromosomes and also some chromosome abnormalities (Dävring & Sunner, 1971). When 2,4,5-T (containing no detectable amount of TCDD) was fed to 2-day old male *D. melanogaster* at concentrations of 0, 250 and 1000 mg/kg of medium for 15 days, the number of sex-linked recessive lethals was significantly increased (Majumdar & Golia, 1974). However, Vogel & Chandler (1974) detected no increase in the frequency of recessive lethal mutations in male *D. melanogaster* fed 2,4,5-T for only 3 days.

When 100 mg/kg bw 2,4,5-T (containing less than 1 mg/kg TCDD) were injected intraperitoneally into mice, no detectable increase in the number of micronuclei in erythrocytes of the bone-marrow was observed 24 hours or 7 days after treatment (Jenssen & Renberg, 1976).

Majumdar & Hall (1973) investigated the effect of 2,4,5-T (containing no detectable TCDD) on the chromosomes of bone-marrow cells of the Mongolian gerbil (*Meriones unguiculatus*). When random-bred males and females, 50-80-days old, received 5 consecutive daily i.p. injections, significant increases in chromatid gaps, chromatid breaks and fragments were observed after total doses of 250 mg/kg bw or more but not after 150 mg/kg bw or less.

2,4,5-T did not increase dominant lethal mutations in mice when given as an i.p. injection of 100 mg/kg bw (Buselmaier *et al.*, 1972).

(b) Man

Occupational exposure

A wide range of toxicological effects have been reported in workers involved in the manufacture of 2,4,5-T from 2,4,5-trichlorophenol [for details of the manufacturing process, see section 2.1(a)] (Bauer *et al.*, 1961; Bleiberg *et al.*, 1964; Jirasek *et al.*, 1973, 1974; Poland *et al.*, 1971). Chloracne, liver disorders, neurological and behavioural changes, fat metabolism disorders and signs of porphyria cutanea tarda are among the more frequently reported effects. In the majority of cases, however, the available data do not distinguish between the possible effects of exposure to 2,4,5-T and those of exposure to associated chemicals or more toxic contaminants such as TCDD (see also monograph on chlorinated dibenzo-dioxins, p. 41).

Chloracne and liver impairment, formerly thought to be caused by chlorophenols, were shown essentially to be due to TCDD (Hofmann, 1957; Kimmig & Schulz, 1957a,b; Schulz, 1957); the actual aetiological cause of porphyria cutanea tarda has not been identified (Poland et al., 1971), and the origin of certain other symptoms, particularly the neurological ones, may also be other frequently associated substances such as 2,4-D or chlorophenols.

An outbreak of chloracne affected 60 workers at the 2,4,5-T factory of the Dow Chemical Company in Midland, Michigan in 1964 (Firestone, 1977).

Of 29 subjects with features of chloracne working in a 2,4-D and 2,4,5-T-producing factory of the Diamond Alkali Co., Newark, New Jersey, US, 11 had increased excretion of uroporphyrins. In 3 cases, a diagnosis of porphyria cutanea tarda was unquestionable; 2 of these had raised serum glutamic-oxaloacetic transaminase levels. Many of the workers, whether or not they had uroporphyrinuria, had hirsutism, hyperpigmentation, increased skin fragility and vesicobullous eruptions on exposed areas of skin (Bleiberg et al., 1964; Firestone, 1977).

Poland et al. (1971) re-examined all of the employees of the same factory in 1969, after the level of TCDD in the 2,4,5-trichlorophenol had been reduced from 10-25 mg/kg to less than 1 mg/kg and found chloracne in 13/73 workers. A number of subjects had hyperpigmentation or facial hypertrichosis, but no definite diagnosis of porphyria could be made, and only one worker had mild uroporphyrinuria. The authors suggested that chloracne and porphyria cutanea tarda are essentially independent syndromes. About 30% of the workers suffered from gastrointestinal symptoms (nausea, vomiting, diarrhoea, abdominal pains or blood in the stools); about 10% of the workers had other systems, such as lower extremity weakness, headache and/or decreased auditory acuity. The severity of chloracne was associated with the degree of hypomania as measured on the Minnesota Multiphasic Personality Inventory hypomanic scale. Serum cholesterol was elevated in 10% of cases, and serum lactic dehydrogenase in 29%. Seven persons (10%) had a white blood cell count of less than $5000/mm^3$.

In a report on the conditions of 64 workers exposed daily to 2-8 mg 2,4,5-T in a manufacturing plant for periods ranging from 1 day to 3 years, Johnson (1971) states [without providing any supporting evidence] that no 'meaningful' differences were observed in [unspecified] clinical assessments in comparison to a control group and that no chromosomal effects were observed in 52 workers whose chromosomes were karyotyped.

In a report of occupational exposure at a factory in the USSR, where production of 2,4,5-T was begun in 1964, 128 workers showed skin lesions, and, among 83 examined, 69 had acne. Many, especially those with the severe skin lesions, also had liver impairment; 18 workers had a neurasthenic syndrome (Telegina & Bikbulatova, 1970).

Similar findings were described by Jirásek et al. (1973, 1974), who reported 76 cases of chloracne between 1965-1968 in a factory in Czechoslovakia producing 2,4,5-T and pentachlorophenol. These effects were attributed to TCDD. Fifty-five patients were submitted to medical follow-ups for over 5 years. Four deaths were observed, 2 of which were from bronchogenic carcinomas (see also monograph on chlorinated dibenzodioxins, p. 41). Some of the workers had symptoms of porphyria cutanea tarda, uroporphyrinuria, abnormal liver tests (bilirubin, serum glutamic-oxaloacetic transaminase, serum glutamic-pyruvic transaminase and bromosulphthalein) and liver enlargement. The majority of patients suffered from severe neurasthenia and depressive syndrome. In 17 subjects, signs of peripheral neuropathy, especially in the lower extremities, were confirmed by electromyographic examinations. More than half of the patients showed raised levels of blood cholesterol and total lipids.

In 1949, an accident occurred at the 2,4,5-T-producing factory of the Monsanto Chemical Company in Nitro, West Virginia, US; 228 people were affected. Symptoms included chloracne, melanosis, muscular aches and pain, fatigue, nervousness and intolerance to cold (see Firestone, 1977).

A similar accident occurred at the 2,4,5-T producing factory of the Phillips Duphar Company in The Netherlands in 1963 (Dalderup, 1974; Hay, 1976). Of 50 people affected, at least 10 still had skin complains in 1976; 4 workers died within 2 years of the accident.

Absorption and excretion

2,4,5-T given orally to human volunteers in doses of 100-150 mg was readily absorbed and gradually eliminated from the blood plasma, showing a first-order elimination rate; more than 80% of the dose was excreted in the urine in an intact form within 72 hours. The daily urinary excretion of 2,4,5-T in exposed workers was found to range from 0.5-3.6 mg/day in 11/21 samples. The corresponding concentrations of 2,4,5-T in the working atmosphere ranged from 0.21-0.67 mg/m^3 (Matsumura, 1970).

Almost all of a single oral dose of 5 mg/kg bw 2,4,5-T (containing less than 0.05 mg/kg TCDD) ingested by 5 human volunteers was absorbed into the body and excreted unchanged in the urine. The concentration of 2,4,5-T in plasma increased rapidly and, after 7 hours, reached a peak of 57 µg/ml; subsequently, the concentration decreased at a first-order rate with a half-life of 23.1 hours. Plasma contained 65% of the 2,4,5-T, almost all of which was reversibly bound to protein (Gehring et al., 1973).

Following oral administration of 2-5 mg/kg bw 2,4,5-T (>99% pure) to human volunteers, the compound was readily absorbed from the gastrointestinal tract and excreted, mainly via the kidneys, without undergoing any metabolic alteration. The half-life of clearance of 2,4,5-T from plasma after oral administration of 5 mg/kg bw was 18.8±3.1 hours (Kohli et al., 1974).

For details of adverse toxicological effects resulting from the spraying of 'Agent Orange' (a 50:50 mixture of the n-butyl esters of 2,4-D and 2,4,5-T, contaminated with up to 30 mg/kg or more TCDD) and other herbicides in Vietnam, see monograph on chlorinated dibenzodioxins, p. 41.

3.3 Case reports and epidemiological studies

Axelson & Sundell (1974) reported that in a cohort study of Swedish railway workers exposed to a variety of herbicides, a significant two-fold excess of all cancers was observed in exposed workers, as compared to the national average. The situation was difficult to evaluate because of the combined exposure of many workers to more than one herbicide. Most of the excess, however, seemed to be due to exposure to 3-amino-1,2,4-triazole (amitrole); within the subgroups that had been exposed to phenoxy acids (2,4-D and/or 2,4,5-T), only a small difference was detected: 5 cancers at all sites observed *versus* 2.8 expected. The authors stated, however, that the use of 2,4-D and 2,4,5-T had probably been higher than that they could trace.

See also monograph on chlorinated dibenzodioxins, p. 41.

4. Comments on Data Reported and Evaluation

4.1 Animal data

2,4,5-T was tested in mice in three studies by oral and subcutaneous administration. All of these studies had limitations due to the small numbers of animals used. Therefore, although an increased incidence of tumours at various sites was observed in one study in which 2,4,5-T (containing less than 0.05 ppm chlorinated dibenzodioxins) was given orally, no evaluation of the carcinogenicity of this compound could be made on the basis of the available data.

4.2 Human data

The results of the single cohort study of a small number of workers exposed to various herbicides, including 2,4-D, 2,4,5-T and 3-amino-1,2,4-triazole (amitrole)[1], are not sufficient to evaluate the carcinogenicity of 2,4,5-T to man (Because 2,4,5-T is contaminated with 2,3,7,8-tetrachlorodibenzo-*para*-dioxin, see also monograph on chlorinated dibenzodioxins, p. 41).

---

[1] See also IARC, 1974.

5. References

Andersen, K.J., Leighty, E.G. & Takahashi, M.T. (1972) Evaluation of herbicides for possible mutagenic properties. J. agric. Fd Chem., 20, 649-656

Anon. (1970) Another herbicide on the blacklist. Nature (Lond.), 226, 309-311

Anon. (1974) EPA exonerates 2,4,5-T. Chemical Week, 3 July, p. 10

Axelson, O. & Sundell, L. (1974) Herbicide exposure, mortality and tumor incidence. An epidemiological investigation on Swedish railroad workers. Work-environm.-hlth, 11, 21-28

Bauer, H., Schulz, K.H. & Spiegelberg, U. (1961) Berufliche Vergiftungen bei der Herstellung von Chlorphenol-Verbindungen. Arch. Gewerbepath. Gewerbehyg., 18, 538-555

Björklund, N.-E. & Erne, K. (1966) Toxicological studies of phenoxyacetic herbicides in animals. Acta vet. scand., 7, 364-390

Bleiberg, J., Wallen, M., Brodkin, R. & Applebaum, I.L. (1964) Industrially acquired porphyria. Arch. Dermatol., 89, 793-797

Böhme, C. & Grunow, W. (1974) Über den Stoffwechsel von 4-(2.4.5-Trichlorphenoxy)-buttersäure bei Ratten. Arch. Toxicol., 32, 227-231

Buselmaier, W., Röhrborn, G. & Propping, P. (1972) Mutagenitäts-Untersuchungen mit Pestiziden im Host-mediated assay und mit dem Dominanten Letaltest an der Maus. Biol. Zbl., 91, 311-325

Chau, A.S.Y. & Terry, K. (1976) Analysis of pesticides by chemical derivatization. III. Gas chromatographic characteristics and conditions for the formation of pentafluorobenzyl derivatives of ten herbicidal acids. J. Ass. off. analyt. Chem., 59, 633-636

Collier, R.H. & Grimes, G.S. (1974) Determination of chlorophenoxy acids in formulations by gas-liquid chromatography of their trimethylsilyl derivatives. J. Ass. off. analyt. Chem., 57, 781-784

Collins, T.F.X. & Williams, C.H. (1971) Teratogenic studies with 2,4,5-T and 2,4-D in the hamster. Bull. environm. Contam. Toxicol., 6, 559-567

Committee on the Effects of Herbicides in Vietnam (1974) The Effects of Herbicides in South Vietnam, Part A, Summary and Conclusions, Washington DC, National Academy of Sciences

Courtney, K.D. & Moore, J.A. (1971) Teratology studies with 2,4,5-trichlorophenoxyacetic acid and 2,3,7,8-tetrachlorodibenzo-p-dioxin. Toxicol. appl. Pharmacol., 20, 396-403

Courtney, K.D., Gaylor, D.W., Hogan, M.D., Falk, H.L., Bates, R.R. & Mitchell, I. (1970) Teratogenic evaluation of 2,4,5-T. Science, 168, 864-866

Dalderup, L.M. (1974) Safety measures for taking down buildings contaminated with toxic materials. II. T. soc. Geneesk., 52, 616-623

Dävring, L. & Sunner, M. (1971) Cytogenic effects of 2,4,5-trichlorophenoxyacetic acid on oogenesis and early embryogenesis in Drosophila melanogaster. Hereditas, 68, 115-122

Dencker, L. (1976) Tissue localization of some teratogens at early and late gestation related to fetal effects. Acta pharmacol. toxicol., 39, Suppl. 1, 59-72

Dougherty, W.H., Coulston, F. & Golberg, L. (1973) Non-teratogenicity of 2,4,5-trichlorophenoxyacetic acid in monkeys (Macaca mulatta). Toxicol. appl. Pharmacol., 25, 442

Drill, V.A. & Hiratzka, T. (1953) Toxicity of 2,4-dichlorophenoxyacetic acid and 2,4,5-trichlorophenoxyacetic acid: a report on their acute and chronic toxicity in dogs. Arch. industr. Hyg. occup. Med., 7, 61-67

Ebron, M. & Courtney, K.D. (1976) Difference in 2,4,5-T distribution in fetal mice and guinea pigs. Toxicol. appl. Pharmacol., 37, 144-145

Emerson, J.L., Thompson, D.J., Gerbig, C.G. & Robinson, V.B. (1970) Teratogenic study of 2,4,5-trichlorophenoxyacetic acid in the rat. Toxicol. appl. Pharmacol., 17, 317

Emerson, J.L., Thompson, D.J., Strebing, R.J., Gerbig, C.G. & Robinson, V.B. (1971) Teratogenic studies on 2,4,5-trichlorophenoxyacetic acid in the rat and rabbit. Fd Cosmet. Toxicol., 9, 395-404

Erne, K. (1966) Distribution and elimination of chlorinated phenoxyacetic acids in animals. Acta vet. scand., 7, 240-256

Fahrig, R. (1974) Comparative mutagenicity studies with pesticides. In: Montesano, R. & Tomatis, L., eds, Chemical Carcinogenesis Essays, Lyon, International Agency for Research on Cancer (IARC Scientific Publications No. 10), pp. 161-181

Fang, S.C., Fallin, E., Montgomery, M.L. & Freed, V.H. (1973) The metabolism and distribution of 2,4,5-trichlorophenoxyacetic acid in female rats. Toxicol. appl. Pharmacol., 24, 555-563

Finkelstein, H. (1969) Preliminary Air Pollution Survey of Pesticides, Raleigh, North Carolina, US Department of Health, Education and Welfare, pp. 49, 52, 130, 136

Firestone, D. (1977) The 2,3,7,8-tetrachlorodibenzo-*para*-dioxin problem: a review. In: Ramel, C., ed., Chlorinated Phenoxy Acids and their Dioxins: Mode of Action, Health Risks and Environmental Effects. Ecol. Bull. (Stockholm), 27 (in press)

Gehring, P.J., Kramer, C.G., Schwetz, B.A., Rose, J.Q. & Rowe, V.K. (1973) The fate of 2,4,5-trichlorophenoxyacetic acid (2,4,5-T) following oral administration to man. Toxicol. appl. Pharmacol., 26, 352-361

Gore, R.C., Hannah, R.W., Pattacini, S.C. & Porro, T.J. (1971) Infrared and ultraviolet spectra of seventy-six pesticides. J. Ass. off. analyt. Chem., 54, 1040-1082

Grasselli, J.G. & Ritchey, W.M., eds (1975) CRC Atlas of Spectral Data and Physical Constants for Organic Compounds, Cleveland, Ohio, Chemical Rubber Co., p. 67

Grunow, W. & Böhme, C. (1974) Über den Stoffwechsel von 2.4.5-T und 2.4-D bei Ratten und Mäusen. Arch. Toxicol., 32, 217-225

Grunow, W., Böhme, C. & Budczies, B. (1971) Renale Ausscheidung von bei Ratten. Fd Cosmet. Toxicol., 9, 667-670

Hall, S.M. (1972) Effects on pregnant rats and their progeny of adequate or low protein diets containing 2,4,5-trichlorophenoxyacetic acid (2,4,5-T) or *p,p*'-DDT. Fed. Proc., 31, 726

Hay, A. (1976) Toxic cloud over Seveso. Nature (Lond.), 262, 636-638

Hofmann, H.T. (1957) Neuere Erfahrungen mit hoch-toxischen Chlorkohlenwasserstoffen. Naunyn-Schmiedeberg's Arch. exp. Path. Pharmakol., 232, 228-230

Hook, J.B., Bailie, M.D., Johnson, J.T. & Gehring, P.J. (1974) *In vitro* analysis of transport of 2,4,5-trichlorophenoxyacetic acid by rat and dog kidney. Fd Cosmet. Toxicol., 12, 209-218

Horwitz, W., ed. (1975) Official Methods of Analysis of the Association of Official Analytical Chemists, 12th ed., Washington DC, Association of Official Analytical Chemists, p. 111

IARC (1974) IARC Monographs on the Evaluation of Carcinogenic Risk of Chemicals to Man, 7, Some Anti-thyroid and Related Substances, Nitrofurans and Industrial Chemicals, pp. 31-43

IARC (1976) IARC Information Bulletin on the Survey of Chemicals Being Tested for Carcinogenicity, No. 6, Lyon, pp. 49, 212

Innes, J.R.M., Ulland, B.M., Valerio, M.G., Petrucelli, L., Fishbein, L., Hart, E.R., Pallotta, A.J., Bates, R.R., Falk, H.L., Gart, J.J., Klein, M., Mitchell, I. & Peters, J. (1969) Bioassay of pesticides and industrial chemicals for mutagenicity in mice: a preliminary note. J. nat. Cancer Inst., 42, 1101-1114

Jenssen, D. & Renberg, L. (1976) Distribution and cytogenetic test of 2,4-D and 2,4,5-T phenoxyacetic acids in mouse blood tissues. Chem.-biol. Interact., 14, 291-299

Jirásek, L., Kalenský, J. & Kubec, K. (1973) Acne chlorina and porphyria cutanea tarda during the manufacture of herbicides. I. Cs. Dermatol., 48, 306-317

Jirásek, L., Kalenský, J. & Kubec, K., Pazderová, J. & Lukáš, E. (1974) Acne chlorina, porphyria cutanea tarda and other manifestations of general intoxication during the manufacture of herbicides. II. Cs. Dermatol., 49, 145-157

Johnson, J.E. (1971) The public health implications of widespread use of the phenoxy herbicides and picloram. Bioscience, 21, 899-905

Johnson, L.D., Waltz, R.H., Ussary, J.P. & Kaiser, F.E. (1976) Automated gel permeation chromatographic cleanup of animal and plant extracts for pesticide residue determination. J. Ass. off. analyt. Chem., 59, 174-187

Khera, K.S. & McKinley, W.P. (1972) Pre- and postnatal studies on 2,4,5-trichlorophenoxyacetic acid, 2,4-dichlorophenoxyacetic acid and their derivatives in rats. Toxicol. appl. Pharmacol., 22, 14-28

Kimmig, J. & Schulz, K.H. (1957a) Berufliche Akne (sog. Chlorakne) durch chlorierte aromatische zyklische Äther. Dermatologica, 115, 540-546

Kimmig, J. & Schulz, K.H. (1957b) Chlorierte aromatische zyklische Äther als Ursache der sogenannten Chlorakne. Naturwissenschaften, 44, 337-338

Kohli, J.D., Khanna, R.N., Gupta, B.N., Dhar, M.M., Tandon, J.S. & Sircar, K.P. (1974) Absorption and excretion of 2,4,5-trichlorophenoxy acetic acid in man. Arch. int. Pharmacodyn., 210, 250-255

Lindquist, N.G. & Ullberg, S. (1971) Distribution of the herbicides 2,4,5-T and 2,4-D in pregnant mice: accumulation in the yolk sac epithelium. Experientia, 27, 1439-1441

Lloyd, J.B. & Beck, F. (1969) The mechanism of teratogenic action of trypan blue. In: Bertelli, A., ed., Proceedings of the International Symposium on Teratology, Como, Italy, 1967, Amsterdam, Excerpta Medica, pp. 145-151

Majumdar, S.K. & Golia, J.K. (1974) Mutation test of 2,4,5-trichlorophenoxyacetic acid on *Drosophila melanogaster*. Canad. J. Genet. Cytol., 16, 465-460

Majumdar, S.K. & Hall, R.C. (1973) Cytogenetic effects of 2,4,5-T on *in vivo* bone marrow cells of Mongolian gerbils. J. Heredity, 64, 213-216

Martin, N., ed. (1968) Pesticide Manual. Basic Information on the Chemicals used as Active Components of Pesticides, 2nd ed., Ombersley, British Crop Production Council, p. 424

Matsumura, A. (1970) The fate of 2,4,5-trichlorophenoxyacetic acid in man. Jap. J. industr. Hlth, 12, 446-451

Muranyi-Kovacs, I., Rudali, G. & Imbert, J. (1976) Bioassay of 2,4,5-trichlorophenoxyacetic acid for carcinogenicity in mice. Brit. J. Cancer, 33, 626-633

Neubert, D. & Dillmann, I. (1972) Embryotoxic effects in mice treated with 2,4,5-trichlorophenoxyacetic acid and 2,3,7,8-tetrachlorodibenzo-*p*-dioxin. Naunyn-Schmiedeberg's Arch. exp. Path. Pharmakol., 272, 243-264

NTIS (National Technical Information Service) (1968a) Evaluation of Carcinogenic, Teratogenic and Mutagenic Activities of Selected Pesticides and Industrial Chemicals, Vol. 1, Carcinogenic Study, Washington DC, US Department of Commerce

NTIS (National Technical Information Service) (1968b) Evaluation of Carcinogenic, Teratogenic and Mutagenic Activities of Selected Pesticides and Industrial Chemicals, Vol. 2, Teratogenic Study in Mice and Rats, Washington DC, US Department of Commerce

Piper, W.N., Rose, J.Q., Leng, M.L. & Gehring, P.J. (1973) The fate of 2,4,5-trichlorophenoxyacetic acid (2,4,5-T) following oral administration to rats and dogs. Toxicol. appl. Pharmacol., 26, 339-351

Pokorny, R. (1941) Some chlorophenoxyacetic acids. J. Amer. chem. Soc., 63, 1768

Poland, A.P., Smith, D., Metter, G. & Possick, P. (1971) A health survey of workers in a 2,4-D and 2,4,5-T plant with special attention to chloracne, porphyria cutanea tarda and psychologic parameters. Arch. environm. Hlth, 22, 316-327

Roll, R. (1971) Untersuchungen über die teratogene Wirkung von 2,4,5-T bei Mäusen. Fd Cosmet. Toxicol., 9, 671-676

Rowe, V.K. & Hymas, T.A. (1954) Summary of toxicological information on 2,4-D and 2,4,5-T type herbicides and an evaluation of the hazards to livestock associated with their use. Amer. J. vet. Res., 15, 622-629

Sauerhoff, M.W., Braun, W.H., Blau, G.E. & Gehring, P.J. (1976) The dose-dependent pharmacokinetic profile of 2,4,5-trichlorophenoxy acetic acid following intravenous administration to rats. Toxicol. appl. Pharmacol., 36, 491-501

Schulz, K.H. (1957) Klinische und experimentelle Untersuchungen zur Ätiologie der Chloracne. Arch. klin. exp. Dermatol., 206, 589-596

Shirasu, Y., Moriya, M., Kato, K., Furuhashi, A. & Kada, T. (1976) Mutagenicity screening of pesticides in the microbial system. Mutation Res., 40, 19-30

Siebert, D. & Lemperle, E. (1974) Genetic effects of herbicides: induction of mitotic gene conversion in *Saccharomyces cerevisiae*. Mutation Res., 22, 111-120

Sjöden, P.-O. & Söderberg, U. (1977) Phenoxyacetic acids: sublethal effects. In: Ramel, C., ed., Chlorinated Phenoxy Acids and their Dioxins. Mode of Action, Health Risks and Environmental Effects. Ecol. Bull. (Stockholm) 27 (in press)

Southwick, L. (1974) 2,4,5-T chronology, an update (1972-1974). Down to Earth, 29, 21-24

Telegina, K.A. & Bikbulatova, L.I. (1970) Affection of the follicular apparatus of the skin in workers occupied in production of butyl ether of 2,4,5-trichlorphenoxyacetic acid. Vestn. Dermatol. Venerol., 44, 35-39

US Department of Agriculture (1971) The Pesticide Review, 1970, Agricultural Stabilization and Conservation Service, Washington DC, US Government Printing Office, p. 2

US Department of Agriculture (1972) The Pesticide Review, 1971, Agricultural Stabilization and Conservation Service, Washington DC, US Government Printing Office, p. 39

US Department of Agriculture (1976) The Pesticide Review, 1972, Agricultural Stabilization and Conservation Service, Washington DC, US Government Printing Office, p. 44

US Department of Commerce (1975) US Exports, Schedule B, Commodity by Country, FT410/December 1975, Washington DC, US Government Printing Office, pp. 2-74

US Food and Drug Administration (1975) *Pesticide Analytical Manual*, Vol. I, *Methods Which Detect Multiple Residues*, Rockville, Maryland, US Department of Health, Education and Welfare

US International Trade Commission (1976a) *Synthetic Organic Chemicals, US Production and Sales of Pesticides and Related Products, 1975 Preliminary*, Washington DC, US Government Printing Office, p. 6

US International Trade Commission (1976b) *Imports of Benzenoid Chemicals and Products, 1974*, ITC Publication 762, Washington DC, US Government Printing Office, p. 97

US Occupational Safety & Health Administration (1976) Air contaminants. *US Code of Federal Regulations*, Title 29, part 1910.93, p. 27

US Tariff Commission (1946) *Synthetic Organic Chemicals, US Production and Sales, 1944*, Report No. 155, Second Series, Washington DC, US Government Printing Office, p. 116

Vogel, E. & Chandler, J.L.R. (1974) Mutagenicity testing of cyclamate and some pesticides in *Drosophila melanogaster*. Experientia, 30, 621-623

Weed Science Society of America (1974) *Herbicide Handbook*, 3rd ed., Champaign, Illinois, pp. 375-378

Wellenstein, G. (1975) Biologische und oeko-toxikologische Probleme bei einer Flug-Begiftung un serer Waelder mit Derivaten der Phenoxyessigsaeure. Qual. Plant. Pl. Fd Hum. Nutr., 25, 1-20

WHO (1971) 1970 Evaluations of some pesticide residues in food. The Monographs. WHO/Food Add./71.42, pp. 459-477

Wilson, J.G., Boutwell, R.K., Davis, D.E., Dost, F.N., Hayes, W.J., Jr, Kalter, H., Loomis, T.A., Schubert, A., Sterling, T.D. & Bowen, D.L. (1971) *Report of the Advisory Committee on 2,4,5-T to the Administrator of the Environmental Protection Agency, May 7*, Washington DC, US Government Printing Office, pp. 44-45, 51-59

Zetterberg, G. (1977) *Experimental results of phenoxy acids on microorganisms*. In: Ramel, C., ed., *Chlorinated Phenoxy Acids and their Dioxins. Mode of Action, Health Risks and Environmental Effects*. Ecol. Bull. (Stockholm), 27 (in press)

Zielinski, W.L., Jr, & Fishbein, L. (1967) Gas chromatographic measurement of disappearance rates of 2,4-D and 2,4,5-T acids and 2,4-D esters in mice. J. agric. Fd. Chem., 15, 841-844

Zweig, G., ed. (1972) *Analytical Methods for Pesticides and Plant Growth Regulators*, Vol. VI, *Gas Chromatographic Analysis*, New York, Academic Press, pp. 630-633

1,2,3-TRIS(CHLOROMETHOXY)PROPANE

1. Chemical and Physical Data

1.1 Synonyms and trade names

Chem. Abstr. Services Reg. No.: 38571-73-2

Chem. Abstr. Name: 1,2,3-Tris(chloromethoxy)propane

Glycerol[tri(chloromethyl)]ether; tris-1,2,3-(chloromethoxy)propane

1.2 Chemical formula and molecular weight

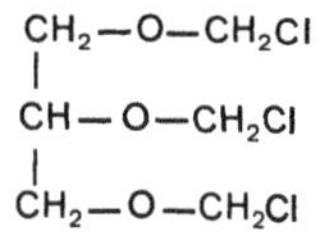

$$\begin{array}{l} CH_2-O-CH_2Cl \\ | \\ CH-O-CH_2Cl \\ | \\ CH_2-O-CH_2Cl \end{array}$$

$C_6H_{11}Cl_3O_3$ Mol. wt: 237.5

1.3 Chemical and physical properties of the pure substance

From Lichtenberger & Martin (1947), unless otherwise specified

(a) Boiling-point: 155°C at 19 mm

(b) Density: $d_4^{17.5}$ 1.3575

(c) Refractive index: $n_D^{17.5}$ 1.4815

(d) Spectroscopy data: Nuclear magnetic resonance spectra are given by Van Duuren et al. (1975).

(e) Stability: Decomposes in moist air

(f) Reactivity: Reacts as an alkylating agent with water and glutathione (Van Duuren et al., 1975)

1.4 Technical products and impurities

No data were available to the Working Group.

2. Production, Use, Occurrence and Analysis

For background information on this section, see preamble, p. 17.

2.1 Production and use

(a) Production

1,2,3-Tris(chloromethoxy)propane was first prepared in 1947 by treating glycerol with paraformaldehyde in the presence of hydrogen chloride to give 1,2,3-tris(chloromethoxy)propane and 4-chloromethoxymethyl-1,3-dioxolan (Lichtenberger & Martin, 1947).

(b) Use

Although 1,2,3-tris(chloromethoxy)propane has been investigated experimentally as a hardening agent for certain epoxy resins (Heslinga & Napjus, 1973), in the creaseproofing of cellulose fabrics (Kocher, 1963) and for use in ion exchangers, it does not appear to have ever been used commercially in either the US or Japan.

2.2 Occurrence

1,2,3-Tris(chloromethoxy)propane is not known to occur in nature.

2.3 Analysis

No data were available to the Working Group.

3. Biological Data Relevant to the Evaluation of Carcinogenic Risk to Man

3.1 Carcinogenicity and related studies in animals

(a) Skin application

Mouse: Fifty 6-8-week old female ICR/Ha Swiss mice were administered 1 mg 1,2,3-tris(chloromethoxy)propane in 0.1 ml cyclohexane on the dorsal skin thrice weekly for up to 502 days. The median survival time of treated animals was 493 days. Six mice developed skin papillomas, the first of which was observed after 328 days, and 3 animals had local squamous-cell carcinomas ($P>0.05$). In 50 control mice treated with cyclohexane alone, the median survival time was greater than 504 days; no skin tumours were observed (Van Duuren et al., 1975).

(b) Subcutaneous and/or intramuscular administration

Mouse: Fifty 6-8-week old female ICR/Ha Swiss mice were given once weekly s.c. injections of 0.3 mg 1,2,3-tris(chloromethoxy)propane in 0.05 ml tricaprylin. The test lasted 569 days, and the median survival time of treated mice was 349 days. Twelve animals developed malignant tumours (10 sarcomas, 2 carcinomas) at the injection site ($P<0.01$). In 50 control mice treated with tricaprylin alone, the median survival time was 436 days; no local malignant tumours occurred (Van Duuren et al., 1975).

(c) Intraperitoneal administration

Mouse: Thirty 6-8-week old female ICR/Ha Swiss mice were given weekly i.p. injections of 0.3 mg 1,2,3-tris(chloromethoxy)propane in 0.05 ml tricaprylin. The test lasted 532 days, and the median survival time of treated mice was 428 days. Five animals developed local sarcomas ($P<0.02$). In 30 controls treated with tricaprylin alone, the median survival time was 513 days; no local malignant tumours occurred (Van Duuren et al., 1975).

3.2 Other relevant biological data

No data were available to the Working Group.

3.3 Case reports and epidemiological studies

No data were available to the Working Group.

4. Comments on Data Reported and Evaluation[1]

4.1 Animal data

1,2,3-Tris(chloromethoxy)propane is carcinogenic in mice, the only species tested, following its subcutaneous or intraperitoneal administration; it produced malignant tumours at the sites of administration. Skin papillomas and a low incidence of skin carcinomas were observed in skin-painting studies in mice.

4.2 Human data

No case reports or epidemiological studies were available to the Working Group.

---

[1]See also the section, 'Animal Data in Relation to the Evaluation of Risk to Man' in the introduction to this volume, p. 15.

5. References

Heslinga, A. & Napjus, P.J. (1973) Hardening an epoxy resin at least two 1,2-epoxy groups. US Patent 3,741,934, 26 June, to Nederlandse Organisatie voor Toegepast-Natuurwetenschappelijk Onderzoek ten behoeve van Nijverheid, Handel en Verkeer

Kocher, F. (1963) Creaseproofing cellulose fabrics. US Patent 3,076,688, 5 February, to Traitements Chimiques des Textiles

Lichtenberger, J. & Martin, L. (1947) Etude sur les éthers chlorométhyliques des polyols. Bull. Soc. chim. Fr., 14, 468-476

Van Duuren, B.L., Goldschmidt, B.M. & Seidman, I. (1975) Carcinogenic activity of di- and trifunctional α-chloro ethers and of 1,4-dichlorobutene-2 in ICR/HA Swiss mice. Cancer Res., 35, 2553-2557

APPENDIX A*

A REPRESENTATIVE LIST OF SYNONYMS AND TRADE NAMES
FOR 2,4-D and 2,4,5-T

Trade Name	Ingredient
A	
Abco Improved W.K-245	(isooctyl ester of 2,4,5-T)
Abco W.K-DT 133	(isooctyl esters of 2,4-D and 2,4,5-T)
Abco W.K-67 2,4-D Weed Killer	(butyl ester of 2,4-D)
Abco WKS-65 Brush Killer	(isooctyl esters of 2,4-D, 2,4,5-T and silvex [2-(2,4,5-trichlorophenoxy)propionic acid])
Acetic acid, (2,4-dichlorophenoxy)-	(2,4-D)
Acetic acid, (2,4,5-trichlorophenoxy)-	(2,4,5-T)
Acide trichloro-2,4 phénoxyacétique	(2,4-D)
Acide trichloro-2,4,5 phénoxyacétique	(2,4,5-T)
Acido(2,4-dicloro-fenossi)-acetico	(2,4-D)
Acido(2,4,5-tricloro-fenossi)-acetico	(2,4,5-T)
Acme Poison Ivy Killer	(dimethylamine salt of 2,4-D + triethylamine salt of 2,4,5-T)
Acme Vegetation Killer	(2,4-D + Prometone [2-methoxy-4,6-bis(isopropylamino)-s-triazine])
Acme Weed-No-More Spotter	(dimethylamine salt of 2,4-D + triethylamine salt of 2,4,5-T)
Agent Orange	(n-butyl esters of 2,4-D and 2,4,5-T)
Agent Purple	(n-butyl esters of 2,4-D and 2,4,5-T + isobutyl ester of 2,4,5-T)
Agent White	(triisopropanolamine salt of 2,4-D + triisopropanolamine)
Agrotect	(2,4-D, form unspecified)
Agway 2,4-D and Silvex Lawn & Weed Killer	(2-ethylhexyl ester of 2,4-D + butoxyethanol ester of silvex [2-(2,4,5-trichlorophenoxy) propionic acid])

---

* Most of these names were provided by the Clinical Toxicology of Commercial Products project, University of Rochester and the Toxicology Information Response Center, Oak Ridge National Laboratory.

Some of these products are no longer manufactured but may still be available.

Agway Weed Killer "66" Improved	(triethanolamine salt of 2,4-D)
Allied Chemical Low Volatile 1-1/3-2/3 Brush Killer	(2,4-D + 2,4,5-T + isooctyl esters 2,4-D and 2,4,5-T
Amchem Amine 2,4-D Low Volatile Ester Weed Killer	(isooctyl ester of 2,4-D)
Amchem Amine 2,4,5-T for Rice	(triethylamine salt of 2,4,5-T)
Amchem 2,4-D-2,4,5-T Low Volatile Ester Brush Killer	(isooctyl esters of 2,4-D and 2,4,5-T)
Amchem 6DT. Low Volatile Ester Brush Killer	(isooctyl esters of 2,4-D and 2,4,5-T)
Amchem Emulsamine Brush Killer	(alkyl C_{12} + C_{14} amine salts of 2,4-D and 2,4,5-T)
Amchem Emulsamine E-3	(dodecylamine salts of 2,4-D + tetradecylamine salts of 2,4-D)
Amchem Isooctyl-DT	(isooctyl esters of 2,4-D and 2,4,5-T)
Amchem Isooctyl-DT6	(isooctyl esters of 2,4-D and 2,4,5-T)
Amchem Isooctyl-T	(isooctyl ester of 2,4,5-T)
Amchem Isooctyl-T6	(isooctyl ester of 2,4,5-T)
Amchem 2,4,5-T Low Volatile Ester Brush Killer	(isooctyl ester of 2,4,5-T)
Amchem 6T Low Volatile Ester Brush Killer	(isooctyl ester of 2,4,5-T)
Amchem Super D Weed one	(diethanolamine salts of 2,4-D and dicamba [3,6-dichloro-2-methoxy-benzoic acid])
Amchem Weed Killer 650	(isopropyl ester of 2,4-D)
Amine 4T	(2,4,5-T, form unspecified)
Amine 4T2	(triethylamine salt of 2,4,5-T)
Amoco Brush Killer	(isooctyl esters of 2,4-D and 2,4,5-T)
Amoco 2,4-D LV Ester	(isooctyl ester of 2,4-D)
Amoco 2,4-D Weed Killer No.5	(butyl and isopropyl esters of 2,4-D)
Amoco 2,4-D Weed Killer No.6B	(butyl ester of 2,4-D)
Amoco 2,4-D Weed Killer No.3E	(butyl and isopropyl esters of 2,4-D)

Amoco 2,4-D Weed Killer No.3-E-M	(butyl and isopropyl esters of 2,4-D)
Amoco 2,4-D Weed Killer No.5-M	(butyl esters of 2,4-D)
Amoco 2,4,5-T Amine	(triethylamine salt of 2,4,5-T)
Amoco 2,4,5-T LV Ester	(isooctyl ester of 2,4,5-T)
Amoxone	(triethanolamine salt of 2,4-D)
Ansar 290D	(triethanolamine salt of 2,4-D + triethanolamine methanearsonate)
Antrol 2,4-D & 2,4,5-T Weed & Brush Killer	(alkanolamine salts [of the ethanol and isopropanol series] of 2,4-D + triethylamine salts of 2,4,5-T)
Antrol Jet Stream Weed Killer	(alkanolamine salts [of the ethanol and isopropanol series] of 2,4-D + butoxypolypropoxypropyl esters of silvex [2-(2,4,5-trichlorophenoxy) propionic acid])
Antrol Squeeze'N Weed	(alkanolamine salts [of the ethanol and isopropanol series] of 2,4-D + butoxypolypropoxypropyl esters of silvex [2-(2,4,5-trichlorophenoxy) propionic acid])
Antrol Wide Stream Chickweed & Clover Killer	(alkanolamine salts [of the ethanol and isopropanol series] of 2,4-D + butoxypolypropoxypropyl esters of silvex [2-(2,4,5-trichlorophenoxy) propionic acid])
Aptrex	(monuron trichloroacetate [3-(*para*-chlorophenyl)-1,1-dimethylurea trichloracetate] + isooctyl ester of 2,4-D)
Aqua-Kleen	(butoxyethanol ester of 2,4-D)
Asgrow Weed-Nix Lawn Food & Weed Killer with 2,4-D and Silvex	(dimethylamine 2,4-dichlorophenoxy-acetate + isooctyl ester of silvex [2-(2,4,5-trichlorophenoxy) propionic acid])
Associated Sales Low Volatile 2,4,5-T Brush Killer	(isooctyl ester of 2,4,5-T)
Associated Sales 4-Pound 2,4-D Ester Weed Killer	(butyl ester of 2,4-D)
Atlacide with 2,4-D	(sodium chlorate + 2,4-D)

B

Balcom's Brush Killer Number 4	(isooctyl ester of 2,4,5-T)
Balcom's G-K-20	(2-ethylhexyl esters of 2,4-D and 2,4,5-T)
Balcom's T-D Special Weed Killer	(isooctyl esters of 2,4-D and 2,4,5-T)
Barber's 2,4-D Ester Weed Killer	(butyl ester of 2,4-D)
Barber's Weed Killer (Amine Formulation)	(dimethylamine salt of 2,4-D)
Barber's Weed Killer (Ester Formulation)	(isopropyl ester of 2,4-D)
Barco Weed Killer (Ester Formulation)	(butyl ester of 2,4-D)
Best 4 Servis Brand Lawn Weed Killer	(dimethylamine salt of 2,4-D)
Blitz 64	(dimethylamine salts of 2,4-D)
Bonide Crabgrass & Broadleaf Weed Killer	(dodecylammonium and octylammonium methanearsonate + octylammonium salt of 2,4-D)
Bonide Dioweed Dust	(triethanolamine salt of 2,4-D)
Bonide Dioweed Liquid	(triethanolamine salt of 2,4-D + 2,4-D)
Bonide Dioweed 40% Liquid	(triethanolamine salt of 2,4-D)
Bonus Type B	(2,4-D + 2-[2-methyl-4-chlorophenoxy]propionic acid)
Breck's Lawn Weed Killer	(butoxyethoxypropanol esters of 2,4-D and 2,4,5-T)
Bridgeport Spot Weed Killer	(isopropyl ester of 2,4-D)
Brulin's Brush Killer	(butyl esters of 2,4-D and 2,4,5,T)
Brulin's 2,4-D Liquid Weed Killer -20%	(triethanolamine salt of 2,4-D)
Brush-Blitz	(isooctyl ester of 2,4,5-T)
Brush Killer 50-50	(butyl esters of 2,4-D and 2,4,5-T)
Brush Killer 155	(dimethylamine salts of trichlorobenzoic acids + triethanolamine salts of 2,4-D and 2,4-dichlorophenoxypropionic acid)
Brush Killer 170	(butoxyethanol esters of 2,4-dichlorophenoxypropionic acid and 2,4-D)

Brush Killer 171	(butoxyethanol esters of 2,4-dichlorophenoxypropionic acid and 2,4-D)
Brush Killer T	(butyl esters of 2,4,5-T)
Brush Killer TX	(isooctyl esters of 2,4,5-T)
Brush Killer X	(isooctyl esters of 2,4-D and 2,4,5-T)
Brush-O-Cide	(isooctyl ester of 2,4-D + 2,4,5-T)
Brush-Off 445 Low Volatile Brush Killer	(2,4,5-T, form unspecified)
Brush-Off No.438 Conc. 2-2 LV Brush Killer	(isooctyl esters of 2,4-D and 2,4,5-T)
Brush-Rhap A-2D-2T	(dimethylamine salt of 2,4-D + triethylamine salt of 2,4,5-T)
Brush-Rhap Amine A-2D-2T	(dimethylamine salt of 2,4-D + triethylamine salt of 2,4,5-T)
Brush-Rhap A-4T	(triethylamine salt of 2,4,5-T)
Brush-Rhap B-2-2	(2,4-D + 2,4,5-T)
Brush-Rhap B-4	(2,4,5-T)
Brush-Rhap B-1.33D - 0.67T	(butyl esters of 2,4-D and 2,4,5-T)
Brush-Rhap B-2D-2T	(butyl esters of 2,4-D and 2,4,5-T)
Brush-Rhap B-4T	(butyl ester of 2,4,5-T)
Brush-Rhap Injection Fluid-B	(2,4,5-T)
Brush-Rhap Injection Fluid Low Volatile 2D-2T	(2-ethylhexyl esters of 2,4-D and 2,4,5-T)
Brush-Rhap Injection Fluid Low Volatile 3D-3T	(2-ethylhexyl esters of 2,4-D and 2,4,5-T)
Brush-Rhap Injection Fluid Low Volatile 4T	(2-ethylhexyl ester of 2,4,5-T)
Brush-Rhap Low Volatile 2D-2T	(2-ethylhexyl esters of 2,4-D and 2,4,5-T)
Brush-Rhap Low Volatile 3D-2T	(2-ethylhexyl esters of 2,4-D and 2,4,5-T)
Brush-Rhap Low Volatile 3D-3T	(2-ethylhexyl esters of 2,4-D and 2,4,5-T)
Brush-Rhap Low Volatile 4T	(2-ethylhexyl ester of 2,4,5-T)
Brush-Rhap Low Volatile 5T	(2-ethylhexyl ester of 2,4,5-T)
Brush-Rhap Low Volatile 6T	(2-ethylhexyl ester of 2,4,5-T)

Brush-Rhap LV-2-2-0	(2,4-D + 2,4,5-T)
Brush-Rhap LV-4-0	(2,4,5-T)
Brush-Rhap LV-40	(isooctyl esters of 2,4,5-T)
Brush-Rhap LV 2D-2T	(2-ethylhexyl esters of 2,4-D and 2,4,5-T)
Brush-Rhap LV Injection Fluid-0	(2,4,5-T)
Brush-Rhap LV-OXY-4T	(2,4,5-T, form unspecified)
Brush-Rhap LV-4T	(2-ethylhexyl ester of 2,4,5-T)
Brush-Rhap LV-6T	(2-ethylhexyl ester of 2,4,5-T)
Brush-Rhap OXY-4T	(butoxyethanol ester of 2,4,5-T)
Butoxyethanol ester of (2,4-dichlorophenoxy) acetic acid	(butoxyethanol ester of 2,4-D)
Butoxyethyl 2,4-dichlorophenoxyacetate	(butoxyethyl salt of 2,4-D)
Butyl 400	(butyl ester of 2,4-D)
Butyl 2,4-D	(butyl ester of 2,4-D)
Butyl dichlorophenoxyacetate	(butyl ester of 2,4-D)
Butyl (2,4-dichlorophenoxy)acetate	(butyl ester of 2,4-D)
Butyl ester 2,4-D	(butyl ester of 2,4-D)
Butyl ester of 2,4-D	(butyl ester of 2,4-D)
Butyl ester of dichlorophenoxyacetic acid	
n-Butylester Kyselini 2,4,5-trichlorfenoxyoctove	(butyl ester of 2,4,5-T)
Butyl 2,4,5-trichlorophenoxyacetate	(butyl ester of 2,4,5-T)
n-Butyl(2,4,5-trichlorophenoxy)acetate	(butyl ester of 2,4,5-T)

C

Certified C-300 Selective Weed Killer	(isooctyl esters of 2,4-D and 2,4,5-T)
Chemform Butoxy Brush Killer	(butoxyethoxypropanol esters of 2,4-D and 2,4,5-T)
Chemical Insecticide's Isopropyl Ester of 2,4-D Liquid Concentrate	(isopropyl ester of 2,4-D)
Chempar Low Volatile Brush Killer No.2	(2,4,5-T + 2,4-D)
Chem-Pels Plus	(isooctyl esters of 2,4-D and 2,4,5-T)

Chem-Weed 2,4,5-T	(butoxyethoxypropanol ester of 2,4,5-T + 2,4,5-T)
Chipco Turf Herbicide "D"	(2,4-D, form unspecified)
Chipco Turf Herbicide "D & T"	(dimethylamine salt of 2,4-D + triethylamine salt of 2,4,5-T)
Chipco Turf Herbicide "T"	(triethylamine salt of 2,4,5-T)
Chipco Turf Kleen	(diethanolamine salts of 2-(2-methyl-4-chlorophenoxy)propionic acid and 2,4-D)
Chipman Amine Brush Killer	(triethylamine salts of 2,4-D and 2,4,5-T)
Chipman Brush Killer 76	(isooctyl esters of 2,4-D and 2,4,5-T)
Chipman Brush Killer 128	(2,4-D + 2,4,5-T, forms unspecified)
Chipman Brush Killer 128 L.V.	(2,4-D + 2,4,5-T, forms unspecified)
Chipman Brush Killer 128 Regular	(2,4-D + 2,4,5-T, forms unspecified)
Chipman 2,4-D Amine 80	(2,4-D, form unspecified)
Chipman 2,4-D Amine No.4	(dimethylamine salt of 2,4-D)
Chipman 2,4-D Butyl Ester 6	(n-butyl ester of 2,4-D)
Chipman 2,4-D Butyl Ester 4E	(butyl ester of 2,4-D)
Chipman 2,4-D Butyl Ester 6E	(butyl ester of 2,4-D)
Chipman 2,4-D Butyl Ester 334E	(butyl ester of 2,4-D)
Chipman 2,4-D Ester 64	(2,4-D ester, form unspecified)
Chipman 2,4-D Ester 128	(2,4-D ester, form unspecified)
Chipman 2,4-D Ester 5% Dust	(2,4-D ester, form unspecified)
Chipman 2,4-D Ester 80 L.V.	(2,4-D ester, form unspecified)
Chipman 2,4-D Gran 20	(isooctyl ester of 2,4-D)
Chipman 2,4-D Low Volatile Ester 6	(isooctyl ester of 2,4-D)
Chipman 2,4-D Low Volatile Ester 4L	(isooctyl ester of 2,4-D)
Chipman 2,4-D Low Volatile Ester 6L	(isooctyl ester of 2,4-D)
Chipman Lawn Weed Killer	(2,4-D [form unspecified] + d-isomer of mecoprop [2-(4-chloro-2-methylphenoxy)propionic acid])
Chipman Low Volatile Brush Killer No.2	(isooctyl esters of 2,4-D and 2,4,5-T)
Chipman Low Volatile Brush Killer No.3	(isooctyl esters of 2,4-D and 2,4,5-T)

Chipman LVE-4L	(isooctyl esters of 2,4,5-T)
Chipman LVE-6L	(isooctyl esters of 2,4,5-T)
Chipman 2,4,5-T Amine 4L	(triethylamine salt of 2,4,5-T)
Chipman 2,4,5-T Low Volatile Ester 4L	(isooctyl ester of 2,4,5-T)
Chipman 2,4,5-T Low Volatile Ester 6L	(isooctyl ester of 2,4,5-T)
Chipman 2,4,5-T 76 (L.V.)	(2,4,5-T, form unspecified)
Chlorocrotyl ester of 2,4-D	(chlorocrotyl ester of 2,4-D)
Chloroxone	(2,4-D, form unspecified)
Clover Killer	(butoxyethanol ester of 2,4,5-T)
Commercial Brush Killer	(isooctyl esters of 2,4-D and 2,4,5-T)
Crop-Guard	(isobutyl and n-butyl esters of 2,4-D)
Crop Rider "45"	(2-ethylhexyl ester of 2,4-D)
Crop Rider 248	(2-ethylhexyl ester of 2,4-D)
Crop Rider Amine 4T	(triethylamine salt of 2,4,5-T)
Crop Rider Amine 4T-2	(triethylamine salt of 2,4,5-T)
Crop Rider 20% Agua Granular	(2-ethylhexyl ester of 2,4-D)
Crop Rider 2.67D	(butyl ester of 2,4-D)
Crop Rider 3.34D	(isopropyl ester of 2,4-D)
Crop Rider 3-34D-2	(isopropyl ester of 2,4-D)
Crop Rider 6D-OS Weed Killer	(butyl ester of 2,4-D)
Crop Rider 6D Weed Killer	(butyl ester of 2,4-D)
Crop Rider LV-6D	(2-ethylhexyl ester of 2,4-D)
Crop Rider 20% Terra Granular	(2-ethylhexyl ester of 2,4-D)
Cross Country Organic Lawn Food with Weed Killer	(sodium salt of 2,4-D)
Cross Country Poison Ivy Killer	(butoxyethoxypropanol esters of 2,4-D and 2,4,5-T)
Cross Country Weedeath	(isopropyl and triethylamine salts of 2,4-D)
Cross Country Weed Killer Spray	(alkanolamine salts of 2,4-D)
Crotilin	(chlorocrotyl ester of 2,4-D)
Crotylin	(chlorocrotyl ester of 2,4-D)

D

D 50	(2,4-D, form unspecified)
Dacamine	(*N*-oleyl 1,3-propylenediamine salt of 2,4-D)
	or
	(*N*-oleyl 1,3-propylenediamine salts of 2,4-D and 2,4,5-T)
Dacamine 4D	(*N*-oleyl 1,3-propylenediamine salt of 2,4-D)
Dacamine 1D/1T	(*N*-oleyl 1,3-propylenediamine salts of 2,4-D and 2,4,5-T)
Dacamine 2D/2T	(*N*-oleyl 1,3-propylenediamine salts of 2,4-D and 2,4,5-T)
Dacamine T	(*N*-oleyl 1,3-propylenediamine salt of 2,4,5-T)
Dacamine 4T	(*N*-oleyl 1,3-propylenediamine salt 2,4,5-T)
2,4-D Acid	(2,4-D)
Dal-E-Rad + 2 Powder	(disodium methanearsonate[hexahydrate] + sodium 2,4-dichlorophenoxy acetate monohydrate)
DB Granular	(disodium tetraborate pentahydrate and decahydrate + 2,4-D)
2,4-D Amine	(dimethylamine salt of 2,4-D)
2,4-D Butyl Ester	(butyl ester of 2,4-D)
2,4-D, *alpha*-chlorocrotyl ester	(chlorocrotyl ester of 2,4-D)
2,4-D dimethylamine salt	(dimethylamine salt of 2,4-D)
Decamine	(2,4-D, form unspecified)
Ded-weed Brush Killer	(2,4,5-T, form unspecified)
Ded-weed for Lawns, New Improved	(isooctyl esters of 2,4-D and 2,4,5-T)
Ded-weed LV-69	(2,4-D, form unspecified)
Ded-weed LV-6 Brush Kil	(2,4,5-T, form unspecified)
Del-Kill Weed Killer 400 Liquid	(mixed aliphatic hydrocarbons + isooctyl ester of 2,4-D + Bromacil [5-bromo-3-*sec*-butyl-6-methyluracil + pentachlorophenol + other phenols)
Del SK 40 Heavy Duty Weed Killer	(alkanolamine salts [of the ethanol and isopropanol series] of 2,4-D)

De-Pester Ded-Weed 50-50 Brush-Kil	(2,4,5-T)
De-Pester Ded-Weed Butyric SB	(4-[2,4-dichlorophenoxy]butyric acid)
De-Pester Ded-Weed for Lawns	(2,4-D + 2,4,5-T + Kerosene)
De-Pester Ded-Weed LV-2	(2,4-D)
De-Pester Ded-Weed LV-6	(2,4,5-T)
De-Pester Ded-Weed LV-9	(2,4,5-T)
De-Pester Ded-Weed ME-4	(butyl ester of 2,4-D)
De-Pester Ded-Weed ME-5	(butyl ester of 2,4-D)
De-Pester Ded-Weed ME-6	(butyl ester of 2,4-D)
De-Pester Ded-Weed ME-9	(butyl ester of 2,4-D)
De-Pester Ded-Weed T6 Brush Kil	(amyl ester of 2,4,5-T)
Destruxol Weed Killer "D"	(isooctyl esters of 2,4-D and 2,4,5-T)
De Witt S-77 Weed Killer	(dimethylamine salts of 2,4-D and 2,4,5-T)
Diamond Alkali Chemicals Crop Rider Amine 4-D	(alkyl and dialkanolamine salts of 2,4-D)
Diamond Alkali Chemicals Crop Rider & Line Rider LV-4D	(2-ethylhexyl ester of 2,4-D)
Diamond Alkali Chemicals 2-2 2-Ethyl Hexyl Brush Killer	(2-ethylhexyl esters of 2,4-D and 2,4,5-T)
Diamond Alkali Chemicals 4 2-Ethyl Hexyl D Weed Killer	(2-ethylhexyl ester of 2,4-D)
Diamond Alkali Chemicals 4-Mixed Amine-D Weed Killer	(alkyl and dialkanolamine salts of 2,4-D)
Diamond Alkali Chemicals Technical 2-Ethyl Hexyl-D	(2-ethylhexyl ester of 2,4-D)
Diamond Alkali Chemicals Technical 2-Ethyl Hexyl-T	(2-ethylhexyl ester of 2,4,5-T)
Diamond Alkali Chemicals The Line Rider	(2-ethylhexyl esters of 2,4-D and 2,4,5-T)
Diamond Shamrock Amine 6D	(dimethylamine salt of 2,4-D)
Diamond Shamrock Amine 2D/2T	(dimethylamine salts of 2,4-D and 2,4,5-T)
Diamond Shamrock Amine 4T	(triethylamine salt of 2,4,5-T)
Diamond Shamrock Butyl 4D	(butyl ester of 2,4-D)
Diamond Shamrock Butyl 6D Weed Killer	(butyl ester of 2,4-D)

Diamond Shamrock Dormant Cane Concentrate LV-6T-OS	(isooctyl ester of 2,4,5-T)
Diamond Shamrock Dormant Cane LV 3D/3T-OS	(isooctyl esters of 2,4-D and 2,4,5-T)
Diamond Shamrock LO-VOL 4D	(isooctyl ester of 2,4-D)
Diamond Shamrock LO-VOL 6D	(isooctyl ester of 2,4-D)
Diamond Shamrock LO-VOL 2D/2T	(isooctyl esters of 2,4-D and 2,4,5-T)
Diamond Shamrock LO-VOL 4T	(isooctyl ester of 2,4,5-T)
Diamond Shamrock LO-VOL 6T	(isooctyl ester of 2,4,5-T)
(2,4-Dichloor-fenoxy)azijnzuur	(2,4-D)
Dichlorophenoxyacetic acid	(2,4-D)
2,4-Dichlorophenoxyactic acid, 4-chlorocrotonyl ester	(chlorocrotonyl ester of 2,4-D)
2,4-Dichlorophenoxyacetic acid, 4-chlorocrotonyl alcohol ester	(chlorocrotonyl alcohol ester of 2,4-D)
2,4-Dichlorophenoxyacetic acid, 2-butenyl ester	(butenyl ester of 2,4-D)
2,4-Dichlorophenoxyacetic acid, butoxyethyl ester	(butoxyethyl ester of 2,4-D)
Dichlorophenoxyacetic acid, butyl ester	(butyl ester of 2,4-D)
2,4-Dichlorophenoxyacetic acid, butyl ester	(butyl ester of 2,4-D)
(2,4-Dichlorophenoxy)acetic acid, butyl ester	(butyl ester of 2,4-D)
(2,4-Dichlorophenoxy)acetic acid, crotyl ester	(crotyl ester of 2,4-D)
(2,4-Dichlorophenoxy)acetic acid Dimethylamine	(dimethylamine salt of 2,4-D)
(2,4-Dichlorophenoxy)acetic acid, isooctyl ester	(isooctyl ester of 2,4-D)
2,4-Dichlorophenoxyacetic acid, isooctyl ester	(isooctyl ester of 2,4-D)
(2,4-Dichlorophenoxy)acetic acid, isopropyl ester	(isopropyl ester of 2,4-D)
2,4-Dichlorophenoxyacetic acid, isopropyl ester	(isopropyl ester of 2,4-D)
(2,4-Dichlorophenoxy)acetic acid, sodium salt	(sodium salt of 2,4-D)

2,4-Dichlorophenoxyacetic acid, sodium salt	(sodium salt of 2,4-D)
2,4-Dichlorphenoxyacetic acid	(2,4-D)
(2,4-Dichlor-phenoxy)-essigsäure	(2,4-D)
Dikonirt	(sodium salt of 2,4-D)
Di-Met Chickweed and Weed Killer	(isooctyl esters of 2,4-D and silvex [2-(2,4,5-trichlorophenoxy) propionic acid])
Di-Met Plus-2, Liquid for Crabgrass and Lawn Weeds	(dodecyl ammonium methanearsonate + octyl ammonium methanearsonate + octyl ammonium salt of 2,4-D)
Di-Met Plus-2, Liquid for Dallis Grass and Lawn Weeds	(dodecyl ammonium methanearsonate + octyl ammonium methanearsonate + octyl ammonium salt of 2,4-D)
Dimethylamine, (2,4-dichlorophenoxy) acetate	(dimethylamine salt of 2,4-D)
Dimethylammonium 2,4-dichlorophenoxy-acetate	(dimethylamine salt of 2,4-D)
Dinoxol	(butoxyethanol esters of 2,4-D and 2,4,5-T)
Dinoxol 64	(butoxyethanol esters of 2,4-D and 2,4,5-T)
Dinoxol Super-6	(butoxyethanol esters of 2,4-D and 2,4,5-T)
2,4-D, isooctyl ester	(isooctyl ester of 2,4-D)
2,4-D, isopropyl ester	(isopropyl ester of 2,4-D)
DMA-4	(dimethylamine salt of 2,4-D)
Dolge E.W.T. Amine Type 2,4-D Weed Killer	(diethanolamine salt of 2,4-D)
Dormant Cane Concentrate	(2-ethylhexyl ester of 2,4,5-T)
Dormone	(2,4-D, form unspecified)
Dow Brush Killer 50-50	(butyl esters of 2,4-D and 2,4,5-T)
Dow Brush Killer TX	(butoxypropyl esters of 2,4,5-T)
Dow Brush Killer X	(isooctyl esters of 2,4-D and 2,4,5-T)
Dow Butyl 265	(butyl esters of 2,4-D)
Dow Butyl 400	(butyl esters of 2,4-D)
Dow 2,4-Dichlorophenoxyacetic Acid, Sodium Salt	(monohydrate sodium salt of 2,4-D)

Dow DMA-4	(dimethylamine salt of 2,4-D)
Dow Formula 40	(alkanolamine salts of 2,4-D)
Dow 2,4,5-T Amine Weed Killer	(triethylamine salt of 2,4,5-T)
2,4-Dow Weed Killer Formula 40	(alkanolamine salts [of the ethanol and isopropanol series] of 2,4-D)
2,4-Dow Weed Killer Formula 40	(alkanolamine salts of 2,4-D)
Dow Weed Killer X	(butoxypropyl ester of 2,4-D)
Dragon Lawn Weed Killer	(2,4-D + dicamba [3,6-dichloro-2-methoxybenzoic acid])
DRO 2,4-D Concentrate	(diethylamine salt of 2,4-D)
Droweed Spot Treatment Kills Lawn Weeds	(propylene glycol butyl ether esters of 2,4-D)
Dro Weedtrol Concentrate	(disodium monomethyl creonate pentahydrate + sodium monohydrate of 2,4-D)
Dupont Lawn Weeder	(propylene glycol and butyl ether esters of 2,4-D)
Du Pont Lawn Weed Killer	(dimethylamine salt of 2,4-D)
Du Pont Turf Food with Weed Killer	(dimethylamine salt of 2,4-D)
Du Pont Weed Killer No.2	(dimethylamine salt of 2,4-D)
D-Weed-O	(isooctyl ester of 2,4-D + Bromacil [5-bromo-3-*sec*-butyl-6-methyluracil] + pentachlorophenol + other chlorophenols)
2,4-Dwuchlorofenoksyoctowy Kwas	(2,4-D)

E

Emulsamine Brush Killer	(dodecyl- and tetradecylamine salts of 2,4-D and 2,4,5-T)
Emulsamine E-3	(dodecyl- and tetradecylamine salts of 2,4-D)
Emulsamine 2,4,5-T	(dodecyl- and tetradecylamine salts of 2,4,5-T)
Emulsavert-D	(2,4-D, form unspecified)
Emulsavert 100	(2,4-D + 2,4,5-T + N,N-dimethyloleylamine salts of 2,4-D and 2,4,5-T)

Emulsavert 248	(2,4-D +2,4,5-T + N,N-dimethyl-oleylamine salts of 2,4-D and 2,4,5-T)
Envert-171	(2,4-D, form unspecified)
Envert-DT	(butoxyethanol esters of 2,4-D and 2,4,5-T)
Envert-T	(butoxyethanol ester of 2,4,5-T)
Esso Herbicide 10	(butyl ester of 2,4-D)
Estasol	(isopropyl ester of 2,4-D)
Estercide T-2	(2,4,5-T, form unspecified)
Estercide T-245	(2,4,5-T, form unspecified)
Esteron 44	(isopropyl ester of 2,4-D)
Esteron 76	(isopropyl and butyl esters of 2,4-D)
Esteron 245	(propylene and polypropylene butyl ether esters of 2,4,5-T)
Esteron 245 (old formulation)	(isopropyl and mixed amyl esters of 2,4,5-T)
Esteron 76 BE	(butyl esters of 2,4-D)
Esteron 76 BE Herbicide	(butyl esters of 2,4-D)
Esteron Brush Killer	(propylene glycol butyl ether esters of 2,4-D and 2,4,5-T)
Esteron Brush Killer (old formulation)	(isopropyl esters of 2,4-D and 2,4,5-T)
Esteron Brush Killer O.B.	(propylene glycol butyl ether esters of 2,4-D and 2,4,5-T)
Esteron 99 Concentrate	(butoxyethanol ester of 2,4-D)
Esteron 245 Concentrate	(propylene glycol butyl ether esters of 2,4,5-T)
Esteron 6E Herbicide	(isooctyl ester of 2,4-D)
Esteron 76-E Weed Killer	(isopropyl and butyl esters of 2,4-D)
Esteron 245 Herbicide	(propylene and polypropylene glycol butyl ether esters of 2,4,5-T)
Esteron 44 Improved Weed Killer	(butyl esters of 2,4-D)
Esteron 245 O.S.	(propylene glycol butyl ether esters of 2,4,5-T)
Esteron Ten-Ten	(propylene glycol butyl ether esters of 2,4-D)

Esteron 44 Weed Killer	(isopropyl and butyl esters of 2,4-D)
Esteron 99 Weed Killer	(propylene glycol butyl ether esters of 2,4-D)
Esteron 99 Weed Killer Concentrate	(propylene glycol butyl ether esters of 2,4-D)
Estone	(ethyl ester of 2,4-D)

F

Feed No Weed	(triethylamine salts of 2,4-D and 2,4,5-T)
Felco Butyl Ester 600 2,4-D Weed Killer	(butyl ester of 2,4-D)
Felco HV2 Weed Killer	(butyl ester of 2,4-D)
Felco HV4 Weed Killer	(butyl ester of 2,4-D)
Felco Low Volatile Ester 600	(isooctyl ester of 2,4-D)
Felco LV 400 Weed Killer	(isooctyl ester of 2,4-D)
Felco Super Brush Killer	(butyl esters of 2,4-D and 2,4,5-T)
Felco 2,4,5-T Brush Killer	(butyl ester of 2,4,5-T)
Fenac Plus	(dimethylamine salts of 2,4-D and 2,3,6-trichlorophenylacetic acid)
Fence Painter Weed Out	(monuron [3-(*para*-chlorophenyl)-1,1-dimethylurea] + sodium salt of 2,4-D + sodium tetraborate)
Fence Rider 22	(butyl esters of 2,4-D and 2,4,5-T)
Fence Rider "45"	(isooctyl esters of 2,4-D and 2,4,5-T)
Fence Rider LV-22	(2-ethylhexyl esters of 2,4-D and 2,4,5-T)
Fence Rider LV-3D/3T	(2-ethylhexyl esters of 2,4-D and 2,4,5-T)
Fence Rider LV-4T Brush Killer	(2-ethylhexyl ester of 2,4,5-T)
Fence Rider LV-6T Brush Killer	(2-ethylhexyl ester of 2,4,5-T)
Fence Rider 3.34-T Brush Killer	(isopropyl ester of 2,4,5-T)
Fence Rider 4T Brush Killer	(butyl ester of 2,4,5-T)
Fence Rider 6T Brush Killer	(butyl ester of 2,4,5-T)
Fernesta	(2,4-D, form unspecified)

Fernimine	(ethanol and isopropyl esters of 2,4-D)
Fernoxene	(sodium salt of 2,4-D)
Fernoxone	(2,4-D, form unspecified)
Ferxone	(2,4-D, form unspecified)
Field-Clean	(isooctyl ester of 2,4-D)
Floratox 4 LB. LV 2,4-D Weed Killer	(isooctyl ester of 2,4-D)
Floratox 428 4-Pound 2,4-D Ester Weed Killer	(butyl ester of 2,4-D)
Floro Tox 2,4-D Amine Weed Killer	(dimethylamine salt of 2,4-D)
Foredex 75	(2,4-D, form unspecified)
Foremost All Season Weed Killer	(mixed aliphatic hydrocarbons + isooctyl ester of 2,4-D + pentachlorophenol + other chlorophenols + bromacil[5-bromo-3-*sec*-butyl-6-methyluracil])
Formula 40	(ethanol and isopropyl esters of 2,4-D)
Forron	(2,4,5-T, form unspecified)
Fortex	(2,4,5-T, form unspecified)
Fruitone A	(2,4,5-T)
FS Amine 400 Weed Killer	(dimethylamine salts of 2,4-D)
FS Ester 400 Weed Killer	(butyl ester of 2,4-D)
FS LV 400 Weed Killer	(isooctyl ester of 2,4-D)

G

GCC-425	(isooctyl esters of 2,4-D, 2,4,5-T and 2-(2,4,5-trichlorophenoxy) propionic acid)
GCC-429	(isooctyl esters of 2,4-D, 2,4,5-T and 2-(2,4,5-trichlorophenoxy) propionic acid)
GCC-165 Weed Killer	(isooctyl ester of 2,4-D + bromacil [5-bromo-3-*sec*-butyl-6-methyluracil] + pentachlorophenol + other chlorophenols)

General Chemical 2,4-D Butyl Ester Weed Killer	(butyl ester of 2,4-D)
General Chemical 2,4-D 3.34 Butyl Ester Weed Killer	(butyl ester of 2,4-D)
General Chemical 2,4-D 4-Butyl Ester Weed Killer	(butyl ester of 2,4-D)
General Chemical 2,4-D 6.00 Butyl Ester Weed Killer	(butyl ester of 2,4-D)
General Chemical 2,4,5-T Amine	(triethylamine salt of 2,4,5-T)
G.L.F. Weed Killer 66 Sequestered	(2,4-D, form unspecified)
Good-Life Weed Woe	(diethanolamine salts of 2-(2-methyl-4-chlorophenoxy)propionic acid, 2,4-D and dicamba [3,6-dichloro-2-methoxy benzoic acid])
Gormel's Brush Killer	(propylene glycol butyl ether esters of 2,4-D and 2,4,5-T)
Gormel's Weed & Clover Killer	(isooctyl esters of 2,4-D and 2,4,5-T)
Gormel's Weed Kil	(alkanolamine salts [of the ethanol and isopropanol series] of 2,4-D)
Green Cross Celatox 50/30	(2,4,5-T + MCP[(4-chloro-2-methylphenoxy)acetic acid])
Green Cross Commercial Weed Killer "96"	(2,4-D + butyl ester of 2,4-D)
Green Cross Ester Weed Killer	(2,4-D)
Green Cross Roadside 2,4-D Low Volatile Weed Killer	(isooctyl ester of 2,4-D)
Green Cross Vegetation Killer	(monuron [3-(*para*-chlorophenyl)-1,1-dimethylurea] + 2,4-D + 2,4,5-T)
Green Cross Weed-No-More	(butyl ester of 2,4-D)
Green Cross Weed-No-More "80"	(2,4-D)
Greenfield Broadleaf Weed & Crab Grass Killer	(trifluralin [a,a,a-trifluoro-2,6-dinitro-*N*,*N*-dipropyl-*para*-toluidine] + disodium methylarsonate + sodium salts of 2,4-D and 2,4,5-T)
Greenfield Crab Grass & Broadleaf Weed Killer	(trifluralin [a,a,a-trifluoro-2,6-dinitro-*N*,*N*-dipropyl-*para*-toluidine] + disodium methylarsonate hexahydrate + isooctyl esters of 2,4-D and 2,4,5-T)
Greenfield Crabgrass & Dandelion Killer	(disodium methanearsonate + trifluralin [a,a,a-trifluoro-2,6-dinitro-*N*,*N*-dipropyl-*para*-toluidine] + sodium salts of 2,4-D and 2,4,5-T)

Greenfield Dandelion & Broadleaf Weed Killer	(isooctyl esters of 2,4-D and silvex [2-(2,4,5-trichlorophenoxy) propionic acid])
Greenfield Dandelion & Chickweed Killer	(isooctyl esters of 2,4-D and silvex [2-(2,4,5-trichlorophenoxy) propionic acid])
Greenfield Two-Way Green Power	(isooctyl esters of 2,4-D and silvex [2-(2,4,5-trichlorophenoxy)propionic acid] + nitrogen + phosphoric acid + soluble potash)
Greenfield Weeds As It Feeds For Lawns	(isooctyl esters of 2,4-D and 2,4,5-T)
Green light Broadleaf Weed Killer	(alkanolamine salts [of the ethanol and isopropanol series] of 2,4-D)
Green Light 2,4-D, 2,4,5-T Weed Killer	(isooctyl esters of 2,4-D and 2,4,5-T)
Green Light Weed Killer	(alkanolamine salts [of the ethanol and isopropanol series] of 2,4-D + triethylamine salt of 2,4,5-T)
Greever's 2,4-D Low Volatile Ester Weed Killer	(isooctyl ester of 2,4-D)
Greever's Low Volatile Brush Killer	(isooctyl esters of 2,4-D and 2,4,5-T)

H

Halts Plus With Dandelion Control	(*S*-(*O,O*-diisopropyl phosphorodithioate)ester of *N*-(2-mercaptoethyl) benzenesulphonamide + 2,4-D + 2(2-methyl-4-chlorophenoxy)propionic acid)
Hedonal	(isooctyl ester of 2,4-D)
Hedonal (The Herbicide)	(2,4-D, form unspecified)
Hedonol	(2,4-D, form unspecified)
Henry Field's Lawn Weed Killer	(isooctyl ester of 2,4-D)
Herbate Ester 80	(isooctyl ester of 2,4-D)
Herbate Ester 128	(2,4-D, form unspecified)
Hercules	(isooctyl esters of 2,4,5-T)
HH Poison Ivy Killer	(triethylamine salt of 2,4,5-T)
Home Use Weed Killer	(alkanolamine salts [of the ethanol and isopropanol series] of 2,4-D)
Hormit	(sodium salt of 2,4-D)

Hormoslyr 64	(2,4-D + 2,4,5-T)
Hub States Selective Weed and Brush Killer Amine Formula 400	(diethylethanolamine salts of 2,4-D and 2,4,5-T)

I

Instemul DA 40	(oleyl amine salt of 2,4-D)
Instemul DA 120 Concentrate	(oleyl amine salt of 2,4-D)
Instemul DTA 22	(oleyl amine salt of 2,4-D + oleyl-linoleyl amine salt of 2,4,5-T)
Instemul DTA 66 Concentrate	(oleyl amine salt of 2,4-D + oleyl-linoleyl amine salt of 2,4,5-T)
Instemul TA 40	(oleyllinoleyl amine salt of 2,4,5-T)
Instemul TA 120 Concentrate	(oleyllinoleyl amine salt of 2,4,5-T)
Inverton 245	(2,4,5-T, form unspecified)
Isooctyl alcohol, (2,4-dichlorophenoxy) acetate	(isooctyl ester of 2,4-D)
Isooctyl 2,4-dichlorophenoxyacetate	(isooctyl ester of 2,4-D)

J

Jet-Weed Killer Power Pellets	(2,4-D + silvex [2-(2,4,5-trichlorophenoxy)propionic acid])

K

Kansel	(2,4-D + dicamba [2-methoxy-3,6-dichlorobenzoic acid]) or (2,4,5-T + propylene glycol butyl ether esters of 2,4,5-T)
Kilbrush 8-16 Ester	(butyl esters of 2,4-D and 2,4,5-T)
Kilex 3	(butyl ester of 2,4,5-T)
Knoxweed	(eptam [S-ethyl dipropylthiocarbamate] + 10 E 2,4-D)

Kro-Foot-Kil	(dimethylamine salts of 2,4-D + phenylmercuric acetate)
Krotilin	(chlorocrotyl ester of 2,4-D)
Krotiline	(chlorocrotyl ester of 2,4-D)

L

Lawn-Keep	(2,4-D, form unspecified)
Lawn Weed Killer	(triethanolamine salt of 2,4-D)
Lawn Weed-Rhap	(2-ethylhexyl esters of 2,4-D and 2,4,5-T)
Lebanon Deluxe Weed and Feed with 2,4-D and Banvel D	(dimethylamine salts of 2,4-D, dicamba [3,6-dichloro-2-methoxy-benzoic acid] and related acids)
Lebanon Weedeth	(dimethylamine salt of 2,4-D, dimethylamine salt of dicamba [3,6-dichloro-2-methoxy-benzoic acid] and related acid)
Limit	(chloro-N,N-diallylacetamide + 2,4-D)
Line Rider 22	(butyl esters of 2,4-D and 2,4,5-T)
Line Rider Amine 4T-2	(alkyl amine salt of 2,4,5-T)
Line Rider Invert D/T	(isooctyl esters of 2,4-D and 2,4,5-T)
Line Rider Invert D/T Concentrate	(isooctyl esters of 2,4-D and 2,4,5-T)
Line Rider Invert T	(isooctyl ester of 2,4,5-T)
Line Rider Invert T Concentrate	(isooctyl ester of 2,4,5-T)
Line Rider LV-21	(isooctyl esters of 2,4-D and 2,4,5-T)
Line Rider LV-4D	(isooctyl ester of 2,4-D)
Line Rider LV-6D	(isooctyl ester of 2,4-D)
Line Rider LV-4T	(2-ethylhexyl ester of 2,4,5-T)
Line Rider LV-6T	(2-ethylhexyl ester of 2,4,5-T)
Line Rider 4T	(butyl ester of 2,4,5-T)
Liqweedate	(2-methoxy-4,6-bis(isopropylamine)-s-triazine + isooctyl esters of 2,4-D and 2,4,5-T)
Liqweedate-2	(2-methoxy-4,6-bis(isopropylamine)-s-triazine + isooctyl ester of 2,4-D)
Lironox	(butyl ester of 2,4-D)

Lithate 2,4-D	(lithium salt of 2,4-D)
Lo-Estasol	(butoxyethanol ester of 2,4-D)
LO-VOL 4T	(2,4,5-T, form unspecified)
L.V. Brush Rhap-4	(isooctyl ester of 2,4,5-T)

M

Machete	(alkanolamine salts [of the ethanol and isopropanol series] of 2,4-D)
Macondray	(2,4-D, form unspecified)
Marico Kill-Weed	(dimethylamine salt of 2,4-D)
Manco Super Kill-Weed	(isooctyl esters of 2,4-D and 2,4,5-T)
Mecopar	(diethanolamine salts of MCPP [2-(2-methyl-4-chlorophenoxy)propionic acid] and 2,4-D)
MFA 40% Butyl Ester Weed Killer	(butyl ester of 2,4-D)
MFA LO-V Super Brush Killer	(octyl esters of 2,4-D and 2,4,5-T)
MFA LO-V 2,4,5-T	(octyl esters of 2,4,5-T)
MFA Super Brush Kill	(butyl esters of 2,4-D and 2,4,5-T)
MFA 2,4,5-T Butyl Ester	(butyl ester of 2,4,5-T)
MFA No.4 Weed Killer	(butyl ester of 2,4-D)
MFA No.6 Weed Killer	(butyl ester of 2,4-D)
Miller's 4# Ester	(butyl ester of 2,4-D)
Miller's 6# Ester	(butyl ester of 2,4-D)
Miller's Lo Vol 4# 2,4-D	(isooctyl ester of 2,4-D)
Milorganite Plus 2,4-D	(2,4-D, form unspecified)
Miracle	(2,4-D, form unspecified)
Monosan	(2,4-D, form unspecified)
Monsanto 2,4-D Amine	(dimethylamine salt of 2,4-D)
Monsanto 2,4-D Butyl Ester	(butyl ester of 2,4-D)
Monsanto 2,4-D Butyl Ester Concentrate	(butyl ester of 2,4-D)
Monsanto 2,4-D Granular	(isooctyl ester of 2,4-D)
Monsanto 2,4-D Isopropyl Ester	(isopropyl ester of 2,4-D)

Monsanto 2,4-D Low Volatile Ester	(isooctyl ester of 2,4-D)
Monsanto 2,4-D 2,4,5-T Amine Brush Killer	(dimethylamine salt of 2,4-D + triethylamine salt of 2,4,5-T)
	or
	(triethylamine salts of 2,4-D and 2,4,5-T)
Monsanto 2,4-D 2,4,5-T Butyl Ester Brush Killer	(butyl esters of 2,4-D and 2,4,5-T)
Monsanto 2,4-D 2,4,5-T Low Volatile Ester Brush Killer	(isooctyl esters of 2,4-D and 2,4,5-T)
Monsanto 2,4,5-T Amine	(triethylamine salt of 2,4,5-T)
Monsanto 2,4,5-T Butyl Ester	(isobutyl and n-butyl esters of 2,4,5-T)
Monsanto 2,4,5-T Low Volatile Ester	(isooctyl ester of 2,4,5-T)
Morselect	(dimethylamine salt of 2,4-D)
Moxone	(2,4-D, form unspecified)
Munichem Muni-Kill	(mixed aliphatic hydrocarbons + isooctyl ester of 2,4-D + bromacil [5-bromo-3-*sec*-butyl-6-methyluracil] + pentachlorophenol + other chlorophenols)

N

Naco LV-4D Weed Killer	(isooctyl ester of 2,4-D)
Nalkil Weed Killer 400 liquid	(isooctyl ester of 2,4-D + bromacil [5-bromo-3-*sec*-butyl-6-methyluracil] + pentachlorophenol + other chlorophenols)
Navy Brand WKB-15	(isooctyl esters of 2,4-D and 2,4,5-T)
Navy Brand WKB-28	(butoxyethoxypropanol esters of 2,4-D and 2,4,5-T)
Niagara Brush-Killer (Ester Form)	(butoxyethanol esters of 2,4-D and 2,4,5-T)
Niagara Commercial Brush Killer	(isooctyl esters of 2,4-D and 2,4,5-T)
Niagara 2,4-D Weed Killer (Amine Form)	(ethanol and propanolamine salts of 2,4-D)
Niagara Estasol	(isopropyl ester of 2,4-D)

NSC 423	(2,4-D, form unspecified)
Nutro Dandelion & Turf Weed Killer	(2,4-D + dicamba [3,6-dichloro-2-methoxybenzoid acid])
Nutro Turf Weed Killer	(ethylhexyl esters of 2,4-D and silvex [2-(2,4,5-trichlorophenoxy) propionic acid])
Nutro Weed Bomb	(2,4-D + MCPP [2-methyl-4-chloro-phenoxy)propionic acid])

O

Olin Butyl Ester 22 Brush Killer	(butyl esters of 2,4-D and 2,4,5-T)
Olin Butyl Ester D4 Weed Killer	(butyl ester of 2,4-D)
Olin Butyl Ester D6 Weed Killer	(butyl ester of 2,4-D)
Olin Butyl Ester D267 Weed Killer	(butyl ester of 2,4-D)
Olin Isopropyl Ester D334 Weed Killer	(isopropyl ester of 2,4-D)
Olin LV Ester 22 Brush Killer	(2-ethylhexyl esters of 2,4-D and 2,4,5-T)
Olin LV Ester D4 Weed Killer	(2-ethylhexyl ester of 2,4-D)
Ortho Brush Killer	(isooctyl esters of 2,4-D and 2,4,5-T)
Ortho 2,4-D LV Ester 4	(isooctyl ester of 2,4-D)

P

Pacific Cooperatives P 2,4-D Amine Weed Killer	(dimethylamine salt of 2,4-D)
Parsons Corn-Tal Weed Killer	(butyl, isopropyl and isooctyl esters of 2,4-D)
Parsons 2,4-D Weed Killer	(dimethylamine salt of 2,4-D)
Parsons 2,4-D Weed Killer Butyl Ester	(butyl ester of 2,4-D)
Parsons 2,4-D Weed Killer Isopropyl Ester	(isopropyl ester of 2,4-D)
Parsons 2,4-D Weed Killer No.40	(dimethylamine salt of 2,4-D)
Parsons Poison Ivy and Brush Killer No.2	(isooctyl esters of 2,4-D and 2,4,5-T)

Parsons 2,4,5-T Brush Killer	(2,4,5-T)
Patterson's Hi-Test Butyl Ester 2,4-D Weed Killer	(butyl ester of 2,4-D)
Patterson's Lawn Weed Killer	(isooctyl esters of 2,4-D and 2,4,5-T)
Patterson's Super Brush Killer	(butyl esters of 2,4-D and 2,4,5-T)
Patterson's Super Brush Killer Low Volatile	(isooctyl esters of 2,4-D and 2,4,5-T)
Patterson's 2,4,5-T Low Volatile & Brush Killer	(isooctyl ester of 2,4,5-T)
Pax Action Weed'N Feed 18-4-4	(alkanolamine salt of 2,4-D + dimethylamine salt of dicamba [3,6-dichloro-2-methoxybenzoic acid] + nitrogen + phosphoric acid + soluble potash)
Pax Total For Lawns 10-6-4	(N-Oleyl 1,3-propylenediamine salt of 2,4-D + dimethylamine salt of 2-(2-methyl-4-chlorophenoxy)propionic acid + dimethyl ester of tetrachloroterephthalic acid + disodium methanearsonate hexahydrate + heptachlor + related compounds + nitrogen + phosphoric acid + potash + S + Fe + Mn + Zn)
Pennamine	(2,4-D, form unspecified)
Pennamine D	(heptylamine salt of 2,4-D)
Phenox	(2,4-D, form unspecified)
Phorfox	(2,4,5-T, form unspecified)
Pielik	(2,4-D, form unspecified)
Pielik E	(sodium salt of 2,4-D)
Pill Kill Kartridges for Dandelions and Broadleaf Weeds	(2,4-D + silvex [2-(2,4,5-trichlorophenoxy)propionic acid])
Planotox	(butoxyethyl ester of 2,4-D)
Plantgard	(2,4-D, form unspecified)
PL Devastate Non-Selective Weed Killer	(isooctyl ester of 2,4-D + bromacil [5-bromo-3-*sec*-butyl-6-methyluracil] + pentachlorophenol + other chlorophenols)
PL Liqui-date	(isooctyl esters of 2,4-D, 2,4,5-T and silvex[2-(2,4,5-trichlorophenoxy)propionic acid])

Plus 2 for Grass	(2,4-D + 2-(2-methyl-4-chlorophenoxy) propionic acid)
Pratt Lawn Weed Killer	(2,4-D + 2,4,5-TP)
Pratt's Crabgrass & Broadleaf Weed Killer	(octyl ammonium methyl arsonate + 2,4-D)
Propi-Rhap Low Volatile 4DP	(2-ethylhexyl ester of 2-(2,4-dichlorophenoxy)propionic acid)
Proturf Broad Spectrum Weedicide	(2,4-D + dicamba [3,6-dichloro-2-methoxybenzoic acid])
Proturf Broad Spectrum Weedicide II	(2,4-D + 2-(2-methyl-4-chlorophenoxy)propionic acid)
Proturf Fertilizer Plus Dicot Weed Control	(2,4-D + dicamba [3,6-dichloro-2-methoxybenzoic acid])
Proturf Fertilizer Plus Dicot Weed Control II	(2,4-D + 2-(2-methyl-4-chlorophenoxy)propionic acid)

R

Real-Kill Spot Weed Killer	(amine salts of 2,4-D, dicamba [3,6-dichloro-2-methoxybenzoic acid] and MCPP [2-(2-methyl-4-chlorophenoxy)propionic acid])
	or
	(amine salts of 2,4-D, dicamba [3,6-dichloro-2-methoxybenzoic acid] and 2,4,5-T)
Reasor-Hill Brush Rhap	(2,4-D + 2,4,5-T)
Red Devil Dry Weed Killer	(2,4-D)
Reddon	(propylene glycol butyl ether esters of 2,4,5-T)
Reddox	(2,4,5-T, form unspecified)
Rhodia 2,4-D Butyl Ester 6L	(butyl ester of 2,4-D)
Rhodia 2,4-D Low Volatile Ester 4L	(isooctyl ester of 2,4-D)
Rhodia Low Volatile Brush Killer No.2	(2,4-D + 2,4,5-T)
R-H Weed Rhap 20	(2,4-D)
Rid-O-Weed	(isopropyl and diisopropanol amine salts of 2,4-D)
Robot Gardener Weed & Crabgrass Killer	(potassium cyanate + 2,4-D)

Roundup Granular	(2-chloro-*N*-isopropylacetanilide + isooctyl ester of 2,4-D)
Roundup Wettable Powder	(2-chloro-*N*-isopropylacetanilide + 2,4-D)

S

Salvik	(2,4-D, form unspecified)
Salvo	(2,4-D, form unspecified)
Science Lawn Weed-Killer	(isooctyl esters of 2,4-D + 2,4,5-T)
Scott's 4-XD Weed Control	(2,4-D)
Security Lawn Weed Killer	(*N*-oleyl 1,3-propylenediamine salt of 2,4-D)
Sesone	(sodium 2,4-dichlorophenoxyethyl sulphate)
Shell 40	(butyl ester of 2,4-D)
"006" Shrub-A-Dub	(isooctyl ester of 2,4-D + bromacil [5-bromo-3-*sec*-butyl-6-methyluracil] + pentachlorophenol + other chlorophenols)
S.I.R.-Ester	(isooctyl esters of 2,4-D and 2,4,5-T)
Sodium 2,4-D	(sodium salt of 2,4-D)
Sodium 2,4-dichlorophenoxyacetate	(sodium salt of 2,4-D)
Spontox	(2,4-D, form unspecified) or (2,4,5-T, form unspecified)
Spritz-Hormit	(sodium salt of 2,4-D)
Stull's Hardwood Spray	(isooctyl ester of 2,4,5-T)
Stull's Low Volatile Brush Killer No.4	(isooctyl esters of 2,4-D and 2,4,5-T)
Stull's Low Volatile Weed Killer	(isooctyl ester of 2,4-D)
Stull's Stu-Ester Low Volatile	(isooctyl ester of 2,4,5-T)
Super Crab-E-Rad + 2	(dodecylammonium methanearsonate + octylammonium methanearsonate + octylammonium salt of 2,4-D)
Super Dal-E-Rad + 2	(dodecylammonium methanearsonate + octylammonium methanearsonate + octylammonium salt of 2,4-D)

Super D Weedone	(diethylamine salts of 2,4-D and dicamba [3,6-dichloro-2-methoxybenzoic acid])
Sure Death 40% Butyl Ester Type Weedkiller	(butyl ester of 2,4-D)
Sure Death 2,4-D Amine Weed Killer	(dimethylamine salt of 2,4-D)
Sure Death Lawn Weed Killer	(2-ethyl 4-methylpentanol and 2-ethylhexanol esters of 2,4-D and 2,4,5-trichlorophenoxypropionic acid)
Sure-Death Low-Vol 2,4-D #4	(2-ethylpentanol and 2-ethylhexanol esters of 2,4-D)
Sure Death No.4 Butyl Ester Weed Killer	(butyl ester of 2,4-D)
Sure Death No.6 Butyl Ester Weed Killer	(butyl ester of 2,4-D)
Sure Death No.6-D Low Vol 2,4-D	(2-ethyl 4 methylpentanol and 2-ethylhexanol esters of 2,4-D)
Sure Death 2,4,5-T Conc.	(2-ethyl 4-methylpentanol and 2-ethylhexanol esters of 2,4,5-T)
Sure Death 2,4,5-T Conc. #4	(butyl ester of 2,4,5-T)
Swift's Gold Bear 40	(triethylamine salt of 2,4-D)
Swift's Gold Bear 2-2 Brush Kill	(isooctyl esters of 2,4-D and 2,4,5-T)
Swift's Gold Bear 55 Brush Kill	(isooctyl ester of 2,4,5-T)
Swift's Gold Bear 44 Ester	(isopropyl ester of 2,4-D)
Swift's Gold Bear Woody Plant Control	(isooctyl esters of 2,4-D and 2,4,5-T)

T

2,4,5-T Amine	(dimethylamine salt of 2,4,5-T)
T-5 Brush Kil	(2,4,5-T, form unspecified)
2,4,5-T, Butoxyethanol ester	(butoxyethanol ester of 2,4,5-T)
2,4,5-T Butyl ester	(butyl ester of 2,4,5-T)
2,4,5-T-dimethylamine salt	(dimethylamine salt of 2,4,5-T)
Techne 40% Butyl Ester Type Weed Killer	(butyl ester of 2,4-D)
Techne Butyl Ester Weed Killer No.4	(butyl ester of 2,4-D)

Techne Butyl Ester Weed Killer No.6	(butyl ester of 2,4-D)
Techne 2,4-D Amine Weed Killer	(dimethylamine salt of 2,4-D)
Techne Low-Vol 2,4-D No.4	(2-ethylpentanol and 2-ethylhexanol esters of 2,4-D)
Techne 2,4,5-T Concentrate No.4	(butyl ester of 2,4,5-T)
Termicide 5-15	(triethanolamine salt of 2,4-D + triethanolamine methanearsonate
T-H Ded-Weed LV-6	(2,4,5-T)
T-H Ded-Weed LV-9	(2,4,5-T)
T-H Ded-Weed ME-6	(butyl ester of 2,4-D)
T-H Ded-Weed ME-9	(butyl ester of 2,4-D)
The Andersons Broadleaf Weed Killer	(dimethylamine salt of 2,4-D + isooctyl ester of silvex [2-(2,4,5-trichlorophenoxy)propionic acid])
The Andersons Weed & Feed	(dimethylamine salt of 2,4-D + isooctyl ester of silvex [2-(2,4,5-trichlorophenoxy)propionic acid])
The Crop Rider	(butyl ester of 2,4-D)
The Line Rider	(2-ethylhexyl esters of 2,4-D and 2,4,5-T)
Thorokil	(2,4-D + bromacil [5-bromo-3-*sec*-butyl-6-methyluracil] + pentachlorophenol)
2,4,5-T, Isooctyl esters	(isooctyl esters of 2,4,5-T)
2,4,5-T Low Volatile Ester 6L	(2,4,5-T, form unspecified)
Tobacco States Brand Ester 210	(isooctyl esters of 2,4-D)
Tobacco States Brand Ester Brush Killer 2-2	(butyl esters of 2,4-D and 2,4,5-T)
Tobacco States Brand Ester 410 Concentrate	(2-ethylhexyl ester of 2,4-D)
Tobacco States Brand Low-Vol Brush Killer 2-20	(isooctyl esters of 2,4-D and 2,4,5-T)
2,4,5-T, Oleic-1,3-propylenediamine salt	(oleic-1,3-propylene-diamine salt of 2,4,5-T)
Tordon 101 Mixture	(triisopropanol amine salts of 2,4-D and 4-amino-3,5,6-trichloropicolinic acid)
Tormona	(2,4,5-T, form unspecified)
2,4,5-T, Propyleneglycol butyl ether esters	(propylene glycol butyl ether esters of 2,4,5-T)

Transamine OA-3D	(*N*,*N*-dimethyloleyllinoleylamine salt of 2,4-D)
Transamine OA-1.5D-1.5T	(*N*,*N*-dimethyloleyllinoleylamine salt of 2,4-D and 2,4,5-T)
Transamine OA-3T	(*N*,*N*-dimethyloleyllinoleylamine salt of 2,4,5-T)
Trelease	(butoxyethanol ester of 2,4,5-T)
Tributon	(2,4-D + 2,4,5-T, forms unspecified)
(2,4,5-Trichloor-fenoxy)-azunzuur	(2,4,5-T)
2,4,5-Trichlorophenoxyacetic acid	(2,4,5-T)
(2,4,5-Trichlorophenoxy)acetic acid	(2,4,5-T)
(2,4,5-Trichlor-phenoxy)-essigsaevre	(2,4,5-T)
Trinixol	(2,4,5-T, form unspecified)
Trinoxol	(butoxyethanol ester of 2,4,5-T)
Trinoxol Super-6	(butoxyethanol ester of 2,4,5-T)
Trioxon	(2,4,5-T, form unspecified)
Trioxone	(butyl ester of 2,4,5-T)
Triple Tonic	(dimethylamine salts and propylene glycol butyl ether esters of 2,4-D + nitrogen + phosphoric acid + soluble potash)
2,4,5-T-Triethylamine salt	(triethylamine salt of 2,4,5-T)
Turf Builder Plus 2	(2,4-D + 2-(2-methyl-4-chloro-phenoxy)-propionic acid)

U

U 46	(2,4-D + 2,4,5-T, forms unspecified)
U-5043	(2,4-D, form unspecified)
U 46 DP	(2,4-D, form unspecified)
Unico Brush Killer	(butyl esters of 2,4-D and 2,4,5-T)
Unico Brush Killer A	(butyl ester of 2,4-D + isooctyl ester of 2,4,5-T)
Unico 2,4-D Ester Weed Killer	(butyl ester of 2,4-D)
Unico Dinitro PE Weed Killer	(alkanolamine salts [of the ethanol and isopropanol series] of 4,6-dinitro-*ortho-sec*-butylphenol)

Unico 2,4-D Lo-V Ester Weed Killer	(2-ethylhexyl ester of 2,4-D)
Unico Lo-V Brush Killer	(2-ethylhexyl esters of 2,4-D and 2,4,5-T)
Unico 2,4,5-T Lo-V Ester Brush Killer	(2-ethylhexyl ester of 2,4,5-T)
Unico Turf Treeter Lawn Weed Killer	(dimethylamine salts of 2,4-D and dicamba [3,6-dichloro-2-methoxybenzoic acid])
U 46 Spezial	(2,4-D + 2,4,5-T, forms unspecified)
Utility Brush Killer No.2	(isooctyl esters of 2,4-D and 2,4,5-T)

V

Vaughan's Liquid K.O.	(octyl ammonium salt of 2,4-D + octyl and dodecyl ammonium methylarsonate)
Veg-I-Kill	(isooctyl ester of 2,4-D + bromacil [5-bromo-3-*sec*-butyl-6-methyluracil] + pentachlorophenol + other chlorophenols)
Veon	(2,4,5-T, form unspecified)
Veon 100	(triethylamine salt of 2,4,5-T)
Veon 245	(triethylamine salt of 2,4,5-T)
Veon BK	(dimethylamine salts of 2,4-D and 2,4,5-T)
Vergemaster	(2,4-D, form unspecified)
Verton CE	(propylene glycol butyl ether esters of 2,4-D and 2,4,5-T)
Verton CE Herbicide	(propylene glycol butyl ether esters of 2,4-D and 2,4,5-T)
Verton D	(2,4-D, form unspecified)
Verton 2D	(propylene glycol butyl ether esters of 2,4-D)
Verton 2-D	(2,4-D, form unspecified)
Verton 4D	(propylene glycol butyl ether esters of 2,4-D)
Verton T	(propylene glycol butyl ether esters of 2,4,5-T)

Verton 2T	(2,4,5-T, form unspecified)
Verton 2-T	(2,4,5-T, form unspecified)
Verton 2T Herbicide	(propylene glycol butyl ether esters of 2,4,5-T)
Vidon 638	(2,4-D, unspecified)
Vi-Par	(diethanolamine salts of 2-(2-methyl-4-chlorophenoxy)-propionic acid and 2,4-D)
Visko-Rhap A-1D	(oleylamine salt of 2,4-D)
Visko-Rhap A-3D	(N,N-dimethyl oleyllinoleylamine salt of 2,4-D)
Visko-Rhap 2,4-D Low Volatile Ester 4L	(isooctyl ester of 2,4-D)
Visko-Rhap H Low Volatile 2T	(2-ethylhexyl ester of 2,4,5-T)
Visko-Rhap Low Drift Herbicides	(2,4-D, form unspecified)
Visko-Rhap Low Volatile 1D-1T	(2-ethylhexyl esters of 2,4-D and 2,4,5-T)
Visko-Rhap Low Volatile 1.5D-1.5T	(2-ethylhexyl esters of 2,4-D and 2,4,5-T)
Visko-Rhap Low Volatile Ester 2D	(2-ethylhexyl ester of 2,4-D)
Visko-Rhap Low Volatile Ester 1D-1T	(2-ethylhexyl esters of 2,4-D and 2,4,5-T)
Visko-Rhap Low Volatile Ester 2T	(2-ethylhexyl ester of 2,4,5-T)
Visko-Rhap Low Volatile 4L	(2,4-D, form unspecified)
Visko-Rhap Low Volatile 2T	(2-ethylhexyl ester of 2,4,5-T)
Visko-Rhap Low Volatile 3T	(2-ethylhexyl ester of 2,4,5-T)
Visko-Rhap Oil-Soluble Amine A-3D	(N,N-dimethyloleyllinoleylamine salt of 2,4-D)

W

Wasco Brush Killer	(2-ethylhexyl esters of 2,4-D and 2,4,5-T)
Weed And Brush Off Amine Formula 400	(diethylethanolamine salts of 2,4-D and 2,4,5-T)
Weed-Ag-Bar	(2,4-D, form unspecified)
Weedar	(2,4-D, form unspecified) or (2,4,5-T, form unspecified)

Weedar 64	(dimethylamine salt of 2,4-D)
Weedar Amine Brush Killer	(dimethylamine salt of 2,4-D + triethylamine salt of 2,4,5-T)
Weedar 2,4,5-T	(triethylamine salt of 2,4,5-T)
Weed-Ban	(amines [form unspecified] of 2,4-D and dicamba[3,6-dichloro-2-methoxybenzoic acid])
Weed-Bane Amine	(2,4-D, form unspecified)
Weed-Bane Ester	(2,4-D, form unspecified)
Weed-B-Gon	(2,4-D, form unspecified)
Weed Broom	(anhydrous disodium methanearsonate + lithium salt of bromacil [5-bromo-3-*sec*-butyl-6-methyluracil] + anhydrous sodium salt of 2,4-D)
Weedez Wonder Bar	(triethylamine salt of 2,4-D)
"006" Weed Killer	(isooctyl ester of 2,4-D + bromacil [5-bromo-3-*sec*-butyl-6-methyluracil] + pentachlorophenol + other chlorophenols)
Weed Killer 646	(butyl ester of 2,4-D)
Weed-Nix Lawn Food With 2,4-D & Banvel D	(dimethylamine salts of 2,4-D, dicamba [3,6-dichloro-2-methoxybenzoic acid] and related acids)
Weed-No-More	(2,4-D ester, form unspecified)
Weedone	(2,4-D, form unspecified) or (2,4,5-T, form unspecified) or (butoxyethanol ester of 2,4,5-T)
Weedone 48	(2,4-D, form unspecified)
Weedone-170	(2,4-D, form unspecified)
Weedone 638	(2,4-D) or (butoxyethanol ester of 2,4-D)
Weedone Aero-Concentrate 96	(butyl ester of 2,4-D)
Weedone Aero-Concentrate E	(butyl ester of 2,4-D)
Weedone Brush Killer 32	(butoxyethanol esters of 2,4-D and 2,4,5-T)
Weedone Brush Killer 64	(butoxyethanol esters of 2,4-D and 2,4,5-T)

Weedone Brush Killer 977	(butoxyethanol esters of 2,4-D and 2,4,5-T)
Weedone Brush Killer 977 Concentrate	(butoxyethanol esters of 2,4-D and 2,4,5-T)
Weedone Concentrate 48	(ethyl ester of 2,4-D)
Weedone Industrial Brush Killer	(butoxyethanol esters of 2,4-D and 2,4,5-T)
Weedone LV4	(butoxyethanol ester of 2,4-D)
Weedone LV-6	(butoxyethanol ester of 2,4-D)
Weedone 2,4,5-T	(2,4,5-T, form unspecified)
Weedone 2,4,5-T Special Air Spray Formula	(butoxyethanol ester of 2,4,5-T)
Weed-Out Lawn Weed Control with 2,4-D and Silvex	(dimethylamine salt of 2,4-D + isooctyl ester of silvex [2-(2,4,5-trichlorophenoxy)propionic acid])
Weed-Rhap	(2,4-D, form unspecified)
Weed-Rhap A-4	(2,4-D)
Weed-Rhap A-4D	(dimethylamine salt of 2,4-D)
Weed-Rhap A-4T	(triethylamine salt of 2,4,5-T)
Weed-Rhap B-4	(2,4-D)
Weed-Rhap B-266	(2,4-D)
Weed-Rhap B-4D	(butyl ester of 2,4-D)
Weed-Rhap B-6D	(butyl ester of 2,4-D)
Weed-Rhap B-2.67D	(butyl ester of 2,4-D)
Weed-Rhap I-3.34	(2,4-D)
Weed-Rhap I-3.34D	(isopropyl ester of 2,4-D)
Weed-Rhap Low Volatile 4D	(2-ethylhexyl ester of 2,4-D)
Weed-Rhap Low Volatile 5D	(2-ethylhexyl ester of 2,4-D)
Weed-Rhap Low Volatile F4D For Mixing With Fertilizer	(2-ethylhexyl ester of 2,4-D)
Weed-Rhap Low Volatile-Granular D	(2-ethylhexyl ester of 2,4-D)
Weed-Rhap LV-4D	(butoxyethanol ester of 2,4-D)
Weed-Rhap LV-4-0	(2,4-D)
Woodbury Pre-Merge Granular 20 2,4-D	(2-ethylhexanol ester of 2,4-D)
Woodbury Woodkill Ester Conc.	(butyl esters of 2,4-D and 2,4,5-T)
Woodkill Ester Concentrate	(butyl esters of 2,4-D and 2,4,5-T)

Z

Zehrung 2,4-D Selective Amine Weed Killer	(dimethylamine salt of 2,4-D)
Zehrung 2,4,5-T Blackberry Vine Killer	(isopropyl ester of 2,4,5-T)
Zehrung Weed Blitz	(triethanolamine salts of 2,4-D and 2,4,5-T)
Zep R-61 Weed Killer	(dimethylamine salts of 2,4-D and 2,4,5-T)

SUPPLEMENTARY CORRIGENDA TO VOLUMES 1 - 14

Corrigenda covering Volumes 1 - 6 appeared in Volume 7, others appeared in Volumes 8, 10, 11, 12 and 13.

Volume 4

p. 265   (e)   *replace* 0.1 mg/kg bw *by* 100 mg/kg bw
          1st line

Volume 14

p. 52   3.1(e)   *replace* Hemalite *by* Nemalite
          1st column

p. 75   3.5   *replace* intestinal *by* interstitial
          2nd line

CUMULATIVE INDEX TO IARC MONOGRAPHS ON THE EVALUATION
OF CARCINOGENIC RISK OF CHEMICALS TO MAN

Numbers underlined indicate volume, and numbers in italics indicate page. References to corrigenda are given in parentheses.

Acetamide	7,*197*
Acriflavinium chloride	13,*31*
Actinomycins	10,*29*
Adriamycin	10,*43*
Aflatoxins	1,*145* (corr. 7,*319*)
	(corr. 8,*349*)
	10,*51*
Aldrin	5,*25*
Amaranth	8,*41*
para-Aminoazobenzene	8,*53*
ortho-Aminoazotoluene	8,*61* (corr. 11,*295*)
4-Aminobiphenyl	1,*74* (corr. 10,*343*)
2-Amino-5-(5-nitro-2-furyl)-1,3,4-thiadiazole	7,*143*
Amitrole	7,*31*
Anaesthetics, volatile	11,*285*
Aniline	4,*27* (corr. 7,*320*)
Apholate	9,*31*
Aramite(R)	5,*39*
Arsenic and inorganic arsenic compounds	2,*48*
Arsenic (inorganic)	
Arsenic pentoxide	
Arsenic trioxide	
Calcium arsenate	
Calcium arsenite	
Potassium arsenate	
Potassium arsenite	
Sodium arsenate	
Sodium arsenite	
Asbestos	2,*17* (corr. 7,*319*)
	14,

Amosite
Anthophyllite
Chrysotile
Crocidolite

Auramine	<u>1</u>,69	(corr. <u>7</u>,319)
Aurothioglucose	<u>13</u>,39	
Azaserine	<u>10</u>,73	
Aziridine	<u>9</u>,37	
2-(1-Aziridinyl)ethanol	<u>9</u>,47	
Aziridyl benzoquinone	<u>9</u>,51	
Azobenzene	<u>8</u>,75	
Benz[c]acridine	<u>3</u>,241	
Benz[a]anthracene	<u>3</u>,45	
Benzene	<u>7</u>,203	(corr. <u>11</u>,295)
Benzidine	<u>1</u>,80	
Benzo[b]fluoranthene	<u>3</u>,69	
Benzo[j]fluoranthene	<u>3</u>,82	
Benzo[a]pyrene	<u>3</u>,91	
Benzo[e]pyrene	<u>3</u>,137	
Benzyl chloride	<u>11</u>,217	(corr. <u>13</u>,243)
Beryllium and beryllium compounds	<u>1</u>,17	

    Beryl ore
    Beryllium oxide
    Beryllium phosphate
    Beryllium sulphate

BHC (technical grades)	<u>5</u>,47	
Bis(1-aziridinyl)morpholinophosphine sulphide	<u>9</u>,55	
Bis(2-chloroethyl)ether	<u>9</u>,117	
N,N-Bis(2-chloroethyl)-2-naphthylamine	<u>4</u>,119	
1,2-Bis(chloromethoxy)ethane	<u>15</u>,31	
1,4-Bis(chloromethoxymethyl)benzene	<u>15</u>,37	
Bis(chloromethyl)ether	<u>4</u>,231	(corr. <u>13</u>,243)
1,4-Butanediol dimethanesulphonate	<u>4</u>,247	
β-Butyrolactone	<u>11</u>,225	
γ-Butyrolactone	<u>11</u>,231	

Cadmium and cadmium compounds   <u>2</u>,74
                                               <u>11</u>,39

  Cadmium acetate
  Cadmium carbonate
  Cadmium chloride
  Cadmium oxide
  Cadmium powder
  Cadmium sulphate
  Cadmium sulphide

Cantharidin   <u>10</u>,79
Carbaryl   <u>12</u>,37
Carbon tetrachloride   <u>1</u>,53
Carmoisine   <u>8</u>,83
Catechol   <u>15</u>,155
Chlorambucil   <u>9</u>,125
Chloramphenicol   <u>10</u>,85
Chlorinated dibenzodioxins   <u>15</u>,41
Chlormadinone acetate   <u>6</u>,149
Chlorobenzilate   <u>5</u>,75
Chloroform   <u>1</u>,61
Chloromethyl methyl ether   <u>4</u>,239
Chloropropham   <u>12</u>,55
Chloroquine   <u>13</u>,47
Cholesterol   <u>10</u>,99
Chromium and inorganic chromium compounds   <u>2</u>,100

  Barium chromate
  Calcium chromate
  Chromic chromate
  Chromic oxide
  Chromium acetate
  Chromium carbonate
  Chromium dioxide
  Chromium phosphate
  Chromium trioxide
  Lead chromate

Potassium chromate
Potassium dichromate
Sodium chromate
Sodium dichromate
Strontium chromate
Zinc chromate hydroxide

Chrysene	<u>3</u>,*159*
Chrysoidine	<u>8</u>,*91*
C.I. Disperse Yellow 3	<u>8</u>,*97*
Citrus Red No. 2	<u>8</u>,*101*
Copper 8-hydroxyquinoline	<u>15</u>,*103*
Coumarin	<u>10</u>,*113*
Cycasin	<u>1</u>,*157* (corr. <u>7</u>,*319*)
	<u>10</u>,*121*
Cyclochlorotine	<u>10</u>,*139*
Cyclophosphamide	<u>9</u>,*135*
Daunomycin	<u>10</u>,*145*
2,4-D and esters	<u>15</u>,*111*
D & C Red No. 9	<u>8</u>,*107*
DDT and associated substances	<u>5</u>,*83* (corr. <u>7</u>,*320*)
DDD (TDE)	
DDE	
Diacetylaminoazotoluene	<u>8</u>,*113*
Diallate	<u>12</u>,*69*
2,6-Diamino-3-(phenylazo)pyridine (hydrochloride)	<u>8</u>,*117*
Diazepam	<u>13</u>,*57*
Diazomethane	<u>7</u>,*223*
Dibenz[*a,h*]acridine	<u>3</u>,*247*
Dibenz[*a,j*]acridine	<u>3</u>,*254*
Dibenz[*a,h*]anthracene	<u>3</u>,*178*
7H-Dibenzo[*c,g*]carbazole	<u>3</u>,*260*
Dibenzo[*h,rst*]pentaphene	<u>3</u>,*197*
Dibenzo[*a,e*]pyrene	<u>3</u>,*201*
Dibenzo[*a,h*]pyrene	<u>3</u>,*207*
Dibenzo[*a,i*]pyrene	<u>3</u>,*215*

Dibenzo[*a,l*]pyrene	*3*,224
1,2-Dibromo-3-chloropropane	*15*,139
ortho-Dichlorobenzene	*7*,231
para-Dichlorobenzene	*7*,231
3,3'-Dichlorobenzidine	*4*,49
trans-1,4-Dichlorobutene	*15*,149
Dieldrin	*5*,125
Diepoxybutane	*11*,115
1,2-Diethylhydrazine	*4*,153
Diethylstilboestrol	*6*,55
Diethyl sulphate	*4*,277
Diglycidyl resorcinol ether	*11*,125
Dihydrosafrole	*1*,170
	10,233
Dihydroxybenzenes	*15*,155
Dimethisterone	*6*,167
Dimethoxane	*15*,177
3,3'-Dimethoxybenzidine (*o*-Dianisidine)	*4*,41
para-Dimethylaminoazobenzene	*8*,125
para-Dimethylaminobenzenediazo sodium sulphonate	*8*,147
trans-2[(Dimethylamino)methylimino]-5-[2-(5-nitro-2-furyl)vinyl]-1,3,4-oxadiazole	*7*,147
3,3'-Dimethylbenzidine (*o*-Tolidine)	*1*,87
Dimethylcarbamoyl chloride	*12*,77
1,1-Dimethylhydrazine	*4*,137
1,2-Dimethylhydrazine	*4*,145 (corr. *7*,320)
Dimethyl sulphate	*4*,271
Dinitrosopentamethylenetetramine	*11*,241
1,4-Dioxane	*11*,247
Disulfiram	*12*,85
Dithranol	*13*,75
Dulcin	*12*,97
Endrin	*5*,157
Eosin	*15*,183
Eosin disodium salt	*15*,183

Epichlorohydrin	11,131
1-Epoxyethyl-3,4-epoxycyclohexane	11,141
3,4-Epoxy-6-methylcyclohexylmethyl-3,4-epoxy-6-methylcyclohexane carboxylate	11,147
cis-9,10-Epoxystearic acid	11,153
Ethinyloestradiol	6,77
Ethionamide	13,83
Ethylene dibromide	15,195
Ethylene oxide	11,157
Ethylene sulphide	11,257
Ethylenethiourea	7,45
Ethyl methanesulphonate	7,245
Ethyl selenac	12,107
Ethyl tellurac	12,115
Ethynodiol diacetate	6,173
Evans blue	8,151
Ferbam	12,121 (corr. 13,243)
2-(2-Formylhydrazino)-4-(5-nitro-2-furyl)thiazole	7,151 (corr. 11,295)
Fusarenon-X	11,169
Glycidaldehyde	11,175
Glycidyl oleate	11,183
Glycidyl stearate	11,187
Griseofulvin	10,153
Haematite	1,29
Heptachlor and its epoxide	5,173
Hexamethylphosphoramide	15,211
Hycanthone	13,91
Hycanthone mesylate	13,92
Hydrazine	4,127
Hydroquinone	15,155
4-Hydroxyazobenzene	8,157
8-Hydroxyquinoline	13,101
Hydroxysenkirkine	10,265
Indeno[1,2,3-cd]pyrene	3,229
Iron-dextran complex	2,161

Iron-dextrin complex	*2,161*	(corr. *7,319*)
Iron oxide	*1,29*	
Iron sorbitol-citric acid complex	*2,161*	
Isatidine	*10,269*	
Isonicotinic acid hydrazide	*4,159*	
Isosafrole	*1,169*	
	10,232	
Isopropyl alcohol	*15,223*	
Isopropyl oils	*15,223*	
Jacobine	*10,275*	
Lasiocarpine	*10,281*	
Lead salts	*1,40*	(corr. *7,319*)
		(corr. *8,349*)
Lead acetate		
Lead arsenate		
Lead carbonate		
Lead phosphate		
Lead subacetate		
Ledate	*12,131*	
Lindane	*5,47*	
Luteoskyrin	*10,163*	
Magenta	*4,57*	(corr. *7,320*)
Maleic hydrazide	*4,173*	
Maneb	*12,137*	
Mannomustine (dihydrochloride)	*9,157*	
Medphalan	*9,167*	
Medroxyprogesterone acetate	*6,157*	
Melphalan	*9,167*	
Merphalan	*9,167*	
Mestranol	*6,87*	
Methoxychlor	*5,193*	
2-Methylaziridine	*9,61*	
Methylazoxymethanol acetate	*1,164*	
	10,131	

Methyl carbamate	*12*,151
N-Methyl-N,4-dinitrosoaniline	*1*,141
4,4'-Methylene bis(2-chloroaniline)	*4*,65
4,4'-Methylene bis(2-methylaniline)	*4*,73
4,4'-Methylenedianiline	*4*,79 (corr. *7*,320)
Methyl iodide	*15*,245
Methyl methanesulphonate	*7*,253
N-Methyl-N'-nitro-N-nitrosoguanidine	*4*,183
Methyl red	*8*,161
Methyl selenac	*12*,161
Methylthiouracil	*7*,53
Metronidazole	*13*,113
Mirex	*5*,203
Mitomycin C	*10*,171
Monocrotaline	*10*,291
Monuron	*12*,167
5-(Morpholinomethyl)-3-[(5-nitrofurfurylidene)-amino]-2-oxazolidinone	*7*,161
Mustard gas	*9*,181 (corr. *13*,243)
1-Naphthylamine	*4*,87 (corr. *8*,349)
2-Naphthylamine	*4*,97
Native carrageenans	*10*,181 (corr. *11*,295)
Nickel and nickel compounds	*2*,126 (corr. *7*,319)
	11 75
Nickel acetate	
Nickel carbonate	
Nickel carbonyl	
Nickelocene	
Nickel oxide	
Nickel powder	
Nickel subsulphide	
Nickel sulphate	
Niridazole	*13*,123
4-Nitrobiphenyl	*4*,113
5-Nitro-2-furaldehyde semicarbazone	*7*,171

1[(5-Nitrofurfurylidene)amino]-2-imidazolidinone	<u>7</u>,181
N-[4-(5-Nitro-2-furyl)-2-thiazolyl]acetamide	<u>1</u>,181
	<u>7</u>,185
Nitrogen mustard (hydrochloride)	<u>9</u>,193
Nitrogen mustard N-oxide (hydrochloride)	<u>9</u>,209
N-Nitrosodi-n-butylamine	<u>4</u>,197
N-Nitrosodiethylamine	<u>1</u>,107 (corr. <u>11</u>,295)
N-Nitrosodimethylamine	<u>1</u>,95
N-Nitrosoethylurea	<u>1</u>,135
N-Nitrosomethylurea	<u>1</u>,125
N-Nitroso-N-methylurethane	<u>4</u>,211
Norethisterone	<u>6</u>,179
Norethisterone acetate	<u>6</u>,179
Norethynodrel	<u>6</u>,191
Norgestrel	<u>6</u>,201
Ochratoxin A	<u>10</u>,191
Oestradiol-17β	<u>6</u>,99
Oestradiol mustard	<u>9</u>,217
Oestriol	<u>6</u>,117
Oestrone	<u>6</u>,123
Oil Orange SS	<u>8</u>,165
Orange I	<u>8</u>,173
Orange G	<u>8</u>,181
Oxazepam	<u>13</u>,58
Oxymetholone	<u>13</u>,131
Oxyphenbutazone	<u>13</u>,185
Parasorbic acid	<u>10</u>,199
Patulin	<u>10</u>,205
Penicillic acid	<u>10</u>,211
Phenacetin	<u>13</u>,141
Phenicarbazide	<u>12</u>,177
Phenobarbital	<u>13</u>,157
Phenobarbital sodium	<u>13</u>,159
Phenoxybenzamine (hydrochloride)	<u>9</u>,223
Phenylbutazone	<u>13</u>,183

Phenytoin	13,201
Phenytoin sodium	13,202
Polychlorinated biphenyls	7,261
Ponceau MX	8,189
Ponceau 3R	8,199
Ponceau SX	8,207
Potassium bis(2-hydroxyethyl)dithiocarbamate	12,183
Progesterone	6,135
Pronetalol hydrochloride	13,227
1,3-Propane sultone	4,253 (corr. 13,243)
Propham	12,189
β-Propiolactone	4,259
n-Propyl carbamate	12,201
Propylene oxide	11,191
Propylthiouracil	7,67
Pyrimethamine	13,233
para-Quinone	15,255
Quintozene (Pentachloronitrobenzene)	5,211
Reserpine	10,217
Resorcinol	15,155
Retrorsine	10,303
Riddelliine	10,313
Saccharated iron oxide	2,161
Safrole	1,169
	10,231
Scarlet red	8,217
Selenium and selenium compounds	9,245
Semicarbazide (hydrochloride)	12,209
Seneciphylline	10,319
Senkirkine	10,327
Sodium diethyldithiocarbamate	12,217
Soot, tars and shale oils	3,22
Sterigmatocystin	1,175
	10,245

Streptozotocin	*4*, 221
Styrene oxide	*11*, 201
Succinic anhydride	*15*, 265
Sudan I	*8*, 225
Sudan II	*8*, 233
Sudan III	*8*, 241
Sudan brown RR	*8*, 249
Sudan red 7B	*8*, 253
Sunset yellow FCF	*8*, 257
2,4,5,-T and esters	*15*, 273
Tannic acid	*10*, 253
Tannins	*10*, 254
Terpene polychlorinates (Strobane$^{(R)}$)	*5*, 219
Testosterone	*6*, 209
Tetraethyllead	*2*, 150
Tetramethyllead	*2*, 150
Thioacetamide	*7*, 77
Thiouracil	*7*, 85
Thiourea	*7*, 95
Thiram	*12*, 225
Trichloroethylene	*11*, 263
Trichlorotriethylamine hydrochloride	*9*, 229
Triethylene glycol diglycidyl ether	*11*, 209
Tris(aziridinyl)-*para*-benzoquinone	*9*, 67
Tris(1-aziridinyl)phosphine oxide	*9*, 75
Tris(1-aziridinyl)phosphine sulphide	*9*, 85
2,4,6-Tris(1-aziridinyl)-*s*-triazine	*9*, 95
1,2,3-Tris(chloromethoxy)propane	*15*, 301
Tris(2-methyl-1-aziridinyl)phosphine oxide	*9*, 107
Trypan blue	*8*, 267
Uracil mustard	*9*, 235
Urethane	*7*, 111
Vinyl chloride	*7*, 291
4-Vinylcyclohexene	*11*, 277

Yellow AB	8,279
Yellow OB	8,287
Zectran	12,237
Zineb	12,245
Ziram	12,259

www.ingramcontent.com/pod-product-compliance
Ingram Content Group UK Ltd.
Pitfield, Milton Keynes, MK11 3LW, UK
UKHW051258180426
11947UKWH00020B/1780